Celiac Disease: Etiology, Diagnosis and Treatment

Celiac Disease: Etiology, Diagnosis and Treatment

Editor: Dallas Lynch

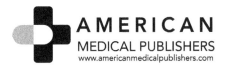

AMERICAN
MEDICAL PUBLISHERS
www.americanmedicalpublishers.com

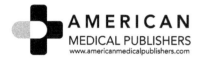

Cataloging-in-Publication Data

Celiac disease : etiology, diagnosis and treatment / edited by Dallas Lynch.
    p. cm.
Includes bibliographical references and index.
ISBN 978-1-63927-624-0
1. Celiac disease. 2. Celiac disease--Etiology. 3. Celiac disease--Diagnosis.
4. Celiac disease--Treatment. I. Lynch, Dallas.
RC862.C44 C45 2023
616.399--dc23

American Medical Publishers,
41 Flatbush Avenue,
1st Floor, New York,
NY 11217, USA

ISBN 978-1-63927-624-0 (Hardback)

Contents

Preface

Celiac disease refers to a type of long-term autoimmune disorder. It majorly affects the small intestine, in which people develop intolerance towards gluten, which is found in foods such as barley, wheat and rye. Classic symptoms of celiac disease include gastrointestinal problems, such as loss of appetite, abdominal distention, chronic diarrhoea and malabsorption. This usually starts from the age of six months to two years. There are several non-classic symptoms, which are common in individuals older than two years. These might include either absent or mild gastrointestinal symptoms, which might infect any part of the human body, or no noticeable symptoms. The diagnosis is generally done through intestinal biopsies and a variety of blood antibody tests, facilitated by particular genetic testing. The disease can be treated by following a mandatory gluten-free diet for lifetime. It helps to recover the intestinal lining and decreases the risk associated with the disease. This book contains some path-breaking studies on celiac disease. It aims to shed light on the etiology, diagnosis and treatment of this disease. This book is appropriate for students seeking detailed information on this medical condition as well as for experts.

This book is a comprehensive compilation of works of different researchers from varied parts of the world. It includes valuable experiences of the researchers with the sole objective of providing the readers (learners) with a proper knowledge of the concerned field. This book will be beneficial in evoking inspiration and enhancing the knowledge of the interested readers.

In the end, I would like to extend my heartiest thanks to the authors who worked with great determination on their chapters. I also appreciate the publisher's support in the course of the book. I would also like to deeply acknowledge my family who stood by me as a source of inspiration during the project.

Editor

Influence of HLA-DQ2.5 Dose on Clinical Picture of Unrelated Celiac Disease Patients

Laura Airaksinen [1], Pilvi Laurikka [1], Heini Huhtala [2], Kalle Kurppa [3,4], Teea Salmi [1,5], Päivi Saavalainen [6], Katri Kaukinen [1,7] and Katri Lindfors [1,*]

[1] Celiac Disease Research Center, Faculty of Medicine and Health Technology, Tampere University, 33520 Tampere, Finland; laura.airaksinen@tuni.fi (L.A.); pilvi.laurikka@tuni.fi (P.L.); teea.salmi@tuni.fi (T.S.); katri.kaukinen@tuni.fi (K.K.)
[2] Faculty of Social Sciences, Tampere University, 33520 Tampere, Finland; heini.huhtala@tuni.fi
[3] Tampere Centre for Child Health Research, Tampere University Hospital and Tampere University, 33521 Tampere, Finland; kalle.kurppa@tuni.fi
[4] Department of Pediatrics, Seinäjoki Central Hospital and University Consortium of Seinäjoki, 60220 Seinäjoki, Finland
[5] Department of Dermatology, Tampere University Hospital, 33521 Tampere, Finland
[6] Research Programs Unit, Immunobiology, and Haartman Institute, Department of Medical Genetics, University of Helsinki, 00014 Helsinki, Finland; paivi.saavalainen@helsinki.fi
[7] Department of Internal Medicine, Tampere University Hospital, 33521 Tampere, Finland
* Correspondence: katri.lindfors@tuni.fi

Abstract: The clinical phenotype of celiac disease varies considerably among patients and the dosage of HLA-DQ2.5 alleles has been suggested to be a contributing factor. We investigated whether HLA-DQ2.5 allele dosage is associated with distinct clinical parameters at the time of diagnosis and with patients' response to a gluten-free diet. The final cohort included 605 carefully phenotyped non-related Finnish celiac disease patients grouped as having 0, 1 or 2 copies of HLA-DQ2.5. Clinical data at the time of diagnosis and during gluten-free diet were collected systematically from medical records and supplementary interviews. An increasing HLA-DQ2.5 dose effect was detected for celiac disease antibody positivity at diagnosis ($p = 0.021$) and for the presence of any first-degree relatives with celiac disease ($p = 0.011$ and $p = 0.031$, respectively). Instead, DQ2.5-negative patients were suffering most often from classical symptoms at diagnosis ($p = 0.007$ between HLA groups). In addition, during follow-up they were most often symptomatic despite a gluten-free diet ($p = 0.002$ between groups). Our results thus suggest that increasing HLA-DQ2.5 dose only has a minor effect on the clinical picture of celiac disease. However, HLA-DQ2.5-negative patients should not be overlooked in clinical practice and particular attention should be paid to this patient group during gluten-free diet.

Keywords: celiac disease; HLA-DQ2.5; dose effect; clinical presentation; gluten-free diet

1. Introduction

Celiac disease is a chronic immune mediated condition driven by the ingestion of dietary gluten. It is characterized by small bowel mucosal damage and autoantibody response to transglutaminase 2 (TG2). The disease can be diagnosed at any age from childhood to older age and there is often a marked diagnostic delay [1,2]. Moreover, there is a substantial variation in the clinical picture of the disease, which may present with gastrointestinal and/or extraintestinal symptoms of varying severity or be completely asymptomatic [3]. Further variation to the disease phenotype is brought by several associated conditions [4]. The only efficient treatment for celiac disease is a strict gluten-free diet

(GFD), which usually results in alleviation of symptoms and normalization of small bowel mucosal morphology. Nevertheless, in a subset of patients, the symptoms and mucosal damage may persist despite a GFD [5,6]. If malabsorption and villous atrophy persist despite strict avoidance of gluten for a minimum of 12 months on GFD and after alternative causes have been excluded, the condition is termed refractory celiac disease (RCD) [7].

Family members of celiac disease patients are at an increased risk of being affected, likely due to their higher frequency of HLA-DQ2.5 or HLA-DQ8, the major determinants contributing to disease susceptibility [8]. HLA-DQ2.5 and DQ8 are heterodimeric molecules present on the surface of antigen presenting cells. In celiac disease, they bind and present deamidated gluten peptides to CD4-positive T cells, leading to the generation of an immune response [9,10]. HLA-DQ2.5 is far more common than HLA-DQ8 as it is present in more than 90% of patients [11]. The HLA-DQ2.5 heterodimer can be encoded by *HLA-DQA1*0501* and *HLA-DQB1*0201* alleles located on the same chromosome (*cis*) or by *DQA1*0505* and *DQB1*0202* on different chromosomes (*trans*). Homozygosity for HLA-DQ2.5 is associated with a particularly high risk for celiac disease [12–14]. This phenomenon has been attributed to the premise that gluten presented by antigen presenting cells in HLA-DQ2.5 homozygous individuals can induce a four-fold higher T cell response than in heterozygous individuals [15]. In addition to the disease risk, the dose of HLA-DQ2.5 has been suggested to affect the phenotype of celiac disease [16]. Earlier research on this issue has nevertheless reported conflicting findings, possibly due to rather small patient cohorts comprising a substantial portion of pediatric patients [16]. Nowadays, the majority of celiac disease diagnoses are made on adults and their clinical picture may be contributed to a larger extent to factors other than the HLA-type. Moreover, earlier research has not excluded patients originating from the same family, thereby increasing the possibility of bias caused by similar genetic background.

We investigated the HLA-DQ2.5 dose effect on various clinical parameters at the time of diagnosis and on patients' response to GFD by exploiting a large and carefully phenotyped cohort of unrelated pediatric and adult celiac disease patients.

2. Materials and Methods

2.1. Patients and Study Design

The study was conducted at Tampere University and Tampere University Hospital. Altogether, 1048 biopsy-proven celiac disease patients were recruited by a nationwide search with the help of national and local celiac societies and by media announcements. The patient information at diagnosis (demographics, clinical and histological data, celiac disease serology, presence of symptoms during childhood, and other concomitant chronic medical conditions as well as family history of celiac disease) was collected from medical records and from supplementary interviews by a physician or a study nurse. In the case of children, the guardian was interviewed. Patients were divided into four different age groups: 0–6 years, 7–20 years, 21–65 years, and >65 years. Diagnostic delay was categorized as 0 (screen-detected patients), <1, 1–5, 5–10 or >10 years. Abdominal symptoms included abdominal pain, diarrhea, loose stools, heartburn, flatulence, constipation, and/or bloating. Malabsorption was defined as weight loss and/or presence of characteristic laboratory abnormalities, such as anemia, hypoalbuminemia, low folate or low vitamin B12. Classical symptoms referred to the presence of both diarrhea and malabsorption [17]. Extraintestinal symptoms included any symptom(s) presenting outside of the gastrointestinal tract, such as dermatitis herpetiformis, infertility, joint pains, and neurological problems. Severity of symptoms was categorized into "no symptoms", "mild symptoms", "moderate symptoms" or "severe symptoms". "First-degree relative" referred to sibling, mother, father or offspring. "Relative" referred to any relative in a family. In addition, follow-up data on self-reported current symptoms, both gastrointestinal and extraintestinal, as well as adherence to GFD, were assessed by interviews. Adherence to GFD was described as either "strict

GFD", "dietary lapses" or "no GFD". In addition, histological and serological data at follow-up were assessed as described below.

In order to avoid false positive findings due to trait correlation between genetically related individuals, only one patient from each family was included (randomly). The final study cohort included 605 celiac disease patients.

The study design, patient recruitment, and collection of patient record data were approved by the Regional Ethics Committee of Tampere University Hospital. All participants gave written informed consent.

2.2. Histology

The results of histological analysis of the small-bowel mucosal biopsies at the time of diagnosis were collected from the pathology reports. In addition, if available, the degree of mucosal recovery on GFD evaluated from possible repeat biopsy was recorded. In both cases, severity of small intestinal mucosal damage was evaluated from several representative and well-orientated biopsy specimens and the degree of diagnostic villous atrophy was classified as partial, subtotal, or total, corresponding approximately to the IIIa, IIIb, and IIIc Marsh–Oberhuber classifications, respectively [18].

2.3. Serology

The results of celiac disease serology at the time of diagnosis were collected from the medical records. A patient was regarded as positive for celiac disease-specific antibodies if he or she was positive for TG2 autoantibodies [19] and/or endomysial autoantibodies (EmA) [20] and/or antireticulin autoantibodies (ARAs, measured in 1980/90s and later replaced by EmA) [21]. ARA and EmA were analyzed using indirect immunofluorescence with rat liver, kidney or stomach tissue (ARA) [21] or human umbilical cord (EmA) [22] as an antigen. Titers 1: ≥5 were considered positive. From serum samples collected at the time of the present study (follow-up data), TG2 antibodies and EmA were determined. TG2 antibodies values were tested by enzyme-linked immunosorbent assay (QUANTA Lite h-tTG IgA, INOVA Diagnostics, San Diego, CA, USA) with the cut-off for positivity being >30 U/L.

2.4. Genetic Analysis

The genotypes corresponding to disease-associated HLA variants, HLA-DQ2.5, HLA-DQ8, and HLA-DQ2.2, were determined using commercial HLA typing kits (Olerup SSP low-resolution kit, Olerup SSP AB, Saltsjöbaden, Sweden or DELFIA® Celiac Disease Hybridization Assay Kit, PerkinElmer Life and Analytical Sciences, Wallac Oy, Turku, Finland) or the TaqMan chemistry based genotyping of the HLA tagging single-nucleotide polymorphisms (SNPs) as previously described [23,24]. In this study, patients carrying alleles *HLA-DQB1*0201* and *HLA-DQA1*0501* in *cis* configuration were considered positive for HLA-DQ2.5. The subjects were divided into three groups according to whether they had zero, one or two copies of HLA-DQ2.5.

2.5. Statistics

Statistical analyses were performed with SPSS Statistics version 23 (IBM Corp, Armonk, NY, USA). Variables were presented as percentages and tested by Chi-square test or Fisher's Exact test, as appropriate. p value < 0.05 was considered significant across all analyses. Statistical analyses were performed for all patients together and for younger patients (<21 years, $n = 124$) and adults ($n = 476$) separately.

3. Results

Altogether, 100 (16.5%) celiac disease patients were negative (X/X group), 401 (66.3%) were heterozygous (DQ2.5/X group), and 104 (17.2%) were homozygous (DQ2.5/DQ2.5 group) for HLA-DQ2.5 (Table 1).

Table 1. Clinical, serological and histological characteristics of 605 celiac disease patients negative (X/X), heterozygous (DQ2.5/X) or homozygous (DQ2.5/DQ2.5) for HLA-DQ2.5 at the time of diagnosis.

	X/X n = 100 % (n)	DQ2.5/X n = 401 % (n)	DQ2.5/DQ2.5 n = 104 % (n)	p
Females	78.0 (78)	73.3 (294)	76.0 (79)	0.589
Age group				0.996 *
0–6 years	7.1 (7)	6.8 (27)	7.7 (8)	
7–20 years	13.1 (13)	13.6 (54)	14.4 (15)	
21–65 years	75.8 (75)	76.1 (302)	73.1 (76)	
>65 years	4.0 (4)	3.5 (14)	4.8 (5)	
Symptoms in childhood	48.9 (43)	43.8 (161)	51.5 (51)	0.334
Diagnostic delay				0.908 *
0 [1]	4.3 (4)	4.9 (18)	3.0 (3)	
<1 year	20.7 (19)	23.6 (86)	25.7 (26)	
1–5 years	37.0 (34)	31.5 (115)	32.7 (33)	
5–10 years	7.6 (7)	10.4 (38)	6.9 (7)	
>10 years	30.4 (28)	29.6 (108)	31.7 (32)	
Classical symptoms [2]	30.0 (30)	16.7 (67)	21.2 (22)	**0.007**
Abdominal symptoms [3]	86.9 (86)	81.3 (322)	81.7 (85)	0.426
Diarrhea	44.7 (42)	37.1 (144)	41.7 (43)	0.337
Anemia	30.3 (30)	28.5 (113)	37.5 (39)	0.209
Extraintestinal manifestations [4]	44.4 (44)	49.5 (196)	47.1 (49)	0.646
Dermatitis herpetiformis	11.0 (10)	17.1 (63)	19.2 (19)	0.270
Severity of symptoms [5]				0.484 *
No symptoms	5.0 (4)	5.9 (17)	4.0 (3)	
Mild	23.8 (19)	25.9 (74)	33.3 (25)	
Moderate	15.0 (12)	12.2 (35)	5.3 (4)	
Severe	56.3 (45)	55.9 (160)	57.3 (43)	
Celiac disease antibody positivity [6,7]	77.8 (49)	86.8 (217)	94.9 (56)	**0.021**
Severity of mucosal damage [8]				0.546 *
Normal morphology	2.4 (2)	3.0 (10)	2.4 (2)	
Partial villous atrophy	27.7 (23)	33.8 (111)	25.3 (21)	
Subtotal/total villous atrophy	69.9 (58)	63.1 (207)	72.3 (60)	

Values in bold face indicate statistically significant difference with p value < 0.05. * Calculated across all variables. Data were available for >90% of patients except for designated parameters where number of cases in different HLA-DQ2.5 dose groups was [5] 80, 286, 75; [7] 63, 250, 59 and [8] 83, 328, 83, respectively. [1] Screen-detected patients. [2] Presence of diarrhea and malabsorption. [3] Abdominal pain, diarrhea, loose stools, heartburn, flatulence, constipation, and/or bloating. [4] Any symptom(s) presenting outside of the gastrointestinal tract, such as dermatitis herpetiformis, infertility, joint pains and neurological problems. [6] Positivity for serum TG2 autoantibodies and/or endomysial autoantibodies and/or antireticulin autoantibodies.

At the time of diagnosis, there was no significant difference in age distribution between the HLA-DQ2.5 dose groups. The proportion of patients suffering from classical symptoms was lowest among heterozygotes and highest among DQ2.5-negative patients (Table 1). No significant differences between the groups were observed in presence of symptoms in childhood, diagnostic delay or the type (abdominal, diarrhea, anemia, extraintestinal) or severity of symptoms (Table 1). The percentage of patients positive for celiac disease-specific autoantibodies was smallest in the HLA-DQ2.5-negative group and greatest in HLA-DQ2.5-homozygous group. The groups were comparable in terms of severity of mucosal damage (Table 1). DQ2.5 homozygotes most often had any relative or a first-degree relative with celiac disease, whereas DQ2.5-negative patients had such relatives the least often (Figure 1A,B).

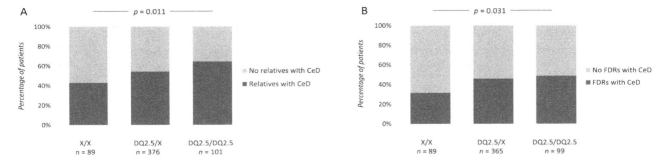

Figure 1. The percentages of patients among different HLA-DQ2.5 dose groups having (**A**) any relatives with CeD and (**B**) having first-degree relatives (FDR) with CeD. Patients are divided into different HLA-DQ2.5 dose groups based on whether they are either negative (X/X), heterozygous (DQ2.5/X) or homozygous (DQ2.5/DQ2.5) for HLA-DQ2.5.

At follow-up (median follow-up time 13 years, range <1–47 years), the DQ2.5-heterozygous patients maintained a strict GFD most often and homozygous patients least often (Table 2). The proportion of patients suffering from self-reported current symptoms was greatest among DQ2.5-negative and smallest among DQ2.5-heterozygous patients. Groups did not differ significantly in terms of antibody positivity, mucosal recovery, concomitant autoimmune diseases or malignancy at the time of the follow-up (Table 2).

Table 2. Clinical, serological and histological characteristics of 605 celiac disease patients negative (X/X), heterozygous (DQ2.5/X) or homozygous (DQ2.5/DQ2.5) for HLA-DQ2.5 at the time of the follow-up.

	X/X $n = 100$	DQ2.5/X $n = 401$	DQ2.5/DQ2.5 $n = 104$	
	% (n)	% (n)	% (n)	p
Adherence to GFD [1]				**0.025** *
Strict GFD [1]	93.8 (91)	97.4 (376)	91.1 (92)	
Dietary lapses	5.2 (5)	2.3 (9)	7.9 (8)	
No GFD [1]	1.0 (1)	0.3 (1)	1.0 (1)	
Self-reported current symptoms [2,3]	44.8 (26)	22.9 (59)	32.3 (20)	**0.002**
Celiac disease antibody positivity [4,5]	28.6 (4)	23.8 (10)	9.1 (1)	0.535
Severity of mucosal damage [6]				0.108 *
Normal morphology	72.9 (35)	55.6 (104)	46.9 (23)	
Partial villous atrophy	25.0 (12)	38.0 (71)	44.9 (22)	
Subtotal/total villous atrophy	2.1 (1)	6.4 (12)	8.2 (4)	
Other illnesses				
Any autoimmune disease [7]	29.8 (28)	23.6 (91)	18.0 (18)	0.155
Type 1 diabetes	3.2 (3)	3.4 (13)	1.0 (1)	0.504
Thyroidal disease	17.9 (17)	14.0 (54)	9.7 (10)	0.248
Malignancy	3.2 (3)	3.9 (15)	5.8 (6)	0.581

Values in bold face indicate statistically significant difference with *p* value < 0.05. * Calculated across all variables. Data were available for >90% of patients except for designated parameters where numbers of cases in different HLA-DQ2.5 dose groups were [3] 58, 258, 62; [5] 14, 42, 11 and [6] 48, 187, 49, respectively. [1] GFD = gluten-free diet. [2] Any type of recurrent gastrointestinal and extraintestinal symptoms. [4] Positivity for serum TG2 and/or endomysial and/or antireticulin autoantibodies. [7] Any autoimmune disease including type 1 diabetes (DM1), thyroidal diseases, IgA nephropathy, Sjögren's syndrome, rheumatoid arthritis, sarcoidosis, psoriasis, vitiligo, and lichen planus.

The results of a subanalysis with adult patients only were parallel to those of the whole cohort. Significant differences between distinct HLA-DQ2.5 dose groups were observed in the presence of classical symptoms and celiac disease-specific antibody positivity at diagnosis ($p = 0.006$ and $p = 0.043$, respectively). Moreover, HLA-DQ2.5 homozygous adults also had more often either any relative or a first-degree relative with celiac disease than did heterozygous or HLA-DQ2.5-negative patients ($p = 0.001$ for any relative and $p = 0.003$ for first-degree relative). For adults at follow-up, significant differences between dose groups were observed in adherence to the GFD and in self-reported current symptoms ($p = 0.016$ and $p = 0.002$, respectively). When children were analyzed separately, no significant differences were found in any of the parameters studied (data not shown).

4. Discussion

It has previously been reported that HLA-DQ2.5 dose is associated with increased risk of celiac disease [14], stronger disease-specific T cell response in vitro [15], and the presence of classical symptoms, particularly in children [16,25]. Here, we observed a dose effect for celiac autoantibody positivity at diagnosis as well as for the presence of any and first-degree relatives with the disease. However, we observed no increase in the presence of classical symptoms with an increasing HLA-DQ2.5 dose; instead, the HLA-DQ2.5-negative group presented most often with this phenotype. In addition, we found no association between HLA-DQ2.5 dose and abdominal symptoms, diarrhea, anemia, extraintestinal manifestations, severity of symptoms or mucosal morphology.

Our finding of an HLA-DQ2.5 dose effect with antibody positivity is rational since the gluten-specific T cells that proliferate and activate more robustly after stimulation in the context of the homozygous HLA-DQ2.5 antigen presenting cells participate in the induction of an anti-TG2 antibody response [26]. Moreover, such a dose effect in patients having a relative with celiac disease likely reflects the presence of the predisposing HLA-DQ2.5 within these families. When comparing our results with those of earlier studies, it is noteworthy that our cohort included mostly adult celiac disease patients, whereas earlier studies were conducted predominantly on pediatric patients [16]. It is possible that the factors affecting the disease phenotype differ between adults and children and also include other determinants besides the HLA-DQ type. The identity of such phenotype-modulating factors remains obscure but may, for instance, include non-HLA genetic variants and/or environmental factors. This assumption is supported by our previous finding that sib pairs with discordant clinical presentation had similar HLA haplotypes more often than pairs with the concordant phenotype did [27]. Interestingly, we have also observed that the diversity and composition of intestinal microbiota varies markedly between different celiac disease phenotypes, this being an interesting issue for further study [28].

HLA-DQ2.5 homozygosity has previously been observed in over 40% of patients with RCD type II (RCDII) in contrast to 20% in uncomplicated celiac disease [29]. RCDII is a severe condition with a poor prognosis [7]. Due to this and the fact that RCDII is very rare in Finland [30], our cohort did not include such cases and we were unable to address the HLA-DQ2.5 dose effect on this parameter. In any case, we found that HLA-DQ2.5 dose is not associated with poorer recovery of the intestinal damage. The investigation of HLA-DQ2.5 dose in RCDII would require a multi-center approach to achieve a sufficient number of patients for statistical power.

We found patients negative for HLA-DQ2.5 to suffer most often from classical symptoms at celiac disease diagnosis. Moreover, they most often experienced symptoms during GFD although their adherence to GFD was excellent. In addition, at follow-up, they did not differ from the other HLA-DQ2.5 groups in terms of celiac disease antibody positivity or small bowel mucosal morphology. A long diagnostic delay has been reported to predispose to persistent symptoms [31], but here patients negative for HLA-DQ2.5 received their diagnoses within the same time limits as the other HLA groups. Alternative explanations for persistent symptoms while on GFD could be altered composition of the small bowel mucosal microbiome [32], small-intestinal bacterial overgrowth [33] or continuous low-grade inflammation in spite of a strict GFD [34]. In any case, our results stress the need to pay special attention to HLA-DQ2.5-negative patients in clinics in order to prevent long-lasting health problems in this patient subset.

4.1. Strengths and Weaknesses

The main strength of our study was a large and well-defined cohort of unrelated adult and pediatric celiac disease patients enabling us to address the effect of HLA-DQ2.5 dose reliably. However, the study was retrospective, which, given its nature may appear as a limitation. In addition, our study considered HLA-DQ2.5 alleles only in the *cis* configuration. Therefore, HLA-DQ2.5/HLA-DQ2.2 genotype was categorized as HLA-DQ2.5-heterozygous in spite of evidence to suggest that this genotype carries an equal risk for celiac disease as HLA-DQ2.5 homozygosity [35]. Moreover, the HLA-DQ2.5-negative group was heterogenous, comprising both the HLA-DQ8-positive cases as well as those without any of the major HLA types predisposing to celiac disease. Further, the small number of pediatric patients inhibited any reliable investigation of the effect of HLA-DQ2.5 dose in this particular subgroup.

4.2. Conclusions

In our cohort with a preponderance of adults, we demonstrated that the effect of HLA-DQ2.5 dose on the clinical picture of celiac disease was only modest. Patients negative for HLA-DQ2.5 were characterized by the most marked seronegativity, by the presence of classic symptoms at diagnosis, and also by symptoms persisting in spite of GFD.

Author Contributions: Conceptualization, L.A., K.K. (Kalle Kurppa), T.S., K.K. (Katri Kaukinen) and K.L.; Data curation, L.A., K.K. (Kalle Kurppa), K.K. (Katri Kaukinen) and K.L.; Formal analysis, L.A., P.L., H.H., P.S. and K.L.; Funding acquisition, L.A., K.K. (Kalle Kurppa), K.K. (Katri Kaukinen) and K.L.; Investigation, L.A., P.L., H.H., P.S. and K.L.; Supervision, K.K. (Katri Kaukinen) and K.L.; Writing—original draft, L.A. and K.L.; Writing—review and editing, L.A., P.L., H.H., K.K. (Kalle Kurppa), T.S., P.S., K.K. (Katri Kaukinen) and K.L. All authors have read and agreed to the published version of the manuscript.

References

1. Gray, A.M.; Papanicolas, I.N. Impact of symptoms on quality of life before and after diagnosis of coeliac disease: Results from a UK population survey. *BMC Health Serv. Res.* **2010**, *10*, 1–7. [CrossRef] [PubMed]
2. Norström, F.; Lindholm, L.; Sandström, O.; Nordyke, K.; Ivarsson, A. Delay to celiac disease diagnosis and its implications for health-related quality of life. *BMC Gastroenterol.* **2011**, *11*. [CrossRef] [PubMed]
3. Di Sabatino, A.; Corazza, G.R. Coeliac disease. *Lancet* **2009**, *373*, 1480–1493. [CrossRef]
4. Caio, G.; Volta, U.; Sapone, A.; Leffler, D.A.; De Giorgio, R.; Catassi, C.; Fasano, A. Celiac disease: A comprehensive current review. *BMC Med.* **2019**, *17*, 1–20. [CrossRef] [PubMed]
5. Midhagen, G.; Hallert, C. High rate of gastrointestinal symptoms in celiac patients living on a gluten-free diet: Controlled study. *Am. J. Gastroenterol.* **2003**, *98*, 2023–2026. [CrossRef] [PubMed]
6. Wahab, P.J.; Meijer, J.W.R.; Mulder, C.J.J. Histologic follow-up of people with celiac disease on a gluten-free diet: Slow and incomplete recovery. *Am. J. Clin. Pathol.* **2002**, *118*, 459–463. [CrossRef]
7. Hujoel, I.A.; Murray, J.A. Refractory Celiac Disease. *Curr. Gastroenterol. Rep.* **2020**, *22*, 18. [CrossRef]
8. Singh, P.; Arora, S.; Lal, S.; Strand, T.A.; Makharia, G.K. Risk of celiac disease in the first- and second-degree relatives of patients with celiac disease: A systematic review and meta-analysis. *Am. J. Gastroenterol.* **2015**, *110*, 1539–1548. [CrossRef]
9. Van De Wal, Y.; Kooy, Y.M.C.; Drijfhout, J.W.; Amons, R.; Koning, F. Peptide binding characteristics of the coeliac disease associated DQ(α1(*)0501, β1(*)0201) molecule. *Immunogenetics* **1996**, *44*, 246–253. [CrossRef] [PubMed]
10. Vartdal, F.; Johansen, B.H.; Friede, T.; Thorpe, C.J.; Stevanović, S.; Eriksen, J.E.; Sletten, K.; Thorsby, E.; Rammensee, H.G.; Sollid, L.M. The peptide binding motif of the disease associated HLA-DQ (α 1(*) 0501, β 1(*) 0201) molecule. *Eur. J. Immunol.* **1996**, *26*, 2764–2772. [CrossRef] [PubMed]
11. Sollid, L.M.; Thorsby, E. HLA susceptibility genes in celiac disease: Genetic mapping and role in pathogenesis. *Gastroenterology* **1993**, *105*, 910–922. [CrossRef]
12. Ploski, R.; Ek, J.; Thorsby, E.; Sollid, L.M. On the HLA-DQ(α1*0501, β1*0201)-associated susceptibility in celiac disease: A possible gene dosage effect of *DQB1*0201*. *Tissue Antigens* **1993**, *41*, 173–177. [CrossRef] [PubMed]
13. van Belzen, M.J.; Koeleman, B.P.C.; Crusius, J.B.A.; Meijer, J.W.R.; Bardoel, A.F.J.; Pearson, P.L.; Sandkuijl, L.A.; Houwen, R.H.J.; Wijmenga, C. Defining the contribution of the HLA region to cis DQ2-positive coeliac disease patients. *Genes Immun.* **2004**, *5*, 215–220. [CrossRef] [PubMed]

14. Margaritte-Jeannin, P.; Babron, M.C.; Bourgey, M.; Louka, A.S.; Clot, F.; Percopo, S.; Coto, I.; Hugot, J.P.; Ascher, H.; Sollid, L.M.; et al. HLA-DQ relative risks for coeliac disease in European populations: A study of the European Genetics Cluster on Coeliac Disease. *Tissue Antigens* **2004**, *63*, 562–567. [CrossRef]

15. Vader, W.; Stepniak, D.; Kooy, Y.; Mearin, L.; Thompson, A.; van Rood, J.J.; Spaenij, L.; Koning, F. The HLA-DQ2 gene dose effect in celiac disease is directly related to the magnitude and breadth of gluten-specific T cell responses. *Proc. Natl. Acad. Sci. USA* **2003**, *100*, 12390–12395. [CrossRef]

16. Bajor, J.; Szakács, Z.; Farkas, N.; Hegyi, P.; Illés, A.; Solymár, M.; Pétervári, E.; Balaskó, M.; Pár, G.; Sarlós, P.; et al. Classical celiac disease is more frequent with a double dose of HLA-DQB102: A systematic review with meta-analysis. *PLoS ONE* **2019**, *14*, e0212329. [CrossRef]

17. Ludvigsson, J.F.; Leffler, D.A.; Bai, J.C.; Biagi, F.; Fasano, A.; Green, P.H.R.; Hadjivassiliou, M.; Kaukinen, K.; Kelly, C.P.; Leonard, J.N.; et al. The Oslo definitions for coeliac disease and related terms. *Gut* **2013**, *62*, 43–52. [CrossRef]

18. Dickson, B.C.; Streutker, C.J.; Chetty, R. Coeliac disease: An update for pathologists. *J. Clin. Pathol.* **2006**, *59*, 1008–1016. [CrossRef]

19. Dieterich, W.; Ehnis, T.; Bauer, M.; Donner, P.; Volta, U.; Riecken, E.O.; Schuppan, D. Identification of tissue transglutaminase as the autoantigen of celiac disease. *Nat. Med.* **1997**, *3*, 797–801. [CrossRef]

20. Chorzelski, T.P.; Sulej, J.; Tchorzewska, H.; Jablonska, S.; Beutner, E.H.; Kumar, V. IgA Class Endomysium Antibodies in Dermatitis Herpetiformis and Coeliac Disease. *Ann. N. Y. Acad. Sci.* **1983**, *420*, 325–334. [CrossRef]

21. Eade, O.E.; Lloyd, R.S.; Lang, C.; Wright, R. IgA and IgG reticulin antibodies in coeliac and non-coeliac patients. *Gut* **1977**, *18*, 991–993. [CrossRef] [PubMed]

22. Sulkanen, S.; Collin, P.; Laurila, K.; Mäki, M. IgA- and IgG-class antihuman umbilical cord antibody tests in adult coeliac disease. *Scand. J. Gastroenterol.* **1998**, *33*, 251–254. [CrossRef] [PubMed]

23. Monsuur, A.J.; de Bakker, P.I.W.; Zhernakova, A.; Pinto, D.; Verduijn, W.; Romanos, J.; Auricchio, R.; Lopez, A.; van Heel, D.A.; Crusius, J.B.A.; et al. Effective detection of human leukocyte antigen risk alleles in celiac disease using tag single nucleotide polymorphisms. *PLoS ONE* **2008**, *3*, e2270. [CrossRef] [PubMed]

24. Koskinen, L.; Romanos, J.; Kaukinen, K.; Mustalahti, K.; Korponay-Szabo, I.; Barisani, D.; Bardella, M.T.; Ziberna, F.; Vatta, S.; Széles, G.; et al. Cost-effective HLA typing with tagging SNPs predicts celiac disease risk haplotypes in the Finnish, Hungarian, and Italian populations. *Immunogenetics* **2009**, *61*, 247–256. [CrossRef] [PubMed]

25. Martínez-Ojinaga, E.; Fernández-Prieto, M.; Molina, M.; Polanco, I.; Urcelay, E.; Núñez, C. Influence of HLA on clinical and analytical features of pediatric celiac disease. *BMC Gastroenterol.* **2019**, *19*, 91. [CrossRef] [PubMed]

26. du Pré, M.F.; Blazevski, J.; Dewan, A.E.; Stamnaes, J.; Kanduri, C.; Sandve, G.K.; Johannesen, M.K.; Lindstad, C.B.; Hnida, K.; Fugger, L.; et al. B cell tolerance and antibody production to the celiac disease autoantigen transglutaminase 2. *J. Exp. Med.* **2020**, *217*. [CrossRef]

27. Kauma, S.; Kaukinen, K.; Huhtala, H.; Kivelä, L.; Pekki, H.; Salmi, T.; Saavalainen, P.; Lindfors, K.; Kurppa, K.; Kauma, S.; et al. The Phenotype of Celiac Disease Has Low Concordance between Siblings, Despite a Similar Distribution of HLA Haplotypes. *Nutrients* **2019**, *11*, 479. [CrossRef]

28. Wacklin, P.; Kaukinen, K.; Tuovinen, E.; Collin, P.; Lindfors, K.; Partanen, J.; Mäki, M.; Mättuö, J. The duodenal microbiota composition of adult celiac disease patients is associated with the clinical manifestation of the disease. *Inflamm. Bowel Dis.* **2013**, *19*, 934–941. [CrossRef]

29. Al-Toma, A.; Goerres, M.S.; Meijer, J.W.R.; Peña, A.S.; Crusius, J.B.A.; Mulder, C.J.J. Human leukocyte antigen-DQ2 homozygosity and the development of refractory celiac disease and enteropathy-associated T-cell lymphoma. *Clin. Gastroenterol. Hepatol.* **2006**, *4*, 315–319. [CrossRef]

30. Ilus, T.; Kaukinen, K.; Virta, L.J.; Pukkala, E.; Collin, P. Incidence of malignancies in diagnosed celiac patients: A population-based estimate. *Am. J. Gastroenterol.* **2014**, *109*, 1471–1477. [CrossRef]

31. Paarlahti, P.; Kurppa, K.; Ukkola, A.; Collin, P.; Huhtala, H.; Mäki, M.; Kaukinen, K. Predictors of persistent symptoms and reduced quality of life in treated coeliac disease patients: A large cross-sectional study. *BMC Gastroenterol.* **2013**, *13*, 75. [CrossRef] [PubMed]

32. Wacklin, P.; Laurikka, P.; Lindfors, K.; Collin, P.; Salmi, T.; Lähdeaho, M.L.; Saavalainen, P.; Mäki, M.; Mättö, J.; Kurppa, K.; et al. Altered Duodenal microbiota composition in celiac disease patients suffering from persistent symptoms on a long-term gluten-free diet. *Am. J. Gastroenterol.* **2014**, *109*, 1933–1941. [CrossRef] [PubMed]

33. Tursi, A.; Brandimarte, G.; Giorgetti, G.M. High prevalence of small intestinal bacterial overgrowth in celiac patients with persistence of gastrointestinal symptoms after gluten withdrawal. *Am. J. Gastroenterol.* **2003**, *98*, 839–843. [CrossRef] [PubMed]

34. Rubio-Tapia, A.; Rahim, M.W.; See, J.A.; Lahr, B.D.; Wu, T.T.; Murray, J.A. Mucosal recovery and mortality in adults with celiac disease after treatment with a gluten-free diet. *Am. J. Gastroenterol.* **2010**, *105*, 1412–1420. [CrossRef]

35. Sollid, L.M. The roles of MHC class II genes and post-translational modification in celiac disease. *Immunogenetics* **2017**, *69*, 605–616. [CrossRef]

2

The Diverse Potential of Gluten from Different Durum Wheat Varieties in Triggering Celiac Disease: A Multilevel In Vitro, Ex Vivo and In Vivo Approach

Federica Gaiani [1,2,†], Sara Graziano [3,†], Fatma Boukid [3,4,†], Barbara Prandi [3,4], Lorena Bottarelli [2,5], Amelia Barilli [6], Arnaldo Dossena [3,4], Nelson Marmiroli [3,7], Mariolina Gullì [3,4,*], Gian Luigi de'Angelis [1,2,*] and Stefano Sforza [3,4,*]

1   Gastroenterology and Endoscopy Unit, University Hospital of Parma, University of Parma, via Gramsci 14, 43126 Parma, Italy; federica.gaiani@unipr.it
2   Interdepartmental Center Biopharmanet-tec, Parco Area delle Scienze, University of Parma, 43124 Parma, Italy; lorena.bottarelli@unipr.it
3   Interdepartmental Center SITEIA.PARMA, Parco Area delle Scienze, University of Parma, 43124 Parma, Italy; sara.graziano@unipr.it (S.G.); fatma.boukid@unipr.it (F.B.); barbara.prandi@unipr.it (B.P.); arnaldo.dossena@unipr.it (A.D.); nelson.marmiroli@unipr.it (N.M.)
4   Department of Food and Drug, Parco Area delle Scienze, University of Parma, 27/A-43124 Parma, Italy
5   Department of Medicine and Surgery, Unit of Pathological Anatomy, University Hospital of Parma, via Gramsci 14, 43126 Parma, Italy
6   Department of Medicine and Surgery, Unit of General Pathology, University of Parma, Via Volturno 39, 43125 Parma, Italy; amelia.barilli@unipr.it
7   Department of Chemistry, Life Sciences, and Environmental Sustainability, University of Parma, Parco Area delle Scienze 11a, 43124 Parma, Italy
*   Correspondence: mariolina.gulli@unipr.it (M.G.); gianluigi.deangelis@unipr.it (G.L.d.); stefano.sforza@unipr.it (S.S.)
†   These authors equally contributed to this work.

Abstract: The reasons behind the increasing prevalence of celiac disease (CD) worldwide are still not fully understood. This study adopted a multilevel approach (in vitro, ex vivo, in vivo) to assess the potential of gluten from different wheat varieties in triggering CD. Peptides triggering CD were identified and quantified in mixtures generated from simulated gastrointestinal digestion of wheat varieties ($n = 82$). Multivariate statistics enabled the discrimination of varieties generating low impact on CD (e.g., Saragolla) and high impact (e.g., Cappelli). Enrolled subjects ($n = 46$) were: 19 healthy subjects included in the control group; 27 celiac patients enrolled for the in vivo phase. Celiacs were divided into a gluten-free diet group (CD-GFD), and a GFD with Saragolla-based pasta group (CD-Sar). The diet was followed for 3 months. Data were compared between CD-Sar and CD-GFD before and after the experimental diet, demonstrating a limited ability of Saragolla to trigger immunity, although not comparable to a GFD. Ex vivo studies showed that Saragolla and Cappelli activated immune responses, although with great variability among patients. The diverse potential of durum wheat varieties in triggering CD immune response was demonstrated. Saragolla is not indicated for celiacs, yet it has a limited potential to trigger adverse immune response.

Keywords: celiac disease; durum wheat; gluten peptides; immune response; ELISA

1. Introduction

Celiac disease (CD) is a chronic autoimmune enteropathy triggered by dietary gluten in genetically predisposed individuals [1]. In Western countries, the prevalence of CD in the general population is about 1%, with regional differences, such as in Finland and Sweden, where prevalence rises to 2–3% [2]. Epidemiologic data have shown a constant increase in incidence of CD not only in countries where a high number of gluten-containing products are the basis of dietary habits, but also in Asian countries such as India [3]. The exact reasons driving this increasing incidence are not yet clear: nowadays, diagnostic techniques are easily available all over the world, and both general practitioners and pediatricians are more and more experienced in suspecting and screening the disease, but certainly global changes in dietary habits related to higher consumption of wheat-based food are playing a role in modifying CD epidemiology [4].

CD development depends on the presence of key genes that regulate the immunological response to dietary gluten and, in particular in subjects bearing human leucocyte antigen (HLA) DQ2/DQ8 haplotypes, gluten represents the key environmental factor triggering the immune response that is the basis of small-intestine mucosal damage, mediated both by innate and adaptive immunity [5,6]. The presence of these alleles is necessary but not sufficient for disease development: although the HLA-DQ2 allele is common in the white population (30% of people are carriers), almost 3% of them will develop CD [6]. On the contrary, 95% of CD patients carry the HLA-DQ2 (DQA1*0501/DQB1*0201) haplotype, while the remaining patients express the HLA-DQ8 (DQA1*0301/DQB1*0302) haplotype [7].

Gluten is a group of glutamine and proline-rich proteins called prolamins, contained in the grains of several cereals, including wheat, rye, barley and oats. In wheat, these proteins are called gliadins or glutenins, based on their monomeric or polymeric structure, and together they form gluten [8]. After gluten ingestion, proteases contained in gastrointestinal secretions hydrolyze glutamine- and proline-rich gluten-composing proteins [9]. However, gluten peptides are not completely hydrolyzed by gastrointestinal enzymes because of their high amounts of proline. Adjuvated by increased permeability of the intestinal mucosa [10], partially hydrolyzed proteins reach the lamina propria, where they are modified by tissue transglutaminase (tTG) by deamidation and transamidation, becoming more affine to major histocompatibility complex class II (MHCII) and initiating lymphocyte activation [9]. Genetic predisposition is necessary to develop CD, indeed HLA-DQ2 and/or HLA-DQ8 alleles code for specific MHC molecules, which are surface receptors on antigen-presenting cells belonging to the immune system. The HLA-DQ2 and HLA-DQ8 proteins have high affinity for deamidated, negatively charged gluten-derived peptides [11]. Although it is not clear how and when the autoimmune reaction driven by gluten is initiated, a high amount of gluten-derived peptides and a high frequency in dietary gluten consumption increases the probability of having substrates to initiate the inflammatory process at the basis of CD.

Several approaches have been followed to better understand CD. In vitro gastrointestinal digestion models have been widely used, with different systems, such as single static, multicompartmental and dynamic. Quite obviously, diverse approaches generated different results, making the comparison between studies not possible [12–14]. A standard model was recently developed to simulate digestive processes [15]. Quantitative tools were afterward required for the quantification of total gluten or the generated peptides associated with CD, such as enzyme-linked immunosorbent assays and proteomics tools [16,17]. The peptides obtained from gliadin digestion trigger the inflammation of the intestinal mucosa due to both the adaptive and the innate immune responses. Intestinal biopsy cultures from celiac patients were demonstrated to be useful in determining innate and adaptive responses to gluten [18]. In particular, interleukin (IL)-15 and interferon (IFN)-γ are part of a more complex network which is responsible of the dysregulation of multiple immune mechanisms in the small intestine, together contributing to CD pathogenesis [19]. It is noteworthy that, even if in vitro and ex vivo approaches have provided great understanding of CD, in vivo studies remain crucial to fully understand how the ingestion of gluten impacts the gastrointestinal tract.

From a multilevel perspective, the present study aims to explore: (i) at the in vitro level, the high diversity in durum wheat varieties on the amount of peptides associated with CD, generated after simulated gastrointestinal digestion, in order to identify a variety with less triggering peptide production, thus lowering the impact on the immune response; (ii) at the ex vivo level, the potential of the above gluten-derived peptides to trigger the production of inflammatory cytokines usually implicated in the initiation of autoimmune inflammation leading to CD and (iii) at the in vivo level, the comparison of a gluten-free diet with a gluten-free diet with a controlled amount of food produced with a selected wheat species, identified as above for being low impact, measuring the immune activation with tTG IgA serum antibodies. The research of a durum wheat variety with low impact on the immune response does not aim to implement a gluten-free diet for celiac subjects, who are not allowed to take gluten, rather it is addressed to the general non-celiac population's dietary habits. The use of wheat varieties that are less stimulating to the immune system, compared to wheat varieties traditionally employed in food production, could bring potential benefits for patients predisposed to celiac disease and not yet manifesting the disorder.

2. Materials and Methods

2.1. In Vitro Study

2.1.1. Material

The durum wheat varieties (*Triticum durum* Desf.; $n = 82$ varieties) utilized in this research were cultivated in the field at the Council for Agricultural Research and Economics–Research Centre for Cereal and Industrial Crops (CREA-CI), Foggia (Italy, 41° 28′ N, 15° 32′ E and 75 m a.s.l.) in a clay–loam soil (typic chromoxerert) in the growing season of 2015–2016. Seeds after harvesting were milled using a laboratory mill (Ika Werke, Staufen, Germany) and stored in plastic bags at 4 °C until analysis. Pasta made with Saragolla wheat and used in this study had a water content of 0.092 ± 0.001%, and a protein content of 10.8 ± 0.3% (wet basis). Immunogenic peptides after in vitro digestion were 1363 ± 66 ppm, and toxic peptides were 461 ± 27 ppm.

2.1.2. In Vitro Gastrointestinal Digestion

Whole wheat flours were subjected to simulated gastrointestinal digestion [15] as follows: (i) 1 g of flour was incubated (2 min; 37 °C under constant gentle mixing) with 1 mL simulated saliva containing porcine amylase (Sigma-Aldrich, St. Louis, MI, USA; 75 U/mL of digesta); (ii) 2 mL simulated gastric juice containing porcine pepsin (Sigma-Aldrich, St. Louis, MI, USA; 2000 U/mL of digesta) was added and incubated (2 h; 37 °C under constant gentle mixing) after pH adjustment to 3; (iii) 4 mL duodenal juice containing porcine pancreatin (SigmaAldrich, St. Louis, MI, USA; 100 U trypsin activity/mL of digesta) and porcine bile (Sigma-Aldrich, St. Louis, MI, USA; 10 mmol/L in the total volume) was added and incubated (2 h; 37 °C under constant gentle mixing) after pH adjustment to 7. Afterward, to inactivate the enzymes, the sample was boiled for 10 min at 95 °C. After centrifugation (3220 g, 4 °C, 45 min), the supernatant (295 µL) was added to 5 µL of internal standard solution (TQQPQQPF(d5)PQQPQQPF(d5)PQ; 1.6 mM); samples were then subjected to reverse phase liquid chromatography coupled to mass spectrometry (RP-UPLC/ESI-MS) to quantify peptides associated with CD [20]. All the samples were digested in duplicate.

2.2. In Vivo Study

In the period between November 2017 and November 2018, all the patients who admitted at the Gastroenterology and Endoscopy Unit of the University Hospital of Parma, Italy, to undergo esophagogastroduodenoscopy for suspected CD were evaluated for inclusion in the present study. The inclusion criteria were age between 2 and 75 years, elevated tTG IgA (UNL (upper limits of normal) = 10 U/mL) and or DPG-AGA IgG (UNL = 10 U/mL). A cohort of patients comparable for demographics and admitted at the Gastroenterology and Endoscopy Unit of the University Hospital of Parma, Italy, for reasons other than suspected CD was considered for inclusion in the control group (CG). These patients were evaluated for eligibility while being referred to the hospital to undergo esophagogastroduodenoscopy for gastroesophageal reflux symptoms, dyspepsia, abdominal pain or weight loss. Their inclusion in the CG was confirmed once duodenal biopsies taken during endoscopy were found to be normal, therefore excluding celiac disease.

Eligible patients and their families were given information describing the study and, subsequently, written consent to participate was gathered. The study protocol was conducted in accordance with the Declaration of Helsinki (1964) and the protocol was approved by the Ethics Committee of Parma (Project POR-FESR 2014–2020) on 25 July 2017. As an ethical requirement, patients were included only if able to sign informed consent (by the legal guardian in case of minors).

Each patient was characterized by demographics and clinical data, including serum levels of hemoglobin, total IgA levels, tTG IgA, DGP-AGA IgG, HLA haplotype for suspected celiac patients, ongoing treatments, first-degree familiarity for CD and comorbidities; all the included patients underwent duodenal biopsies to ascertain CD in suspected patients and to rule it out in controls. Specifically, all controls underwent one biopsy in the descending duodenum and one biopsy in the bulb, while for suspected celiac patients four biopsies in the descending duodenum and one in the bulb were taken, in accordance with current guidelines for diagnosis [21]. Moreover, all the included patients underwent three additional biopsies taken from the descending duodenum for the in vitro study.

After diagnosis of CD was ascertained by histologic examination and graded in accordance with Marsh–Oberhüber classification [22], celiac patients were divided in two cohorts on a voluntary basis. The first cohort followed a gluten-free diet including a daily portion (40–70 g of pasta based on the age of the considered patient) of experimental pasta made with Saragolla wheat flour (CD-Sar cohort) for three months; pasta was provided by the investigators. The second cohort followed a complete and rigorous gluten-free diet (CD-GFD cohort). Both the CD-Sar and the CD-GFD cohorts underwent serum dosage of the same parameters described at the enrollment after three months of the diet. Experimental pasta samples used were produced at the pilot plant of Barilla (Parma, Italy) following the conventional industrial processing diagram of pasta production. None of the patients either in the CD-GFD group nor in the CD-Sar group had ever followed a gluten-free diet before inclusion in the study. Nutritional counseling was provided by gastroenterologists after diagnosis of CD and before the start of the study, to maximize compliance to the diet (either totally gluten-free or gluten-free with a portion of Saragolla wheat pasta).

Data extracted from demographics, antibody serum levels before and after three months of the diet, HLA typing and histological examination were compared among groups.

2.3. Ex Vivo Study

All the included patients underwent three additional biopsies taken from the descending duodenum for the ex vivo study. Freshly isolated biopsies were placed in the wells of a tissue culture plate containing DMEM/F12 supplemented with 10% heat-inactivated fetal calf serum, 100 U/mL penicillin and 100 mg/mL streptomycin. From each patient, one mucosa biopsy was cultured with the medium (control), one was cultured in the medium after the addition of 5% of the in vitro digested flour of Cappelli and one was cultured after the addition of 5% of the in vitro digested flour of Saragolla. The culture plate was placed in an organ culture chamber, gassed with a mixture of 95% O_2 and 5% CO2, and incubated at 37 °C for 4 h. As demonstrated by previous works [23], significant differences in the cytokine production were already measurable after 120 min of biopsy incubation with digested gliadin. So, the incubation period was set to 4 h to maximize the possibility to observe eventual differences in the cytokine production among the samples. At the end of the culture period, supernatant fluid from the cultured specimens was collected and stored at −70 °C until used. IL-15 and IFN-γ were determined in the supernatants by ELISA using the Quantikine® ELISA Human IL-15 Immunoassay and Human IFN-γ Immunoassay (R&D Systems, Inc., Minneapolis, MN 55413, USA), following the manufacturer's instructions.

2.4. Statistical Analysis

Significant differences among the generated peptides after digestion were found using analysis of variance (ANOVA) with a confidence interval of 95% ($p \leq 0.05$). Principal component analysis based on unsupervised features (peptides generated after in vitro digestion) was performed based on the correlation matrix. For the evaluation of significant differences of the output of in vivo and ex vivo results, the non-parametric Wilcoxon–Mann–Whitney test was used ($p \leq 0.05$). All the statistical analyses were determined using the program SPSS for Windows (Version 24.0, SPSS Inc., Chicago, IL, USA).

3. Results

3.1. In Vitro Results

The peptides identified could be subdivided into two groups, according to the literature [24–26]: peptides triggering the adaptive and innate immune responses. Seven immunogenic peptides derived from γ-gliadin were identified as being involved in the adaptive immune response ("immunogenic peptides", IPs). IP sequences are described in Figure 1. All IP sequences contained the motif DQ2.5-glia-γ4c (QQPQQPFPQ) [27]. Three peptides deriving from α-gliadin were identified as being involved in the innate immune response ("toxic peptides", TPs). TP sequences are described in Figure 1. The sequence of these peptides contained the motifs PSQQ, QQQP, QQPY or QPYP able to trigger the innate immune response. The quantification of these peptides showed significant differences, as illustrated in Figure 1 and based on statistical data (Supplementary Table S1). Full characterization of the 82 varieties can be found in Taranto et al. (2020) [28]. Such a high variability might be attributed to high genetic variability among the studied varieties (i.e., matrix properties including protein structure and starch–protein interactions), which greatly influence digestive enzyme accessibility to gluten [29,30].

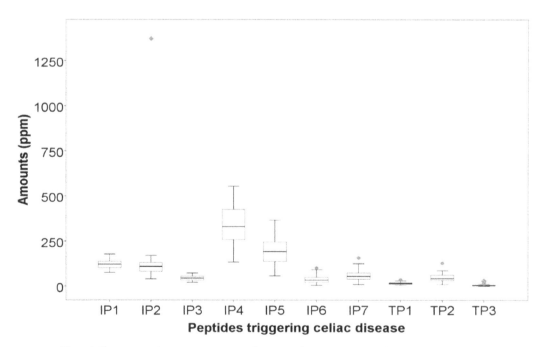

Figure 1. Variability in the amounts of peptides associated with celiac disease. IP1: TQQPQQPFPQ; IP2: SQQPQQPFPQPQ; IP3: QAFPQQPQQPFPQ; IP4: TQQPQQPFPQQPQQPFPQ; IP5: PQTQQPQQPFPQFQQPQQPFPQPQQP; IP6: FPQQPQLPFPQQPQQPFPQPQQPQ; IP7: QQPQQPFPQPQQTFPQQPQLPFPQQPQQPF. TP1: LQPQNPSQQQPQ; TP2: RPQQPYPQPQPQ. TP3: LQPQNPSQQQPQEQVPL.

Principal component analysis (PCA) was therefore performed to enable a better picture. Figure 2A displays the two-dimensional scattering plot of the quantity of peptides associated with CD. The first two principal components (PCs) explained 83% of the total variability. The first component explained 60% as a function of the major part of the identified peptides (IP1, IP2, IP3, IP4, IP5, IP6, IP7, TP1 and TP2); whereas the second component explained only 23% as a function of TP3 (Figure 2A). The projection of the studied durum wheat samples on the factorial space (Figure 2B) showed important variability among the 82 varieties, confirming the high genetic diversity of the studied collection.

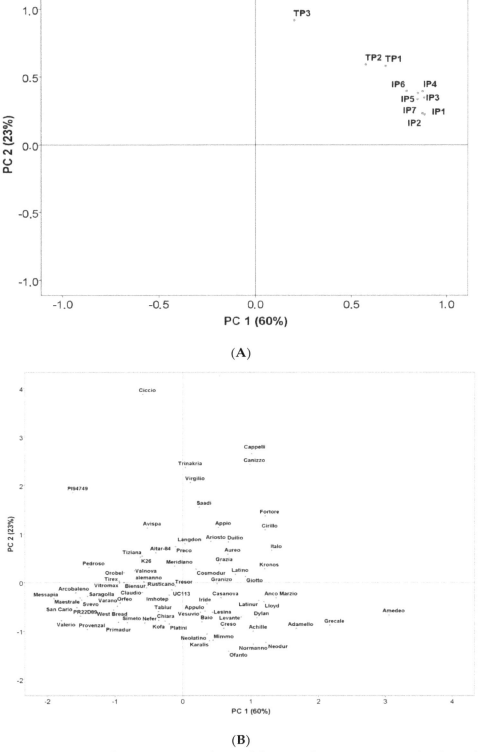

(A)

(B)

Figure 2. (**A**) Principal component analysis of durum wheat epitopes involved in celiac disease (CD). Biplot of the two first principal components based on the durum wheat epitopes involved in CD. Abbreviations IP1: TQQPQQPFPQ; IP2: SQQPQQPFPQPQ; IP3: QAFPQQPQQPFPQ; IP4: TQQPQQPFPQQPQQPFPQ; IP5: PQTQQPQQPFPQFQQPQQPFPQPQQP; IP6: FPQQPQLPFPQQPQQPFPQPQQPQ; IP7: QQPQQPFPQPQQTFPQQPQLPFPQQPQQPF. TP1: LQPQNPSQQQPQ; TP2: RPQQPYPQPQPQ. TP3: LQPQNPSQQQPQEQVPL. (**B**) Principal component analysis of durum wheat epitopes involved in CD. Rotated principal scores of the durum wheat varieties projected into the first two principal components.

Using PCA (Figure 2B), we were also able to locate varieties with a low amount of triggering peptides after digestion, thus with a potentially low impact on CD (Group 1) and those with a high amount of triggering peptides after digestion, thus with high impact (Group 2). As shown in Figure 2B, two groups of wheat varieties were clearly identified: high in CD-triggering peptides (total peptides between 900 ppm and 2700 ppm) and low in CD-triggering peptides (total peptides <600 ppm). The selection of Saragolla and Cappelli was based on the amount of peptides, Saragolla (513 ppm peptides generated after digestion) was selected as representative of Group 1, and Cappelli (1488 ppm peptides generated after digestion) as representative of Group 2, to be used in the following analyses. Both varieties are widely cultivated in Italy and utilized to produce monovarietal flours for pasta; Saragolla is a modern variety, released in 2004, while Cappelli is an old one, released in 1915.

3.2. In Vivo Results

Overall, 46 patients with ages between 3 and 69 years were recruited: 19 non-celiac patients were included in the control group (CG), while 27 celiac patients were divided into the CD-Sar group (11 patients) and CD-GFD group (16 patients). All the patients included in the CD-Sar group were minors (aged between 3 and 17 years), while among patients included in CD-GFD group, 13 were minors and three were adults (aged 45, 20 and 25 years). Characteristics of the included patients are described in Table 1.

Table 1. Clinical characteristics of the included subjects.

Parameter	Total (*n* = 46)	CD-Sar (*n* = 11)	CD-GFD (*n* = 16)	CG (*n* = 19)
Age, years (mean (range))	(3–69)	8.27 (3–17)	12.96 (5–45)	29.42 (5–69)
Sex: M	18 (39.13%)	5 (45.45%)	3 (18.75%)	10 (52.63%)
F	28 (60.87%)	6 (54.55%)	13 (81.25%)	9 (47.37%)
BMI (mean (range))	(11.16–29.35)	16.41 (12.5–23.18)	16.4 (12–21.5)	19.58 (11.16–29.35)
Comorbidities:				
none	43 (93.49%)	11 (100%)	14 (87.5%)	18 (94.74%)
atopy	1 (2.17%)	0	1 (6.25%)	0
autoimmune thyroiditis	1 (2.17%)	0	1 (6.25%)	0
hematologic disorders	1 (2.17%)	0	0	1 (5.26%)
Ongoing treatments:				
none	40 (86.96%)	11 (100%)	13 (81.25%)	16 (84.21%)
PPI/ranitidine	3 (6.52%)	0	1 (6.25%)	2 (10.53%)
prokinetics	1 (2.17%)	0	0	1 (5.26%)
levothyroxine	1 (2.17%)	0	1 (6.25%)	0
oral contraceptives	1 (2.17%)	0	1 (6.25%)	0
Symptoms:				
none	9 (19.56%)	2 (18.18%)	7 (43.75%)	0
diarrhea	6 (13.04%)	1 (9.09%)	4 (25%)	1 (5.26%)
abdominal pain	14 (30.43%)	5 (45.45%)	6 (37.5%)	3 (15.79%)
growth delay/weight loss	7 (15.22%)	2 (18.18%)	3 (18.75%)	2 (10.53%)
constipation	3 (6.52%)	2 (18.18%)	1 (6.25%)	0
reflux symptoms/pyrosis	9 (19.56%)	0	0	9 (47.37%)
nausea/dyspepsia	4 (8.7%)	0	0	4 (21.05%)

Table 1. *Cont.*

Parameter	Total ($n = 46$)	CD-Sar ($n = 11$)	CD-GFD ($n = 16$)	CG ($n = 19$)
Familiarity for CD:				
yes	7 (15.22%)	4 (36.36%)	3 (18.75%)	0
no	39 (84.78%)	7 (63.64%)	13 (81.25%)	19 (100%)
tTG IgA (mean (range))	n/a	79.68 (13–173)	85.11 (9.8–275)	n/a
DPG-AGA IgG (mean (range))	n/a	77.6 (3.3–302)	38.5 (3.3–82)	n/a
Hb (g/dL) (mean (range))	n/a	12.17 (7.4–14)	12.9 (11.5–15)	n/a
HLA haplotype:				
DQB1*02 ho/DQ8-	n/a	3 (27.3%)	1 (6.25%)	n/a
DQB1*02 he/DQ8+		1 (9%)	0	
DQB1*02 he/DQ8-		2 (18.2%)	6 (37.5%)	
DQB1*02 -/DQ8+		3 (27.3%)	0	
n/a		2 (18.2%)	9 (56.25%)	
Marsh (histology):				
0	19 (41.31%)	0	0	19 (100%)
1	3 (6.52%)	2 (18.18%)	1 (6.25%)	0
3 (a or b or c)	24 (52.17%)	9 (81.82%)	15 (93.75%)	0

Abbreviations: CD-Sar, group of celiac patients undergoing a gluten-free diet with pasta produced with Saragolla wheat; CD-GFD, group of celiac patients undergoing a gluten-free diet; CG, control group; M, males; F, females; BMI, body mass index; PPI, proton pump inhibitor; tTG IgA, antibody anti-transglutaminase, class IgA; DPG-AGA IgA, antibody anti-deaminated peptide of gliadin, class IgG; HLA, Human Leukocyte Antigen; Hb, hemoglobin; ho, homozygous; he, heterozygous. Familiarity stands for first-degree familiarity.

Most of the recruited patients were females (60.87%), who represented most patients in the CD-GFD group, while sexes were equally distributed among the CD-Sar and CG. In all groups, most of the patients had no comorbidities and were on no medications. The distribution of symptoms of presentation was inhomogeneous and only a few celiac patients presented with typical CD (e.g., diarrhea, weight loss). At recruitment, tTG IgA levels were elevated and suspicious for CD, with comparable titers between the CD-Sar group and CD-GFD group. None of the patients diagnosed with celiac disease presented selective IgA deficiency. First-degree familiarity for celiac CD was negative in most celiac patients, and in all cases in the control group. Overall, HLA haplotype distribution was inhomogeneous and did not show significant differences ($p = 0.085$) between groups. Regarding diagnosis of CD, histology of duodenal biopsies was investigated in all groups, showing a complete normality in the CG, and the highest degree of pathognomonic histologic characteristics for CD both in the CD-Sar and CD-GFD groups, with duodenal biopsies classified as Marsh 3 grade in 81.82% and 93.75% of patients, respectively. For all celiac patients, no other histologic lesions were detected in gastric and esophageal biopsies, except for one patient, who was demonstrated to be affected by eosinophilic esophagitis. This patient was included in the CD-Sar group. Overall, the CD-Sar and CD-GFD groups demonstrated comparable clinic characteristics.

The effect of the inclusion in the diet of pasta prepared with Saragolla wheat flour on immune activation was then compared to the GFD, by the determination of antibody serum levels before and after 3 months of the diet. Overall, two patients included in the CD-Sar cohort and eight patients included in the CD-GFD cohort refused to undergo the second antibody determination after 3 months of the diet. Results are shown in Table 2.

Specifically, tTG IgA variation (Δ) after the administered diet was determined and compared between the CD-Sar and CD-GFD groups, showing no significant differences (p=0.06). Results are shown in Table 2.

The influence of diet on immune activation was mainly determined by tTG IgA variation, although DPG-AGA IgG and hemoglobin serum levels were also investigated, showing similarly no differences between groups (Table 2).

Table 2. Variation of serum CD antibodies and hemoglobin values before and after 3 months of diet. Comparison between CD-Sar and CD-GFD.

Laboratory Test	CD-Sar (*n* = 11)	CD-GFD (*n* = 16)	Δ Sar-GFD
tTG IgA: T0 (mean (range))	79.68 (13–173)	85.11 (9.8–275)	
3 M (mean (range))	51.32 (7.1–114)	10.6 (2.8–24)	$p = 0.06$
n/a T0	0	0	
n/a 3 M	2 (18.2%)	8 (50%)	
DPG-AGA IgG: T0 (mean (range))	77.6 (3.3–302)	38.5 (3.3–82)	
3 M (mean (range))	20.8 (1.5–128)	6.65 (1.5–21)	$p = 0.62$
n/a T0	4 (26.4%)	8 (50%)	
n/a 3 M	3 (27.3%)	10 (52.6%)	
Hb: T0 (mean (range))	12.17 (7.4–14)	12.9 (11.5–15)	
3 M (mean (range))	12.28 (9–14.4)	13.5 (11.4–15.2)	$p = 0.97$
n/a T0 (%)	1 (9.1%)	3 (%)	
n/a 3 M (%)	3 (27.3%)	8 (50%)	

Abbreviations: CD-Sar, group of celiac patients undergoing a gluten-free diet with pasta produced with Saragolla wheat; CD-GFD, group of celiac patients undergoing a gluten-free diet; tTG IgA, antibody anti-transglutaminase, class IgA; DPG-AGA IgA, antibody anti-deaminated peptide of gliadin, class IgG; Hb, hemoglobin; T0, at the start of the study, time 0; 3 M, after three months of experimentation; n/a, not available.

In the patient diagnosed as celiac and affected by eosinophilic esophagitis, it was also possible to compare duodenal biopsies before and after three months of the diet with Saragolla wheat, as the patient needed to repeat endoscopy after therapy with proton pump inhibitors, accordingly to international guidelines [31]. As shown in Figures 3 and 4, diet with Saragolla wheat pasta did not modify duodenal histology, and it did not worsen the Marsh grade, which was 3a both at diagnosis and after three months of the diet. The comparison between the gluten-free diet with Saragolla wheat and the completely gluten-free diet was carried out for a limited period of time (3 months) with the only aim to observe if the immune response of celiac patients continued to be triggered by Saragolla wheat as by a traditional wheat-containing diet, or if this selected wheat variety had a limited potential to trigger autoimmunity, in terms of tTG titer. Yet, we specify that the cohort of celiac patients undergoing the gluten-free diet with Saragolla was necessary, as celiac patients are the only subjects in which an immune response is measurable by using antibody titers (tTG IgA). We also specify that the diet including Saragolla was stopped after three months for celiac patients, as it is not suitable for them to achieve remission of the disease.

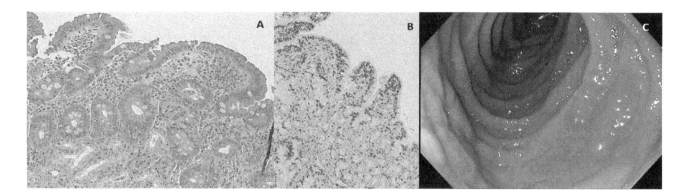

Figure 3. Duodenal mucosa before experimental diet. (**A**) Hematoxylin–eosin 4× magnification, duodenal mucosa before experimental diet. Celiac disease classified as Marsh 3a; (**B**) immunohistochemical coloration for CD3+ lymphocytes, duodenal mucosa before experimental diet; (**C**) endoscopic appearance of the duodenal mucosa before experimental diet.

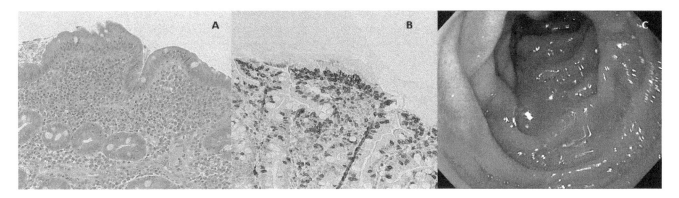

Figure 4. Duodenal mucosa after experimental diet. (**A**) Hematoxylin–eosin 4× magnification, duodenal mucosa after experimental diet. Celiac disease classified as Marsh 3a; (**B**) immunohistochemical coloration for CD3+ lymphocytes, duodenal mucosa after experimental diet; (**C**) endoscopic appearance of the duodenal mucosa after experimental diet.

3.3. Ex Vivo Results

Overall, 43 patients were subjected to three additional duodenal biopsies which were utilized for the ex vivo treatments with the products of the in vitro digestion of rice flour (GF) and Saragolla (Sar) and Cappelli (Cap) wheat flours. In many studies, organ culture experiments have been performed by using digested gliadin fractions because many more components are present in digested flour that could interfere with the results of the organ culture system [32,33]. However, using a digested flour is much closer to what physiologically happens in the human body than the selected peptide fraction. The biopsies utilized were from 16 non-celiac individuals (CG group) and 27 celiac patients (CD group). After the different treatments, the level of IL-15 and IFN-γ were measured by an ELISA test. In general, high individual variability was observed, for both IL15 and IFN- γ levels. Therefore, the values of IL-15 and of IFN-γ measured in biopsies treated with Sar or Cap were normalized with respect to GFD (Table 3).

Table 3. Cytokine level measured by ELISA test in biopsies treated with the product of in vitro digestion of rice flours (GF) and wheat flours of Saragolla (Sar) or Cappelli (Cap). The values reported are normalized with respect to GF.

	IL-15 Normalized (Mean (Range))	IFN-γ Normalized (Mean (Range))
Control Group	$n = 15$	$n = 14$
Sar/GF	0.97 (0.07–3.53)	0.90 (0.48–1.31)
Cap/GF	1.20 (0.12–2.95)	1.29 (0.52–4.97)
Celiac Group	$n = 16$	Sar $n = 22$-Cap $n = 23$
Sar/GF	1.48 (0.36–2.51)	1.87 (0.19–17.06)
Cap/GF	1.43 (0.64–2.71)	0.93 (0.12–3.03)

Abbreviations: ELISA, enzyme-linked immunosorbent assay; IL-15, interleukin 15; IFN-γ, interferon γ; n/a, not available.

The effect of the Sar and Cap treatments was not significantly different in CG for both IL-15 and IFN-γ levels. However, Cap treatment determined an increase in IL-15 (20%) and IFN-γ (29%) levels, differently from the Sar treatment. Regarding the CD group, in 15 cases, the treatment with either Sar or Cap digestion products determined an increase in the amount of IL-15 of 48 and 43%, respectively, as compared with the GF treatment. In 12 cases, the IL-15 levels were similar in response to all the treatments with the in vitro digestion products. As for the IFN-γ levels measured in the CD group, Sar treatment determined an increase of about 87% with respect to GF treatment. For one celiac patient affected by eosinophilic esophagitis, it was also possible to compare duodenal biopsies before and after three months of the diet with Saragolla pasta. The results obtained showed that IL-15 levels remained stable in response to each treatment even after the diet; interestingly, the IFN-γ level increased after the treatment with Cap, but not with Sar, in biopsies taken after three months of the diet (Table 4).

Table 4. Cytokine level measured by ELISA test in biopsies treated with the product of in vitro digestion of rice flours (GF) and wheat flours of Saragolla (Sar) or Cappelli (Cap). The values reported are normalized with respect to GF. Comparison of duodenal biopsies of one patient before and after three months of the diet with Saragolla pasta.

Timing	IFN Normalized		IL-15 Normalized	
	Sar	Cap	Sar	Cap
before	4.85	n/a	0.55	0.84
after	0.53	3.03	1.05	0.74

Abbreviations: ELISA, enzyme-linked immunosorbent assay; IL-15, interleukin 15; IFN-γ, interferon γ.

4. Discussion

In recent decades, CD has changed from a rare disease to a more and more diagnosed disorder through the worldwide population, not only in Western countries, but also among Eastern populations such as India, where gluten consumption is limited, although increasing [3]. Even if the disease is well known in terms of pathognomonic histologic lesions and clinical manifestations, and the diagnostic approach is standardized all over the world, little is known about the mechanisms of initiation of the autoimmune response. Gluten is recognized as the main trigger of inflammation, and, at present, a completely gluten-free diet is the only effective treatment for celiac patients, and potentially the only way to avoid the initiation of the immune response. Nevertheless, based on dietary habits, especially in Western countries, a rigorous gluten-free lifelong diet is not always easy to follow. On the other hand, no effective preventive method of the onset of CD has been discovered.

Starting from this background, the interest of this study was to investigate if selected wheat varieties had a different impact on the onset of the immune response leading to manifest CD.

The pre-clinical in vitro phase was crucial to select the wheat variety, which produced the lowest number of immunogenic peptides. An important collection of durum wheat varieties was in vitro digested and analyzed by liquid chromatography coupled to mass spectrometry for their peptides triggering immune and innate responses. The identification of CD-triggering peptides after simulated gastrointestinal digestion and untargeted MS analysis revealed that the identified peptides belong mainly to γ-gliadin and α-gliadin. These findings are consistent with previous observations [20,34]. A high variability, determined by one-way analysis of variance (ANOVA), and further confirmed by multivariate analysis (PCA), was evident in the analyzed samples, suggesting that different varieties might bear strong differences in their potential to trigger CD. Two groups were identified, classified as "high" and "low" in CD-triggering peptides. Results revealed that Saragolla (Group 1, low impact) and Cappelli (Group 2, high impact) are the median of groups 1 and 2, respectively. Furthermore, Saragolla was also used for the next in vivo experiments. Although a challenge with pasta exclusively made with Cappelli variety would have been advisable, ethical concerns prevented this possibility.

Obviously, Saragolla wheat, as for all gluten-containing wheat species, cannot be integrated in a gluten-free diet, as demonstrated by the comparison between duodenal histology before and after the experimental diet (Figures 3 and 4), as the typical lesions of CD are neither healed nor improved by this type of diet. The choice to administrate the experimental diet to celiac patients was led by the need for testing immunogenicity in a population which was certainly reactive to gluten peptides, and therefore celiac, but also sensitive to a reduction of exposure to the inflammatory trigger in terms of a reduction of specific antibody production. This method allowed us to avoid a gluten challenge in a cohort of celiac patients already on a gluten-free diet, and therefore in remission, as it would have raised ethical concerns. We started from a high and certainly pathological titer, considering that the absence of immune stimulus leads to a decrease in antibodies, and we evaluated how much the Saragolla diet detaches itself from the stimulation of the usual mix of grains and how much it can be assimilated into a gluten-free diet. Since tTG titer is not a reliable indicator of the severity of histologic lesions but an epiphenomenon of the autoimmune process at the basis of CD depending on the ability of each CD patient's immune system to elevate antibodies [35], the evaluation of the tTG-IgA level improvement was not evaluated as absolute numbers, but as percent variation from the starting level (Δ).

The effects of Saragolla diet on histology could be measured only for one patient requiring a second endoscopy and, therefore, these results are isolated and do not allow us to draw strong conclusions. Nevertheless, our study demonstrated that Saragolla wheat did not worsen previous histologic lesions, which was quite surprising, but perfectly in line with our in vitro findings, demonstrating that Saragolla wheat produces, upon digestion, a low amount of CD-triggering peptides. As a controlled amount of gluten was administered through the Saragolla pasta, we did not expect the histological lesions of this patient to heal, but this patient remained clinically stable during the three months of experimentation, at Marsh 3a grade, and did not worsen to Marsh 3c grade. Moreover, the tTG IgA value decreased from 15 U/mL to 8.6 U/mL. Although a second duodenal biopsy would have been methodologically important to complete the clinical consequences of the Saragolla diet for all the patients included in the CD-Sar cohort, it would have needed a second invasive exam against any clinical indications, which would have been ethically inappropriate. Therefore, the comparison between tTG IgA values before and after the experimental diet was considered appropriate. Importantly, the gluten-free diet integrated with Saragolla wheat pasta did not worsen the immune response, as shown by the improvement or steadiness of antibody titers, which, albeit not pathogenic, are strongly linked to an ongoing autoimmune process. Overall, during the study, tTG IgA values demonstrated high variability both at the time of recruitment and after the three months of the diet, especially in the CD-Sar cohort, which highlight that antibody titers should never be considered as an absolute value, but always considered by means of variation of the value in time, probably due to a variability among patients in gluten tolerance and the ability of the immune system to produce specific autoantibodies.

The time period of three months for the experimentation is certainly limited, but it was chosen as an appropriate compromise between the need to observe variation of the immune response by means of antibody titer variation and ethical concerns regarding the deliberate intake of gluten among patients diagnosed as celiac (CD-Sar cohort) without exposing patients to the risk of deteriorating clinical conditions.

Of note, the study was not conducted as blind nor as double-blind, and therefore lacks a cohort undergoing placebo. Every patient included in the CD-Sar group needed to add in the diet a portion of pasta provided by the researchers, therefore it would have been hard to blind this specific action. Among the weak points of the study, celiac patients enrolled were not randomly assigned to either the CD-GFD cohort or CD-Sar cohort. This choice was made to guarantee the best possible compliance of the patients to the diet, who were willing to actively participate in either cohort. The impossibility to blind the inclusion in groups was a weak point of the study, although the effect of either a completely gluten-free diet or the "Saragolla diet" was measured rigorously by dosing tTG IgA titers before and after three months of the diet in both groups. Moreover, nutritional counseling was provided by gastroenterologists after the diagnosis of celiac disease and before the start of the diet, in order to maximize the compliance to the diet, therefore allowing the results of antibody titer dosage to show the real evolution of the immune response under the diet.

Based on the above results, it might be possible to deduce that the immune response is significantly less stimulated by Saragolla wheat, compared to what is known in the literature when common wheat varieties or gliadin extracts are used [33,36]. Actually, if we consider the natural history of CD, a celiac patient who is not following a strict gluten-free diet will continue having rises in tTG IgA values until the environmental trigger is eliminated, which is gluten, as an epiphenomenon of the perpetuation of the immune response trigger. Therefore, the trend shown by tTG IgA in the CD-Sar cohort highlighted a limited ability of Saragolla wheat to activate autoimmunity. The variation in antibody titer was unfortunately affected by a percentage of patients who dropped out during the follow-up, as shown in Table 2. Anyway, the obtained results allowed us to compare cohorts reliably, from a methodological perspective.

Even though Saragolla wheat administration is not indicated for celiac patients, it could be extremely interesting to hypothesize its employment in potentially at-risk individuals, such as first-degree relatives of celiac patients or those patients affected by autoimmune diseases related to CD (Down syndrome, Hashimoto thyroiditis, diabetes mellitus type 1, etc.).

Certainly, the hypothesis to prevent CD onset by introducing less immune-reactive durum wheat varieties in the general population's diet has not been proven yet. Anyway, the present study shows for the first time in the literature an experimental basis for this hypothesis, which will have to be confirmed in larger cohorts to be considered appliable to the general population, but is not contradicted by our results. Moreover, no previous comprehensive study has ever been reported on this topic, because it is very challenging to design and conduct clinical trials using food produced with monovarietal flours, which is one of the strong methodological points of our study.

The hypothesis of using Saragolla wheat, or varieties with similar characteristics, for the production of monovarietal flours and products with low immunogenicity might be considered. The possibility to spread, in large-scale commercial distribution, this kind of product, could, theoretically, reduce the burden of the best-known environmental trigger of CD, with a consequent lower incidence of the disease itself.

This concept can be compared to the use of hydrolyzed milk in neonates, which has a reduced antigenic burden compared to conventional milk; it can be employed in the diet of unweaned babies with a familiarity for atopy, reducing the risk of cow's milk protein allergy, a fearsome consequence of the early contact between the neonate's intestine and heterologous proteins [35,37]. Although it is a theoretical assumption, the most evident benefit of the use of a less immunogenic wheat in the diet should be noted in Western countries, whose dietary habits are characterized by an important quantity of gluten-containing food.

5. Conclusions

The results of the present study demonstrate a limited ability of selected wheat varieties such as Saragolla to trigger the immune response, as the basis of CD in vitro, in vivo and ex vivo. The aim of this work was not to make gluten-free pasta but to demonstrate a minor impact of certain wheat varieties. However, the final target of a diet based on selected wheat varieties are not celiac patients, but those subjects at risk of CD. Although Saragolla cannot be applied in the gluten-free diet, in a future perspective, its employment could be hypothesized in large-scale commercial distribution, with the aim to reduce the burden of the environmental trigger of CD, therefore potentially reducing its incidence in the general population. This hypothesis has not been proven yet, but the present study provides for the first time in the literature an experimental basis to support it, which anyway will have to be confirmed in larger cohorts to better explore the feasibility of this solution. However, these first results are encouraging, demonstrating that this approach deserves further investigation.

Author Contributions: Conceptualization, F.G., M.G., G.L.d., S.S.; methodology, A.D., N.M., M.G., G.L.d., S.S.; software, F.B.; validation, M.G., S.S., G.L.d.; formal analysis, A.B., S.G., F.B., B.P., M.G.; investigation, F.G., F.B., B.P., S.G., L.B.; data curation, F.G., L.B., B.P., F.B., S.G.; writing—original draft preparation, F.G., S.G., F.B., B.P.; writing—review and editing, A.D., N.M., M.G., G.L.d., S.S.; supervision, A.D., N.M., M.G., G.L.d., S.S.; project administration, S.S., A.D., N.M.; funding acquisition, S.S. All authors have read and agreed to the published version of the manuscript.

Acknowledgments: The plant set was kindly provided by E. Francia, Department of Life Sciences, University of Modena and Reggio Emilia, Italy. The authors are grateful to Barilla S.p.A and in particular to Giancarlo Addario and Marco Silvestri for producing and providing food used for the experimental diet. The authors are grateful to all the enrolled patients and their families, to Enrico Maria Silini and Letizia Gnetti of Histology and Pathologic Anatomy of the University Hospital of Parma for the preparation and interpretation of slides of duodenal biopsies.

References

1. Ludvigsson, J.F.; Leffler, D.A.; Bai, J.C.; Biagi, F.; Fasano, A.; Green, P.H.R.; Hadjivassiliou, M.; Kaukinen, K.; Kelly, C.P.; Leonard, J.N.; et al. The Oslo definitions for coeliac disease and related terms. *Gut* **2013**, *62*, 43–52. [CrossRef] [PubMed]

2. Mustalahti, K.; Catassi, C.; Reunanen, A.; Fabiani, E.; Heier, M.; McMillan, S.; Murray, L.; Metzger, M.-H.; Gasparin, M.; Bravi, E.; et al. The prevalence of celiac disease in Europe: Results of a centralized, international mass screening project. *Ann. Med.* **2010**, *42*, 587–595. [CrossRef] [PubMed]

3. Kochhar, R.; Sachdev, S.; Kochhar, R.; Aggarwal, A.; Sharma, V.; Prasad, K.K.; Singh, G.; Nain, C.K.; Singh, K.; Marwaha, N. Prevalence of coeliac disease in healthy blood donors: A study from north India. *Dig. Liver Dis.* **2012**, *44*, 530–532. [CrossRef] [PubMed]

4. Catassi, C.; Gatti, S.; Fasano, A. The new epidemiology of celiac disease. *J. Pediatr. Gastroenterol. Nutr.* **2014**, *59* (Suppl. 1), S7–S9. [CrossRef] [PubMed]

5. Maiuri, L.; Ciacci, C.; Ricciardelli, I.; Vacca, L.; Raia, V.; Auricchio, S.; Picard, J.; Osman, M.; Quaratino, S.; Londei, M. Association between innate response to gliadin and activation of pathogenic T cells in coeliac disease. *Lancet* **2003**, *362*, 30–37. [CrossRef]

6. Sciurti, M.; Fornaroli, F.; Gaiani, F.; Bonaguri, C.; Leandro, G.; Di Mario, F.; De'Angelis, G.L. Genetic susceptibilty and celiac disease: What role do HLA haplotypes play? *Acta Biomed.* **2018**, *89*, 17–21.

7. Stepniak, D.; Koning, F. Celiac Disease—Sandwiched between Innate and Adaptive Immunity. *Hum. Immunol.* **2006**, *67*, 460–468. [CrossRef]

8. Shewry, P.R.; Halford, N.G.; Belton, P.S.; Tatham, A.S. The structure and properties of gluten: An elastic protein from wheat grain. *Philos. Trans. R. Soc. Lond B Biol. Sci.* **2002**, *357*, 133–142. [CrossRef]

9. Balakireva, A.V.; Zamyatnin, A.A. Properties of Gluten Intolerance: Gluten Structure, Evolution, Pathogenicity and Detoxification Capabilities. *Nutrients* **2016**, *8*, 644. [CrossRef]

10. Barilli, A.; Gaiani, F.; Prandi, B.; Cirlini, M.; Ingoglia, F.; Visigalli, R.; Rotoli, B.M.; De'Angelis, N.; Sforza, S.; De'Angelis, G.L.; et al. Gluten peptides drive healthy and celiac monocytes toward an M2-like polarization. *J. Nutr. Biochem.* **2018**, *54*, 11–17. [CrossRef]

11. Engström, N.; Saenz-Méndez, P.; Scheers, J.; Scheers, N. Towards Celiac-safe foods: Decreasing the affinity of transglutaminase 2 for gliadin by addition of ascorbyl palmitate and ZnCl2 as detoxifiers. *Sci. Rep.* **2017**, *7*, 77. [CrossRef] [PubMed]

12. Vensel, W.H.; Dupont, F.M.; Sloane, S.; Altenbach, S.B. Effect of cleavage enzyme, search algorithm and decoy database on mass spectrometric identification of wheat gluten proteins. *Phytochemistry* **2011**, *72*, 1154–1161. [CrossRef] [PubMed]

13. Colgrave, M.L.; Byrne, K.; Howitt, C.A. Food for thought: Selecting the right enzyme for the digestion of gluten. *Food Chem.* **2017**, *234*, 389–397. [CrossRef] [PubMed]

14. Zou, W.; Sissons, M.; Gidley, M.J.; Gilbert, R.G.; Warren, F.J. Combined techniques for characterising pasta structure reveals how the gluten network slows enzymic digestion rate. *Food Chem.* **2015**, *188*, 559–568. [CrossRef]

15. Minekus, M.; Alminger, M.; Alvito, P.; Ballance, S.; Bohn, T.; Bourlieu, C.; Carriere, F.; Boutrou, R.; Corredig, M.; Dupont, D.; et al. A standardised static in vitro digestion method suitable for food—an international consensus. *Food Funct.* **2014**, *5*, 1113–1124. [CrossRef]

16. Koerner, T.B.; Abbott, M.; Godefroy, S.B.; Popping, B.; Yeung, J.M.; Diaz-Amigo, C.; Roberts, J.; Taylor, S.L.; Baumert, J.L.; Ulberth, F.; et al. Validation procedures for quantitative gluten ELISA methods: AOAC allergen community guidance and best practices. *J. AOAC Int.* **2013**, *96*, 1033–1040. [CrossRef]

17. Martinez-Esteso, M.J.; Norgaard, J.; Brohee, M.; Haraszi, R.; Maquet, A.; O'Connor, G. Defining the wheat gluten peptide fingerprint via a discovery and targeted proteomics approach. *J. Proteom.* **2016**, *147*, 156–168. [CrossRef]

18. Gianfrani, C.; Maglio, M.; Aufiero, V.R.; Camarca, A.; Vocca, I.; Iaquinto, G.; Giardullo, N.; Pogna, N.; Troncone, R.; Auricchio, S.; et al. Immunogenicity of monococcum wheat in celiac patients. *Am. J. Clin. Nutr.* **2012**, *96*, 1339–1345. [CrossRef]

19. Abadie, V.; Jabri, B. IL-15: A central regulator of celiac disease immunopathology. *Immunol. Rev.* **2014**, *260*, 221–234. [CrossRef]

20. Prandi, B.; Mantovani, P.; Galaverna, G.; Sforza, S. Genetic and environmental factors affecting pathogenicity of wheat as related to celiac disease. *J. Cereal Sci.* **2014**, *59*, 62–69. [CrossRef]

21. Husby, S.; Koletzko, S.; Korponay-Szabo, I.R.; Mearin, M.L.; Phillips, A.; Shamir, R.; Troncone, R.; Giersiepen, K.; Branski, D.; Catassi, C.; et al. European Society for Pediatric Gastroenterology, Hepatology, and Nutrition guidelines for the diagnosis of coeliac disease. *J. Pediatr. Gastroenterol. Nutr.* **2012**, *54*, 136–160. [CrossRef] [PubMed]

22. Oberhuber, G. Histopathology of celiac disease. *Biomed. Pharmacother.* **2000**, *54*, 368–372. [CrossRef]

23. Hollon, J.; Puppa, E.L.; Greenwald, B.; Goldberg, E.; Guerrerio, A.; Fasano, A. Effect of gliadin on permeability of intestinal biopsy explants from celiac disease patients and patients with non-celiac gluten sensitivity. *Nutrients* **2015**, *7*, 1565–1576. [CrossRef] [PubMed]

24. Gianfrani, C.; Auricchio, S.; Troncone, R. Adaptive and innate immune responses in celiac disease. *Immunol. Lett.* **2005**, *99*, 141–145. [CrossRef] [PubMed]

25. Schuppan, D.; Junker, Y.; Barisani, D. Celiac disease: From pathogenesis to novel therapies. *Gastroenterology* **2009**, *137*, 1912–1933. [CrossRef] [PubMed]

26. Arentz-Hansen, H.; McAdam, S.N.; Molberg, O.; Fleckenstein, B.; Lundin, K.E.; Jorgensen, T.J.; Jung, G.; Roepstorff, P.; Sollid, L.M. Celiac lesion T cells recognize epitopes that cluster in regions of gliadins rich in proline residues. *Gastroenterology* **2002**, *123*, 803–809. [CrossRef]

27. Sollid, L.M.; Qiao, S.W.; Anderson, R.P.; Gianfrani, C.; Koning, F. Nomenclature and listing of celiac disease relevant gluten T-cell epitopes restricted by HLA-DQ molecules. *Immunogenetics* **2012**, *64*, 455–460. [CrossRef]

28. Taranto, F.; D'Agostino, N.; Rodriguez, M.; Pavan, S.; Minervini, A.P.; Pecchioni, N.; Papa, R.; De Vita, P. Whole Genome Scan Reveals Molecular Signatures of Divergence and Selection Related to Important Traits in Durum Wheat Germplasm. *Front. Genet.* **2020**, *11*, 217. [CrossRef]

29. Boukid, F.; Prandi, B.; Faccini, A.; Sforza, S. A Complete Mass Spectrometry (MS)-Based Peptidomic Description of Gluten Peptides Generated During In Vitro Gastrointestinal Digestion of Durum Wheat: Implication for Celiac Disease. *J. Am. Soc. Mass Spectrom.* **2019**, *30*, 1481–1490. [CrossRef]

30. Taranto, F.; D'Agostino, N.; Catellani, M.; Laviano, L.; Ronga, D.; Milc, J.; Prandi, B.; Boukid, F.; Sforza, S.; Graziano, S. Characterization of Celiac Disease-Related Epitopes and Gluten Fractions, and Identification of Associated Loci in Durum Wheat. *Agronomy* **2020**, *10*, 1231. [CrossRef]

31. Lucendo, A.J.; Molina-Infante, J.; Arias, A.; von Arnim, U.; Bredenoord, A.J.; Bussmann, C.; Dias, J.A.; Bove, M.; Gonzalez-Cervera, J.; Larsson, H.; et al. Guidelines on eosinophilic esophagitis: Evidence-based statements and recommendations for diagnosis and management in children and adults. *United Eur. Gastroenterol. J.* **2017**, *5*, 335–358. [CrossRef] [PubMed]

32. Bracken, S.C.; Kilmartin, C.; Wieser, H.; Jackson, J.; Feighery, C. Barley and rye prolamins induce an mRNA interferon-gamma response in coeliac mucosa. *Aliment. Pharmacol. Ther.* **2006**, *23*, 1307–1314. [CrossRef] [PubMed]

33. Carroccio, A.; Di Prima, L.; Noto, D.; Fayer, F.; Ambrosiano, G.; Villanacci, V.; Lammers, K.; Lafiandra, D.; De Ambrogio, E.; Di Fede, G.; et al. Searching for wheat plants with low toxicity in celiac disease: Between direct toxicity and immunologic activation. *Dig. Liver Dis.* **2011**, *43*, 34–39. [CrossRef] [PubMed]

34. Prandi, B.; Faccini, A.; Tedeschi, T.; Cammerata, A.; Sgrulletta, D.; D'Egidio, M.G.; Galaverna, G.; Sforza, S. Qualitative and quantitative determination of peptides related to celiac disease in mixtures derived from different methods of simulated gastrointestinal digestion of wheat products. *Anal. Bioanal. Chem.* **2014**, *406*, 4765–4775. [CrossRef] [PubMed]

35. Ludvigsson, J.F.; Ciacci, C.; Green, P.H.; Kaukinen, K.; Korponay-Szabo, I.R.; Kurppa, K.; Murray, J.A.; Lundin, K.E.A.; Maki, M.J.; Popp, A.; et al. Outcome measures in coeliac disease trials: The Tampere recommendations. *Gut* **2018**, *67*, 1410–1424. [CrossRef]

36. Grover, J.; Chhuneja, P.; Midha, V.; Ghia, J.E.; Deka, D.; Mukhopadhyay, C.S.; Sood, N.; Mahajan, R.; Singh, A.; Verma, R.; et al. Variable Immunogenic Potential of Wheat: Prospective for Selection of Innocuous Varieties for Celiac Disease Patients via in vitro Approach. *Front. Immunol.* **2019**, *10*, 84. [CrossRef]

37. Vandenplas, Y. Prevention and Management of Cow's Milk Allergy in Non-Exclusively Breastfed Infants. *Nutrients* **2017**, *9*, 731. [CrossRef]

3

Molecular Biomarkers for Celiac Disease: Past, Present and Future

Aarón D. Ramírez-Sánchez [1,†]🆔, Ineke L. Tan [1,2,†]🆔, B.C. Gonera-de Jong [3], Marijn C. Visschedijk [2], Iris Jonkers [1]🆔 and Sebo Withoff [1,*]

[1]   Department of Genetics, University of Groningen, University Medical Center Groningen, 9700 RB Groningen, The Netherlands; a.d.ramirez.sanchez@umcg.nl (A.D.R.-S.); i.l.tan@umcg.nl (I.L.T.); i.h.jonkers@umcg.nl (I.J.)
[2]   Department of Gastroenterology and Hepatology, University of Groningen, University Medical Center Groningen, 9700 RB Groningen, The Netherlands; m.c.visschedijk@umcg.nl
[3]   Department of Pediatrics, Wilhelmina Hospital Assen, 9401 RK Assen, The Netherlands; Gieneke.Gonera@wza.nl
*   Correspondence: s.withoff@umcg.nl
†   These authors contributed equally to this work.

Abstract: Celiac disease (CeD) is a complex immune-mediated disorder that is triggered by dietary gluten in genetically predisposed individuals. CeD is characterized by inflammation and villous atrophy of the small intestine, which can lead to gastrointestinal complaints, malnutrition, and malignancies. Currently, diagnosis of CeD relies on serology (antibodies against transglutaminase and endomysium) and small-intestinal biopsies. Since small-intestinal biopsies require invasive upper-endoscopy, and serology cannot predict CeD in an early stage or be used for monitoring disease after initiation of a gluten-free diet, the search for non-invasive biomarkers is ongoing. Here, we summarize current and up-and-coming non-invasive biomarkers that may be able to predict, diagnose, and monitor the progression of CeD. We further discuss how current and emerging techniques, such as (single-cell) transcriptomics and genomics, can be used to uncover the pathophysiology of CeD and identify non-invasive biomarkers.

Keywords: celiac disease; new biomarkers; diagnosis; follow-up; non-invasive

1. Introduction

Celiac disease (CeD) is a complex immune-mediated disorder triggered by dietary gluten in genetically predisposed individuals. The estimated worldwide prevalence of CeD is very high (1–1.5%) [1]. The disease is characterized by inflammation and villous atrophy of the small intestine that can lead to gastrointestinal complaints, malnutrition, and malignancies. The clinical spectrum of CeD is, however, broad and can include extra-intestinal symptoms, such as anemia, fatigue and dermatitis herpetiformis [2]. These factors make CeD complicated to diagnose, and it is estimated that only 1/3 to 1/9 of all CeD patients are properly diagnosed [3]. Once diagnosed, the only available treatment for CeD is a strict life-long, gluten-free diet (GFD).

The most recent guidelines recommend starting the diagnostic process for CeD in (1) patients with symptoms suggestive of CeD, (2) individuals with laboratory abnormalities previously associated with CeD (e.g., those indicative of malabsorption), or (3) other risk groups such as first-degree family members of CeD patients, patients with Type I Diabetes Mellitus, and patients with Down Syndrome [4,5]. Concerning these recent recommendations, serological testing for the presence of antibodies against gliadin and deamidated gliadin peptide has been replaced by testing for Immunoglobulin A (IgA) antibodies against tissue transglutaminase (anti-TG2) and endomysium (anti-EMA), which both display higher sensitivity and specificity [4]. The diagnostic procedure also differs between adults and children. Regarding adults, serology is combined with histopathological evaluation of small-intestinal biopsies [4], and it is important to include a duodenal bulb biopsy to increase the diagnostic yield [6]. CeD disease status is subsequently scored based on decreased villous height-to-crypt depth ratio (villous atrophy and crypt hyperplasia) and the influx of intraepithelial lymphocytes (IELs). The histological classification used for CeD is called the Marsh classification [7]. Regarding children, high antibody titers (anti-TG2 $\geq$ 10 times the upper limit of normal and positive anti-EMA in a second blood sample) are sufficient to establish CeD, which makes the diagnosis less invasive by eliminating the need for duodenal-endoscopy [5]. Children with anti-TG2 levels < 10 times the upper limit of normal still require a biopsy to confirm CeD.

Since more than 99% of CeD patients are human leukocyte antigen (HLA)-DQ2- or HLA-DQ8-positive, HLA-genotyping does not have added value for diagnostic purposes, since positive serology correlates almost perfectly with the presence of these HLA-types [8]. Moreover, these HLA haplotypes also occur in the general population with a frequency of approximately 40% [9,10]. However, due to its requirement for the development of CeD, HLA-genotyping can be used to rule out CeD, for example in first-degree relatives of CeD patients or in individuals who self-diagnose with CeD and start a GFD [4,5].

During this review, we summarize the strategies that are used to identify potential novel molecular biomarkers for CeD diagnosis and follow-up. To enable an understanding of how diagnostic CeD biomarkers might be involved in CeD etiology, we first summarize the immunopathology of CeD.

2. CeD Immunopathology

As a complex disease, the pathophysiology of CeD involves a combination of environmental, genetic, and immunological factors, and possibly also microbial factors (Figure 1).

The most important environmental factor involved in CeD is gluten exposure [11,12]. Glutens are storage proteins commonly found in grains that are widely used in the Western diet (wheat, barley, and rye). Due to their high proline content, gluten proteins are inefficiently degraded into peptides in the small intestine, where they traverse the intestinal barrier and reach the lamina propria by transcellular or paracellular routes (Figure 1A) [13]. Regarding the lamina propria, gliadin peptides are deamidated by tissue transglutaminase 2 (TG2) and can be taken up by antigen-presenting cells. Specific deamidated gliadin molecules have a very high affinity for the CeD-associated HLA-DQ2 and -DQ8 molecules, which leads to the generation and activation of a pool of gluten-specific CD4+ T cells [14–16]. Activated gluten-specific T cells then respond and produce the pro-inflammatory cytokines interleukin (IL)-21 and interferon-gamma (IFN-γ) [17]. Furthermore, IL-15, which is a hallmark for CeD, is upregulated in both the epithelial barrier and the lamina propria. Together, these cytokines orchestrate a cascade that leads to increased stress in intestinal epithelial cells, migration of CD8+ cells to the epithelial layer, and activation of B cells. Upon arrival in the epithelial layer, the CD8+ T cells (designated CD8+ intraepithelial lymphocytes (IELs)) are effectively "licensed to kill" epithelial cells, thereby damaging the villous structure of the small intestine (villous atrophy) [17]. Gluten-specific T cells also promote the activation of B cells, which develop into plasma cells, thereby producing the auto-antibodies that are used as the biomarkers in CeD serology tests (Figure 1A) [4,18]. Moreover, a recently proposed hypothesis suggests that B cells may have an antigen-presenting role in CeD [18,19].

Although gluten peptides play a critical role in CeD immunopathology, not all CeD patients develop CeD upon their first intake of gluten. It has been postulated that viral (e.g., reovirus and norovirus [20,21]) and/or fungal infections (Candida [22]) create the environment for an anti-gluten response to be elicited. Bacterial microbiota also has been implicated in CeD but may act in a different way than viruses. Duodenal microorganisms have different capacities to degrade gluten. Pseudomonas aeruginosa, a bacteria enriched in the duodenum of CeD patients for example, produces elastases that can degrade and modify the gluten to produce gliadin peptides that are highly immunogenic [23], which may explain how the microbiota can cause imbalance in the immune homeostasis (Figure 1A). Additionally, it has been shown that some bacterial protein fragments can elicit a stronger activation of gluten-specific T cells by binding to HLA-DQ2 [24,25]. However, there is currently no evidence for which microbes might produce these peptides in CeD patients.

Genetics plays a pivotal role in CeD. The HLA-DQ2 and/or -DQ8 haplotypes are required to mount the specific response against gliadin peptides. However, ~40% of the Western population are DQ2/DQ8 carriers, even though only 3% of DQ2/DQ8 carriers develop CeD [10,26,27]. DQ2/DQ8 carriership, thus, is essential for the development of CeD, but carriership is not the cause. Thus far, genome-wide association studies have identified more than 40 non-HLA risk loci associated with CeD [28,29]. Together, these loci and the HLA loci explain more than 40% of the heritability of CeD [30]. Many of the genes in these loci are immune genes [31]. Since most of the non-HLA CeD single-nucleotide polymorphisms (SNPs) are located in the non-coding genome, they are likely to contribute to CeD pathology by affecting the expression of genes involved in the biological pathways that are perturbed in CeD. Although a single SNP might affect only the risk of developing CeD to a small extent, a combination of multiple SNPs and loci may affect downstream central hub genes that could implicate novel biomarkers and therapeutic targets [31,32]. Accompanying the recent publication of data from large case–control genome-wide association studies and population controls, such as the UK biobank, is the now possible ability to calculate genetic risk scores that combine the additive risk of multiple CeD risk-SNPs into one score to indicate the risk of developing CeD [10,33,34]. Indeed, a genetic risk score based on only 46 SNPs differed significantly between CeD patients and controls, which makes genetic risk scores easier to interpret and implement in future clinical applications than the whole-genome panels that are used in case–control studies [34].

It is a challenge to clearly identify the individual contributions of environmental, immunological, and genetic factors to CeD, as none of the currently known factors are sufficient to explain CeD risk completely. It seems that all these factors are part of an interconnected puzzle that causes loss of tolerance to gluten and the subsequent clinical manifestations of CeD. Fundamental studies can help to unravel CeD pathogenesis and identify key players and biomarkers for early detection, monitoring and control of CeD.

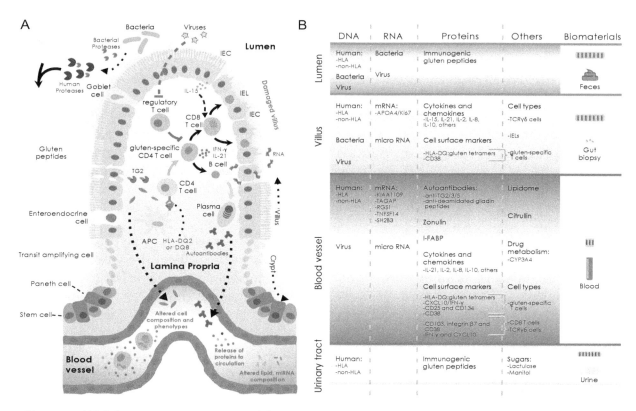

Figure 1. (**A**) Schematic representation of the immunopathology of Celiac Disease (CeD). Dietary gluten is partially degraded by human and microbial proteases. These peptides pass the epithelial layer (IEC: Intestinal epithelial cell) by paracellular or transcellular transport. Upon entering, tissue transglutaminase 2 (TG2) deamidates the gluten peptides, which are then processed by antigen presenting cells (APCs) and presented to CD4+ T cells in the context of human leukocyte antigen (HLA)-DQ2 or HLA-DQ8. After a process of selection, gluten-specific CD4+ T cells propagate and orchestrate the immune response by producing specific cytokines such as interleukin (IL)-21 and interferon-gamma (IFN-γ). Combined with IL-15, these cytokines promote the development of B cells into antibody-producing plasma cells and the activation of intraepithelial lymphocytes (IELs), which acquire cytotoxic properties to attack intestinal epithelial cells, thereby causing villus atrophy. The immune response in CeD causes modifications observable in blood such as release of immune- or damage-related markers (highlighted in red). Figure adapted from Moerkens and Mooiweer et al., [35]. (**B**) CeD biomarkers currently under study categorized by different compartments (rows, left) and separated by biotype (columns). Biomarkers that can be analyzed in easily collected biomaterials rather than invasive biopsies are more desired for diagnostics (rows, right).

3. Novel Developments in Diagnosis

Rapid screening of high-risk populations is expected to decrease the number of undetected CeD cases [36]. Recently, effort has been invested in developing point-of-care tests that allow for quick, non-invasive, cost-effective, user-friendly diagnosis, for instance a test based on detection of IgA anti-TG2 antibodies in finger prick blood [37,38]. Unfortunately, the clinical studies performed thus far show that the accuracy and, especially, the sensitivity of these tests need to be optimized before widespread implementation [4,5,37,39].

Novel developments in endoscopic techniques now can capture the location and extent of villous atrophy more directly. These approaches include chromoendoscopy (mucosal staining with a specific dye), confocal endomicroscopy (microscopic visualization during upper-endoscopy) and non-invasive techniques such as capsule endoscopy, and they have been reviewed extensively elsewhere [40].

4. Why Do We Need Novel Biomarkers?

To date, CeD diagnosis relies on serology and on biopsies acquired in an invasive manner. Despite diagnostic advances, there are several reasons to keep searching for additional novel biomarkers to improve CeD diagnostics and follow-up.

(1) Serological tests can lead to false-negative or false-positive results.

Current serological tests can yield false negatives in IgA-deficient patients. About 2–3% of all CeD patients display IgA-deficiency, a 10-fold higher incidence than in the general population [41]. False-positive results have been observed in several other (auto-)immune related diseases, such as primary biliary cholangitis, and in enteric infections [4,42,43]. Moreover, there is a patient group coined 'potential CeD patients' who have positive serology but no villous atrophy who, therefore, may not need to follow a GFD [44,45]. However, the estimated cumulative incidence of children with potential CeD who develop villous atrophy within the 12-year follow-up after first seropositivity is around 43% [45].

(2) Prevention of severe small-intestinal damage.

Anti-TG2 only appears in circulation after the villous structure of the small intestine is affected. Novel biomarkers that enable the detection of CeD-onset (for instance in high-risk individuals) could lead to rapid initiation of a GFD. This would prevent full-blown disease and could be helpful for distinguishing which potential CeD patients will progress to CeD and which will not.

(3) GFD adherence and response is difficult to monitor.

It is difficult to adhere a strict lifelong GFD. Added to the social consequences of a GFD, unintentional gluten intake is common when following a GFD due to cross-contact from various sources, including dietary supplements and even playdough [46]. Currently, GFD adherence is monitored by dietetic review and serology. However, unintentional gluten intake, and the challenges of monitoring gluten intake in young children, make it difficult to interpret dietetic reviews and the serological markers, and even the absence of clinical symptoms, correlate poorly with mucosal healing [47–50]. Regarding cases with persistent symptoms but without elevated anti-TG2, it would be useful to have additional biomarkers that could exclude dietary lapses as a cause of symptoms. Also, in the case of intentional gluten intake, for example during puberty, additional biomarkers possibly could reflect gluten intake with or without mucosal damage without elevated levels of anti-TG2. Novel tools that allow sensitive and rapid gluten monitoring, ideally by patients themselves, would help to avoid certain foods and behaviors.

(4) Comorbidities and complications.

Although the most severe complaints may improve within several weeks after starting a GFD, mucosal recovery is only achieved in about 50% of CeD patients after one year of GFD, even when a strict diet is followed [48,51]. The persistence of intestinal damage is associated with a higher rate of CeD-associated complications such as bone abnormalities and malignancies [48,51]. Currently, we have no biomarkers that predict the onset of co-morbidities in CeD patients, such as dermatitis herpetiformis, other immune-mediated diseases (e.g., Type I Diabetes or thyroid diseases), or severe complications such as refractory CeD or enteropathy-associated T cell lymphoma.

(5) Clinical trial evaluation for the development of new treatments.

Assessing villous damage in biopsies is currently the method of choice to evaluate treatment response to novel drugs for CeD; however, non-invasive markers for mucosal damage or infiltration of IELs would help in clinical trials to evaluate treatment response [52].

To summarize, the search for novel biomarkers is crucial to improving early diagnosis, decreasing diagnostic burden, testing treatment efficacy, and improving follow-up and monitoring of CeD comorbidities after the start of a GFD. Ideally, these biomarkers should be detectable in a material that can be obtained in a non-invasive or minimally invasive manner, such as blood, feces, or urine.

5. Non-Invasive and Minimally Invasive Biomarkers

Regarding the next sections, we discuss potential novel non-invasive and minimally invasive biomarkers for diagnosis and follow-up of CeD and give an overview of how state-of-the-art techniques could lead to a better understanding of CeD pathology and to novel biomarkers. An overview of the biomarkers discussed is presented in Figure 1B and Table 1.

5.1. Cytokines, Chemokines and Other Proteins Detectable in Blood

Cytokines and chemokines are key players in the immunopathology of CeD. It is important to realize that the key driving cytokines or chemokines that are involved in disease initiation, maintenance, and/or progression may not be detectable in blood. It is possible that these biomarkers are produced in narrow windows of time or they might be diluted to undetectable levels in circulation. Nevertheless, some of these proteins are relevant for diagnostics because they reveal specific signature changes in CeD that can highlight different stages of disease progression.

Basal levels of some cytokines are increased in patients with active CeD compared to patients on a GFD and using healthy controls. Previous reports describe that the increased serum levels of some cytokines (such as IL-4, IL-10, IL-1α, IL-1β, IL-8 and IL-21) seen in CeD patients are correlated with IgA anti-TG2 titers and villous atrophy, making them candidates for diagnostic biomarkers [53,54]. Remarkably, the levels of some cytokines, such as IL-8, remain high for a long time after initiation of a GFD. This may be linked to the long recovery time of the duodenum and may present a way to detect CeD in patients already on a GFD.

New techniques to perform targeted high- or medium-throughput proteomics, such as the Olink platform [55], now make it possible to measure multiple protein markers using a small volume of sample. Using these techniques, circulating IL-2, IL-8 and IL-17A were detected in blood within two or three hours after gluten challenge in CeD patients but not in individuals with self-reported gluten sensitivity [56,57], probably reflecting rapid activation of 'primed' gluten-specific T cells upon antigen exposure. Although the authors found that cytokine response varied broadly among patients, 19 of 26 CeD patients (73%) versus just one of 67 self-reported gluten sensitivity patients (1.5%) were confirmed as IL-2 responders upon gluten challenge [58]. Interestingly, the patients with the highest levels of cytokines in the bloodstream also displayed the most severe symptoms [56,57].

To conclude, using the rapid rise of cytokines as a biomarker upon gluten-challenge may reduce the duration of current diagnostics methods that rely on two- to six-week long gluten challenges for an accurate result from serology or biopsy tests [4]. Gluten-related cytokine responses also may be useful clinical biomarkers for assessing patient recovery after CeD-mediated villous atrophy.

Table 1. Overview of current and future biomarkers for celiac disease (CeD).

Based on Detection of:	Functional Group	Molecular Biomarker	Detectable in:	Comments	Practical Considerations
DNA	HLA-DQ2 or DQ8	HLA-DQ2 or DQ8	Virtually any human tissue	Useful in situations with expected false-negative serology. Negative HLA-DQ2/DQ8 excludes CeD reliably without need of gluten challenge. Positive test requires additional tests.	PCR-based tests available.
	Non-HLA loci	Risk variants	Virtually any human tissue	>40 risk loci identified, mostly in non-coding regions. Prognostic value of genomic risk scores need to be evaluated (who will develop CeD and who will not). Future studies: crucial to find associated genes and pathways to elucidate pathogenesis, potential new biomarkers and treatments.	Research in discovery phase. SNP based tests need to be developed if genomic risk score is proven to have sufficient diagnostic value.
Microbial DNA/RNA	Microbiome	Not yet available	Feces, brush biopsy	Enrichment for pro-inflammatory bacteria (Proteobacteria) and depletion of beneficial ones (Bifidobacterium and Lactobacillus). Studies necessary on the diagnostic/prognostic value of individual combined abundance of specific bacteria.	Research in preliminary discovery phase.
Viral DNA/RNA	Virome	Not yet available	Feces, brush biopsy, blood	Potential role in triggering the CeD by disturbing the oral tolerance. Associations found with CeD in reovirus, rotavirus, enterovirus, adenovirus, hepatitis C virus, hepatitis B virus, and some strains of Epstein-Barr virus and Cytomegalovirus. Studies necessary on the diagnostic/prognostic value of individual combined abundance of specific viruses.	Research in preliminary discovery phase.
RNA	Bulk mRNA	KIAA1109, TAGAP, RGS1, TNFSF14, and SH2B3	Blood	Transcripts overexpressed in RNA form PBMCs of CeD patients 9 months before diagnosis.	Potential use as predictor markers, further validation necessary before clinical application.
		APOA4:Ki67	Small intestinal biopsy	Biomarker for villous-to-crypt ratio in transcriptome data of biopsies, that eliminates observer variation in reviewing histological slides. Could help in basis (large-scale) transcriptome studies where no measured villous-to-crypt ratio is available and in clinical trials.	Requires small intestinal biopsy. Suitable to implement in clinical drug trials.
	Small non-coding RNAs	MicroRNAs	Small intestinal biopsy, blood	Differences detected between controls and CeD. Diagnostic and prognostic value to be determined.	Research in discovery phase.
Proteins	Antibodies	anti-TG2 IgA	Blood, saliva	Very high sensitivity/specificity for active CeD. Not reliable if individual is on GFD or has IgA deficiency. Less useful for follow up.	Currently used as a serological tool of choice in clinics. Saliva based and rapid on site point-of-care tests are under investigation.

Table 1. *Cont.*

Based on Detection of:	Functional Group	Molecular Biomarker	Detectable in:	Comments	Practical Considerations
		anti-TG2 IgG	Blood	IgG based tests (anti-TG2/anti-DGP) tests of choice in case of IgA-deficiency.	IgG based tests; have more inter-test variability than IgA-anti-TG2.
		Anti-Deamidated gliadin peptides (DGP) IgG	Blood	See IgG anti-TG2	See IgG anti-TG2.
		anti-EMA IgA	Blood	Used in combination with IgA anti-TG2 to confirm CeD in the non-biopsy approach.	Implemented in clinics. The indirect immunofluorescence test is more laborious and subjective than ELISA based anti-TG2.
		anti-TG3	Blood, skin biopsy	Diagnosis of Dermatitis Herpetiformis	Further validation is necessary before clinical applications.
		anti-TG6	Blood	Diagnosis of Gluten ataxia	Further validation is necessary before clinical applications.
	Cytokines and chemokines	IL-15	Small intestinal biopsy	Hallmark of CeD, involved in the T cell response. Elevated in CeD. Expressed on the surface of cells that are mainly located in gut.	Requires small intestinal biopsy.
		IL-21	Blood, small intestinal biopsy	Together with IL-15, involved in the T cell response. Elevated serum basal levels in CeD. Correlated with anti-TG2 titers.	Further validation is necessary before clinical application.
		IL-2	Blood, small-intestinal biopsy	Involved in the T cell response. Distinguishes CeD cases from self-reported gluten sensitivity patients. Increased within 2 h after gluten-challenge in CeD. Elevated serum titers is associated with worse symptoms. Distinguishes CeD cases from self-reported gluten sensitivity patients.	Further validation is necessary before clinical application. Requires a short (hours) gluten-challenge test.
		IL-8	Blood, small-intestinal biopsy	Involved in the T cell response. Elevated serum basal levels in CeD. Correlated with anti-TG2 titers. Increased within 2 h after gluten-challenge. Elevated serum titers are associated with worse symptoms. Takes more than one year of GFD to diminish to normal levels.	Further validation is necessary before clinical application. Can be used after a short gluten-challenge test, or as a long-term marker of recovery.
		IL-10	Blood, small-intestinal biopsy	Correlated with anti-TG2 titers. Elevated serum basal levels in CeD.	Further validation is necessary before clinical application. Requires a short (hours) gluten-challenge test.

Table 1. *Cont.*

Based on Detection of:	Functional Group	Molecular Biomarker	Detectable in:	Comments	Practical Considerations
		IL-17A	Blood, small-intestinal biopsy	Produced by T cells, mainly. Increased within 2 h after gluten-challenge. Elevated serum titers are associated with worse symptoms.	Further validation is necessary before clinical application. Requires a short (hours) gluten-challenge test.
		IL-1a	Blood	Elevated serum basal levels in CeD. Correlated with anti-TG2 titers.	Further validation is necessary before clinical application. Requires a short (hours) gluten-challenge test.
		IL-1b	Blood	Elevated serum basal levels in CeD. Correlated with anti-TG2 titers. Take more than one year of GFD to diminish to normal levels.	Further validation is necessary before clinical application. Potential use to assess the recovery of villus atrophy in long-term.
		IL-4	Blood	Elevated serum basal levels in CeD. Correlated with anti-TG2 titers.	Further validation is necessary before clinical application. Requires a short (hours) gluten-challenge test. Requires a short gluten-challenge test.
		Others	Blood	CCL20, IL-6, CXCL9, IFNγ, IL-10, IL-22, TNFα, CCL2, and amphiregulin.	Research in discovery phase.
	Peptides	Immunogenic gluten peptides	Urine, feces	Indicates presence of (unintended) gluten intake. Better marker for dietary adherence than IgA anti-TG2.	Can be detected in urine 3h after gluten intake, after 3 days in feces. Point-of-care at home tests are in clinical trials.
	Others	I-FABP	Blood	Non-invasive marker of villous atrophy. Indicates damage to small-intestinal enterocytes. Might be useful to identify patients that do not require additional biopsies to complement anti-TG2 if anti-TG2 is increased, but not >10x the upper limit of normal levels.	Note that elevated I-FABP is not specific to CeD, but occurs also in other enteropathies. Still, as a marker for intestinal damage is ready to be validated and implemented for clinical purposes.
		Zonulin	Blood	Marker for the intestinal barrier integrity.	Detectable by ELISA, but specificity and intra-individual fluctuations make it an unsuitable biomarker.

Table 1. *Cont.*

Based on Detection of:	Functional Group	Molecular Biomarker	Detectable in:	Comments	Practical Considerations
Cell-types	Gluten specific T-cells	HLA-DQ:gluten tetramers	Blood, small-intestinal biopsies	Complex used to identify gluten specific T cells by using their affinity to gluten epitopes.	Requires FACS, which is labor intensive, making it a less attractive biomarker for clinical applications.
		CXCL10, IFN-γ	Blood	Alternative to HLA-DQ:gluten tetramers to identify gluten specific T cells.	Uses ELISPOT, which is relatively easy to implement, but the test is not as specific as using tetramers.
		CD25, CD134	Blood	Alternative to HLA-DQ:gluten tetramers to identify gluten specific T cells.	Uses ELISPOT and FACS, which makes its use more difficult, thereby being less attractive in clinical applications.
		CD38	Blood, small-intestinal biopsies	Marker for subset of gluten specific T cells. Distinguish CeD on GFD patients. Capable of indicating a first exposure or a re-exposure to gluten.	Requires FACS, which is labor intensive, making it a less attractive biomarker for clinical applications.
	CD8 T cells	CD8	Blood	Relevant cells for CeD immunopathology, involved in the cellular mediated immunology.	Can be detected in blood by FACS after a short gluten challenge, being suitable candidates to diagnose CeD on GFD prospective patients.
	TCRγδ cells	TCRγδ	Blood, small-intestinal biopsies	Relevant cells for CeD immunopathology, used in the biopsy assessment. Cell count is highly increased in active CeD.	Requires FACS, which is labor intensive making it a less attractive biomarker for clinical application.
Metabolome	Lipidome	Not yet available	Blood	Lipid profile potential prognostic marker: Differences in lipidome detectable in a high risk cohort between children that will develop CeD versus those that will not, before the introduction of gluten. Might be useful to identify those patients that require intensive follow up with serology.	Research still in a preliminary, discovery phase.
	Amino acids	Citrulline	Blood	Non-invasive marker of villous atrophy. Amino acid specifically present in small-intestinal enterocytes. Circulating citrulline in blood is a proxy of small-intestinal enterocyte mass.	Note that elevated citrulline is not specific to CeD, but occurs in a range of diseases associated with small-intestinal damage. Still worthwhile to compare diagnostic yield with I-FABP, as citrulline might become a better predictor of villous atrophy.

Table 1. *Cont.*

Based on Detection of:	Functional Group	Molecular Biomarker	Detectable in:	Comments	Practical Considerations
	Drug metabolization	Metabolization rate drugs processed by CYP3A4	Blood	Non-invasive marker of villous atrophy. Indicates the expression of CYP3A4 in the small intestine and therefore a marker of presence of small intestinal epithelial damage.	Requires the administration of drugs. Grapefruit juice can influence the results. Likely not specific for CeD.
Sugars	Large sugars	Lactulose/Mannitol ratio	Urine	Indication of small-intestinal barrier function, different between CeD and controls.	Less attractive biomarker due to variation in the reliability of the tests. Still the only marker for intestinal integrity that can be measured non-invasively.

Abbreviations listed in the Table 1: human leukocyte antigen (HLA)); Polymerase chain reaction (PCR); single-nucleotide polymorphisms (SNP); peripheral blood mononuclear cells (PBMC); gluten-free diet (GFD); tissue transglutaminase (TG); endomysium (EMA); Immunoglobulin (Ig); interleukin (IL); fluorescence-activated cell sorting (FACS); Intestinal fatty-acid binding protein (I-FABP).

5.2. Cellular Composition of the Peripheral Blood Mononuclear Cell (PBMC) Fraction and Gene and/or Protein Expression

Differences in the composition of the peripheral blood mononuclear cell (PBMC) compartment in blood, or alterations in the expression profiles of these cells, may provide biomarkers for CeD. Cell types that are highly specific for CeD, such as gluten-specific T cells, but rare or not present in healthy individuals are of special interest [59].

Gluten-specific T cells can be observed at very low counts in circulation, an issue that can be overcome by enriching and/or staining them with HLA-DQ:gluten tetramers (a complex of four subunits of HLA-DQ2 binding to a gluten peptide) and subsequent fluorescence-activated cell sorting (FACS). Detection of gluten-specific T cells in circulation is a proposed marker for CeD that can detect CeD after the start of a GFD [59,60].

The HLA-DQ: gluten tetramer method requires staining and sorting the cells (FACS), which is labor-intensive and difficult to implement on a large scale. Therefore, there have been efforts to find non-invasive proxies for the number of circulating gluten-specific T cells in CeD using easier and less expensive methods that can be implemented on a larger scale. This includes the combined measurement of certain plasma cytokines (like C-X-C Motif Chemokine Ligand 10 (CXCL10)/ IFN-γ) by ELISA and the detection of the presence of CD25/CD134 positive cells with enzyme-linked immunospot (ELISPOT) [61].

The detection of surface markers in CeD-associated cell types also can provide valuable supplementary information. Regarding gluten-specific T cells, Zühlke et al., demonstrated that the expression of CD38 can distinguish CeD patients on a GFD and indicate a re-exposure to gluten [62]. Phenotyping of surface cell markers of CD8+ and gamma-delta ($\gamma\delta$) T cells is also a good alternative for diagnosing CeD in individuals who are already on a GFD. López–Palacios et al., showed, after a short three-day gluten challenge, both cell types co-expressed CD103, integrin $\beta7$ and CD38 in 15 out of 15 CeD patients but only in one of 35 controls [61]. Even with the necessity of a laborious technique like FACS, these biomarkers may have potential for monitoring the efficacy of drugs to treat CeD without the need for an invasive biopsy.

RNA extracted from peripheral blood cells reflects the cellular composition and state of blood and, thus, may contain non-invasive markers for CeD diagnosis. Although RNA is sensitive to degradation, it is easier and cheaper to detect than proteins because this usually requires less input material and test accuracy does not rely on the specificity of antibodies. Concerning CeD patients, an increase in Tumor Necrosis Factor Ligand Superfamily 13B (TNFSF13B) messenger RNA (mRNA) levels and a decrease in TNF Receptor Superfamily Member 9 (TNFRSF9) mRNA levels in whole blood has been observed [63]. Remarkably, in a longitudinal cohort of high-risk individuals, five genes (KIAA1109, T Cell Activation RhoGTPase Activating Protein (TAGAP), Regulator of G Protein Signaling 1 (RGS1), TNFSF14, and SH2B Adaptor Protein 3 (SH2B3)) were overexpressed in PBMCs of CeD patients at least nine months before CeD diagnosis. Based on expression of these genes, it was possible to classify CeD cases and controls in 95.5% of patients (*n* = 22) [64]. These predictive markers may be helpful for identifying individuals at high risk of CeD earlier than current serological markers, which could prevent mucosal damage and symptoms because patients could initiate a GFD earlier.

To conclude, detection of CeD-specific cell types in circulation or recognition of specific markers at protein- and RNA-levels may allow for earlier diagnosis of CeD than current serological methods and allow for diagnosis without the need for a duodenal biopsy in individuals already following a GFD.

5.3. (Circulating) micro-RNAs

MicroRNAs (miRNAs) have been put forward as disease- or disease stage–specific biomarkers. MiRNAs are short RNAs (19–24 nucleotides) that play a role in post-transcriptional gene regulation [65]. The miRNA transcriptome can be disturbed in disease-affected tissues, and disease-specific differences have been measured in extracellular body fluids such as blood, saliva and urine [66–68].

Several miRNA studies have shown the potential of miRNAs as biomarkers for CeD. Studies on duodenal biopsies showed that the miRNA profiles of CeD patients differ significantly from those of controls [69–75]. Only a few studies are available on circulating miRNA profiles in plasma or serum samples [71,74–76], but there are indications that circulating miRNAs are differentially expressed between CeD cases and controls. MicroRNA-21 is upregulated in both duodenal biopsies and circulation, for example [71,74,75].

The function of extracellular miRNAs is under debate. It is feasible that miRNAs in circulation are a consequence of tissue damage, but it also has been suggested that miRNA-containing vesicles play a role in the immune synapse and they might act as "micro-hormones" and function elsewhere in the body [77,78]. This second hypothesis is supported by the findings that miRNAs are selectively packaged in extracellular vesicles and miRNAs secreted by a donor cell type can be taken up by other cells and regulate gene-expression [79–81]. Thus, future studies also should assess the advantages of using miRNAs as potential prognostic markers for CeD.

5.4. Microbiome and Virome

5.4.1. Microbiome

Growing evidence supports the hypothesis that the gut microbiome plays an important role in CeD pathogenesis. Generally, it has been shown that "beneficial" microbes, such as some species of Bifidobacterium and Lactobacillus, are decreased in the duodenum of CeD patients, while pro-inflammatory bacteria, such as Proteobacteria, are more prevalent when compared to healthy individuals [82]. Olivares et al., showed that children at high risk of developing CeD (HLA-DQ2 carriers with a first-degree relative affected by CeD) exhibit a different fecal microbiome composition than low risk (non-HLA-DQ2/DQ8 carriers with a first-degree relative affected by CeD) and healthy individuals [83]. Analysis of stool samples from pre-diagnosis early timepoints in infants who later developed CeD ($n = 10$) and children who remained healthy ($n = 10$) suggested that the HLA-DQ2 haplotypes may alter the early trajectory of gut microbiota and influence the maturation of the immune system [84].

Although gut microbiome dysbiosis may have potential for prediction of CeD, multiple environmental factors such as diet, age, sex, and use of antibiotics and other drugs also can affect microbiome composition. Therefore, potential biomarkers from the microbiome need exploration in larger cohorts.

5.4.2. Virome

Like bacteria, viruses may act as protectors or triggers in CeD development. Potentially protective viruses include rubella, Epstein–Barr virus, cytomegalovirus, and herpes simplex type 1 virus [85]. Viruses that have been associated negatively with CeD include reovirus, rotavirus, enterovirus, adenovirus, hepatitis C virus, hepatitis B virus, and some strains of Epstein–Barr virus and cytomegalovirus [86,87]. Remarkably, exposure to specific viruses, such as reo- and rotaviruses, early in life is associated with a higher risk for CeD, suggesting that previous infections with this virus may have triggered CeD onset in some patients [20,88,89].

Viruses may affect mechanisms involved in oral tolerance to dietary antigens. Oral tolerance is the state in which the immune system accepts the intake of innocuous antigens found in food without mounting a rejection response [88,90]. Bouziat et al., showed in a mouse model how reoviruses can induce T helper type 1-associated immunity toward dietary antigens, thereby causing loss of oral tolerance, in line with observations from experiments with noroviruses [20,21].

To conclude, the exploration of the gut microbiome and the virome in larger and longitudinal studies may help to identify markers for disease onset and progression of CeD.

5.5. Lipids and Lipid Processing Genes as Markers for CeD

Digestion and absorption of lipids in the small intestine is disturbed in CeD because the surface area of the small intestine is reduced due to villous atrophy [91]. Studying the circulating lipidome and other proxies of disturbed lipid uptake and metabolism, therefore, might provide interesting biomarker candidates for CeD.

Recently, two independent prospective and longitudinal studies in children at high risk for CeD reported that lipid profiles were significantly different in serum samples of participants who developed CeD during follow-up compared to the participants who did not develop CeD [92,93]. Changes in phosphatidylcholines were observed in CeD patients early in life, even before the introduction of dietary gluten. The authors postulated that these differences are independent of the degree of villous atrophy and suggested that unknown genetic factors could be the cause. To contrast, a previous longitudinal study reported that the lipid profile at four months of age did not differ between the children who did develop CeD and those who did not [94]. Thus, candidate lipid biomarkers need to be validated on a larger scale before they are clinically applicable.

Considering small-intestinal biopsies of patients with CeD, there is significant deregulation of key genes or proteins involved in lipid metabolism pathways [91,95–97]. These include Fatty Acid Binding Protein 2 (FABP2 or I-FABP) and Apolipoprotein A4 (APOA4), which are currently being studied as potential biomarkers for CeD. When damaged, intracellular I-FABP is released by small intestinal epithelial cells and can be detected in circulation. Plasma I-FABP has been shown to be increased in CeD patients compared to controls and correlates with the degree of villous atrophy [98,99]. Moreover, after a two-week gluten challenge in patients with CeD, I-FABP levels increased in 80% of participants (mean 1.8-fold increase) [100]. Although the exact specificity/sensitivity of I-FABP as a CeD biomarker fluctuates, in most studies I-FABP has high specificity but lower sensitivity [98,99]. However, because increased I-FABP levels are associated with a range of enteropathies, specificity is expected to be lower if controls with gastrointestinal complaints other than CeD are included in specificity studies. Thus far, anti-TG2 serology remains the more reliable diagnostic biomarker in the studies where I-FABP also is measured [98,99]. Nonetheless, I-FABP might be useful for avoiding diagnostic biopsies in patients who have elevated anti-TG2 levels but who do not fulfill the criteria for serological diagnosis (anti-TG2 level > 10 times the upper limit of normal) [98]. Future independent studies are necessary to validate the added value of I-FABP in CeD diagnostics and to assess whether it could be used in early prediction or follow-up of CeD.

5.6. Citrulline as a Marker for Mucosal Damage

Plasma citrulline is derived specifically from small-intestinal enterocytes [101]. During a recent study of 131 adult CeD patients, plasma citrulline levels exhibited a comparable specificity to plasma I-FABP and a higher sensitivity to detect villous atrophy, making this an interesting biomarker candidate for monitoring villous atrophy [99].

5.7. CYP3A4 Metabolization as a Marker for Mucosal Damage

Cytochrome P450 3A4 (CYP3A4), which is highly expressed in epithelial cells along the small-intestinal tract, is a member of the Cytochrome P450 enzyme family that metabolizes a range of commonly used drugs including simvastatin, a cholesterol synthesis inhibitor. CYP3A4 reduction or inhibition leads to a reduction in the metabolism of specific CYP3A4 substrates [102,103]. Considering biopsies of CeD patients, CYP3A4 is decreased [96,97,104,105], leading to a reduction in the metabolization of substrates [102,103]. Morón et al., showed, after oral simvastatin intake, the maximum serum level of simvastatin was significantly higher in active CeD ($n = 18$) compared to healthy controls ($n = 11$), and patients on a GFD ($n = 25$) had simvastatin levels comparable to healthy controls [103]. CYP3A4 metabolizing capacity, therefore, might be an interesting non-invasive proxy for villous atrophy, although this requires taking serum samples following administration of drugs metabolized by CYP3A4, making this method less suitable for children.

5.8. Intestinal Permeability Measurements as Proxy for Intestinal Barrier Function

Intestinal barrier function is impaired in CeD, leading to an increased permeability compared to controls, and there have been efforts to use these observations as a biomarker for CeD [106].

Zonulin is a protein that regulates tight-junctions and can disturb intestinal barrier function. It was proposed as a marker for intestinal barrier integrity and is a drug target in clinical trials for CeD (AT-1001, larazotide acetate) [107–110] (Available online: https://clinicaltrials.gov/ct2/show/NCT03569007). Some studies suggest that zonulin is indeed higher in serum of patients with CeD versus controls, but serum values do not change upon start of the GFD, making zonulin unsuitable for monitoring in follow-up [108,111,112]. The current zonulin detection method also has limitations, including fluctuations within the same individual in time, and the low specificity for zonulin of some commercially available ELISA kits [112–114].

Non-invasive tests for intestinal permeability, such as the lactulose–mannitol ratio measured in urine, are based on the principle that large sugars like lactulose cannot pass the intestinal barrier under normal conditions but can pass if the integrity of the barrier is affected. The results of these permeability tests have been shown to differ between CeD patients and controls [111]. However, the reliability of these tests has been shown to be variable and, therefore, are not recommended as clinical biomarkers for CeD [4,106,115,116]. Nonetheless, sugar-based permeability tests in urine are the only completely non-invasive tests available to measure intestinal permeability and, thus, remain valuable in fundamental studies.

5.9. Gluten Peptides as Biomarkers for GFD Adherence

Immunogenic gluten peptides are interesting markers to measure dietary compliance. ELISA-based tests that detect immunogenic gluten peptides in feces, serum, or urine are sensitive enough to detect small quantities of gluten in the diet [117–120]. Immunogenic gluten peptides can be detected frequently in the stool of patients on a GFD [119]. These studies indicate that unnoticed dietary lapses are common, even in patients who report strict GFD adherence. Furthermore, 70% of patients positive for gluten peptides tested negative for anti-TG2 IgA, which suggests that these dietary lapses are not detected when only measuring anti-TG2 IgA [117,119]. Immunogenic gluten peptides in feces can be detected approximately three days after a gluten challenge. Immunogenic gluten peptides in urine show up sooner, but also disappear more quickly, which suggests that measuring gluten in urine might be more useful for identifying which dietary products contain gluten [118]. Currently, clinical trials [NCT03462979 clinicaltrials.gov] are testing the use of point-of-care immunogenic gluten peptide tests at home.

5.10. Antibodies against Tissue Transglutaminases to Detect Skin and Neurological Manifestations of CeD

Serological antibodies against tissue transglutaminase 3 (TG3) and 6 (TG6) have been suggested as biomarker candidates for extra-intestinal manifestations of CeD. Rapid diagnosis of dermatitis herpetiformis (by anti-TG3) and of gluten-induced neurological manifestations such as ataxia (anti-TG6) would be valuable but need further investigation before being implemented in the clinical setting [4,121–124].

6. Duodenal Biopsies as Source for Novel Biomarkers

Although there is considerable interest in identifying CeD biomarkers that can be found in samples that can be collected in a non-invasive manner, it is also clear that the disease focus is on the small intestine. Due to this, fundamental research is focusing on small-intestinal samples of CeD patients and on the cell types present therein. Novel high-throughput techniques are currently being applied to uncover pathogenic pathways that are altered in the small intestine of CeD, including (single-cell) transcriptomics, medium and high-throughput proteomics, and cytometry by time-of-flight (CyTOF).

It is hoped that these techniques open new avenues that lead to novel biomarkers for CeD diagnostics and monitoring.

6.1. Transcriptomic Studies: Markers for Small-Intestinal Damage

Transcriptome studies of intestinal biopsies of CeD patients have revealed genes and pathways that are altered by disease which, therefore, have potential as markers for small intestinal damage and function.

The transcriptome of the small-intestine can be used as a marker for the villous-to-crypt-ratio measured in histopathological slides [125,126]. The ratio of two genes, APOA4:Ki67, correlates well with the degree of villous atrophy, for example. APOA4 is a lipid-processing gene highly expressed in intestinal villi, whereas Ki67 is a broadly used cellular proliferation marker expressed in the intestinal crypts [69,95,104,127]. Measuring these genes in biopsies could help to reduce observer variation in reviewing histological slides and allow assessment of villous atrophy in (public) RNA-sequencing data for which the villous-to-crypt ratio is not available.

Added to the examples discussed above of how deregulated pathways in CeD, such as drug-metabolization, have led to biomarkers for CeD, there are other pathways/genes identified by transcriptome studies that might be worth exploring as non-invasive markers. Lactase (LCT) has a lower expression in CeD biopsies [95,97,104]. LCT encodes for the enzyme that breaks down lactose, and lactase activity can be measured reliably by a non-invasive hydrogen breath test [128]. Lactose malabsorption is common in CeD, and there are indications that this phenotype improves upon adopting a GFD [128,129]. Furthermore, among the upregulated immune-related genes in CeD biopsies, some can be measured in feces. These include the gene S100A9, which forms the heterodimer calprotectin, and the antimicrobial peptide lipocalin (LCN2, also known as NGAL (Neutrophil Gelatinase-Associated Lipocalin)), both of which are used as fecal biomarkers for disease activity in inflammatory bowel disease [104,116,130–132]. Deregulation of these genes is not specific for CeD but might be a potential proxy for small-intestine health, either individually or combined with other markers for mucosal damage.

6.2. Single Cells to Multi-Dimensions

The proteome or transcriptome profile of bulk samples, such as small-intestine biopsies or blood of CeD patients, is mainly driven by the cell type–composition of each tissue. However, the more abundant cells may overshadow the expression of rare cells present in tissues. Therefore, the use of high-throughput techniques, especially those that allow the characterization of single cells, is essential in the study of complex diseases.

Classically, FACS has been used to study cell surface markers and internal proteins in single cells. To date, FACS allows the analysis of up to 20 proteins at the same time in millions of cells. Recently, CyTOF has emerged as a technology that combines the principle of FACS and mass spectrometry. CyTOF allows the study of around 40 surface markers in millions of cells [133]. Recently, van Unen et al., applied this technology to gut biopsies and PBMCs of CeD patients, refractory CeD patients, and Crohn's disease patients and pinpointed differences between the three patient groups [134].

Another emerging approach is single-cell RNA sequencing (scRNAseq) [135], which characterizes the transcriptome at a single-cell level. While the number of cells that can be analyzed simultaneously by scRNAseq is low compared to FACS and CyTOF (thousands to millions, respectively), the number of markers that can be analyzed increases to thousands of genes. ScRNAseq also does not require prior knowledge about which markers to use. Considering the context of CeD, Atlasy et al., identified an Natural Killer T–like cell subset that was absent in the duodenum from CeD patients and CeD-specific transcriptome changes in T cells, myeloid cells, and mast cells [136].

ScRNAseq also can be combined with methods that detect other layers of data in the same cell. Some examples of multilayer techniques include the characterization of cell surface markers (CITE-seq [137]), whole genome screening of open (active) chromatin (single-cell RNA/ATAC-seq [138]), actual position in the tissue by spatial transcriptome reconstruction, or mass cytometry imaging [139–141]. All these advances hold promise as the foundation for a multidimensional understanding of complex diseases. Henceforth, combining these high-throughput multi-omics studies with new model systems for CeD, like organ-on-chip technology [35], can help identify potential biomarkers in the pathogenesis of CeD.

7. Conclusions and Future Perspectives

During this review we have discussed non-invasive biomarker candidates that may complement current diagnostics and monitoring of CeD. Some of these markers are already being validated and/or implemented in the clinic. We also briefly highlighted how modern high-throughput techniques can help find new targets for diagnostics, monitoring, and drug development.

The current serological markers, TG2- and EMA-antibodies, are the cornerstone of the diagnosis due to their high specificity/sensitivity. However, simultaneously measuring additional markers for intestinal damage or function, such as citrulline or I-FABP, could identify cases with villous damage in future, thereby reducing or replacing the need for invasive biopsies in cases with borderline serology. Even if the individual biomarker candidates discussed here turn out to be more general markers of intestinal damage or inflammation, and nonspecific for CeD, efforts should be made to assess the diagnostic value of using combinations of these biomarkers for CeD.

Currently, there are no biomarkers to predict who will develop CeD. Genetics may provide part of the key. Genetic screening already has the potential to identify those individuals at highest risk for CeD, and new algorithms are being tested to increase the predictive power of genetic risk scores [34]. Future studies also should focus on whether genetic risk scores have added value over the use of serology alone, and whether genetic risk scoring would help to identify individuals who would benefit from serological screening for CeD at specific points in their lives. Many of the other markers described here such as the lipid profile and changes in circulating cell types or gene/protein expression, are also worth investigating as predictive tools for CeD.

Previously mentioned, one of the disadvantages of current diagnostics based on antibodies is that they cannot be used to diagnose patients already following a GFD. The option to establish the diagnosis in patients who are on a GFD after a single dose of gluten by measuring specific circulating cytokines is worth exploring because it eliminates the need for a longer gluten challenge, which may cause intestinal damage and symptoms. Measuring cytokines also could be a quick assay to assess the response to a gluten challenge after administration of adjuvant treatments in clinical trials. This would have huge benefits for assessing drug efficacy in CeD, since invasive duodenal biopsies would not be required to assess how patients are responding to a gluten challenge.

Hereafter, even dietary lapses and unintentional exposures might be detectable by measuring gluten peptides in urine, as studies so far have shown that these are quicker and more sensitive markers than anti-TG2.

Next steps would be to further explore the heterogeneity of CeD to identify markers that could help to predict who will develop complications associated with CeD or other immune-mediated diseases. We would like to emphasize that fundamental studies investigating the pathogenesis of CeD are essential in working toward more personalized diagnostics, monitoring, and treatment of CeD. Results of current and future fundamental research have yielded and will yield interesting non-invasive markers for CeD.

Author Contributions: Conceptualization, A.D.R.-S., I.L.T., I.J., S.W., M.C.V., B.C.G.-d.J.; Writing—Original Draft Preparation, A.D.R.-S., I.L.T.; Writing—Review & Editing, I.J., S.W., M.C.V., B.C.G.-d.J.; Visualization, A.D.R.-S.; Supervision, I.J., S.W. All authors have read and agreed to the published version of the manuscript.

Acknowledgments: We would like to thank Kate Mc Intyre for editing the manuscript. We would like to acknowledge Renée Moerkens and Joram Mooiweer for providing and allowing the adaptation of their figures.

References

1. Singh, P.; Arora, A.; Strand, T.A.; Leffler, D.A.; Catassi, C.; Green, P.H.; Kelly, C.P.; Ahuja, V.; Makharia, G.K. Global Prevalence of Celiac Disease: Systematic Review and Meta-analysis. *Clin. Gastroenterol. Hepatol.* **2018**, *16*, 823–836.e2. [CrossRef] [PubMed]

2. Spijkerman, M.; Tan, I.L.; Kolkman, J.J.; Withoff, S.; Wijmenga, C.; Visschedijk, M.C.; Weersma, R.K. A large variety of clinical features and concomitant disorders in celiac disease—A cohort study in The Netherlands. *Dig. Liver Dis.* **2016**, *48*, 499–505. [CrossRef] [PubMed]

3. Fueyo-Díaz, R.; Magallón-Botaya, R.; Masluk, B.; Palacios-Navarro, G.; Asensio-Martínez, A.; Gascón-Santos, S.; Olivan-Blázquez, B.; Sebastián-Domingo, J.J. Prevalence of celiac disease in primary care: The need for its own code. *BMC Health Serv. Res.* **2019**, *19*, 1–9. [CrossRef] [PubMed]

4. Al-Toma, A.; Volta, U.; Auricchio, R.; Castillejo, G.; Sanders, D.S.; Cellier, C.; Mulder, C.J.; Lundin, K.E.A. European society for the study of coeliac disease (ESsCD) guideline for coeliac disease and other gluten-related disorders. *United Eur. Gastroenterol. J.* **2019**, *7*, 583–613. [CrossRef]

5. Husby, S.; Koletzko, S.; Korponay-Szabó, I.; Kurppa, K.; Mearin, M.L.; Ribes-Koninckx, C.; Shamir, R.; Troncone, R.; Auricchio, R.; Castillejo, G.; et al. European society paediatric gastroenterology, hepatology and nutrition guidelines for diagnosing coeliac disease 2020. *J. Pediatr. Gastroenterol. Nutr.* **2020**, *70*, 141–156. [CrossRef]

6. McCarty, T.R.; O'Brien, C.R.; Gremida, A.; Ling, C.; Rustagi, T. Efficacy of duodenal bulb biopsy for diagnosis of celiac disease: A systematic review and meta-analysis. *Endosc. Int. Open* **2018**, *6*, E1369–E1378. [CrossRef]

7. Peña, A.S. What is the best histopathological classification for celiac disease? Does it matter? *Gastroenterol. Hepatol. Bed Bench* **2015**, *8*, 239–243.

8. Karell, K.; Louka, A.S.; Moodie, S.J.; Ascher, H.; Clot, F.; Greco, L.; Ciclitira, P.J.; Sollid, L.M.; Partanen, J. HLA types in celiac disease patients not carrying the DQA1 *05-DQB1 *02 (DQ2) heterodimer: Results from the European genetics cluster on celiac disease. *Hum. Immunol.* **2003**, *64*, 469–477. [CrossRef]

9. Abadie, V.; Sollid, L.M.; Barreiro, L.B.; Jabri, B. Integration of genetic and immunological insights into a model of celiac disease pathogenesis. *Annu. Rev. Immunol.* **2011**, *29*, 493–525. [CrossRef]

10. Romanos, J.; Rosén, A.; Kumar, V.; Trynka, G.; Franke, L.; Szperl, A.; Gutierrez-Achury, J.; Van Diemen, C.C.; Kanninga, R.; Jankipersadsing, S.A.; et al. Improving coeliac disease risk prediction by testing non-HLA variants additional to HLA variants. *Gut* **2014**, *63*, 415–422. [CrossRef]

11. Sollid, L.M.; Jabri, B. Triggers and drivers of autoimmunity: Lessons from coeliac disease. *Nat. Rev. Immunol.* **2013**, *13*, 294–302. [CrossRef] [PubMed]

12. Andrén Aronsson, C.; Lee, H.S.; Hård Af Segerstad, E.M.; Uusitalo, U.; Yang, J.; Koletzko, S.; Liu, E.; Kurppa, K.; Bingley, P.J.; Toppari, J.; et al. Association of gluten intake during the first 5 years of life with incidence of celiac disease autoimmunity and celiac disease among children at increased risk. *JAMA-J. Am. Med. Assoc.* **2019**, *322*, 514–523. [CrossRef] [PubMed]

13. Schumann, M.; Siegmund, B.; Schulzke, J.D.; Fromm, M. Celiac disease: Role of the Epithelial Barrier. *Cell. Mol. Gastroenterol. Hepatol.* **2017**, *3*, 150–162. [CrossRef] [PubMed]

14. Ting, Y.T.; Dahal-Koirala, S.; Kim, H.S.K.; Qiao, S.W.; Neumann, R.S.; Lundin, K.E.A.; Petersen, J.; Reid, H.H.; Sollid, L.M.; Rossjohn, J. A molecular basis for the T cell response in HLA-DQ2.2 mediated celiac disease. *Proc. Natl. Acad. Sci. USA* **2020**, *117*, 3063–3073. [CrossRef] [PubMed]

15. Broughton, S.E.; Petersen, J.; Theodossis, A.; Scally, S.W.; Loh, K.L.; Thompson, A.; van Bergen, J.; Kooy-Winkelaar, Y.; Henderson, K.N.; Beddoe, T.; et al. Biased T cell receptor usage directed against human leukocyte antigen DQ8-restricted gliadin peptides is associated with celiac disease. *Immunity* **2012**, *37*, 611–621. [CrossRef]

16. Arentz-Hansen, H.; Körner, R.; Molberg, Ø.; Quarsten, H.; Vader, W.; Kooy, Y.M.C.; Lundin, K.E.A.; Koning, F.; Roepstorff, P.; Sollid, L.M.; et al. The intestinal T cell response to α-gliadin in adult celiac disease is focused on a single deamidated glutamine targeted by tissue transglutaminase. *J. Exp. Med.* **2000**, *191*, 603–612. [CrossRef]

17. Jabri, B.; Sollid, L.M. T Cells in Celiac Disease. *J. Immunol.* **2017**, *198*, 3005–3014. [CrossRef]

18. Høydahl, L.S.; Richter, L.; Frick, R.; Snir, O.; Gunnarsen, K.S.; Landsverk, O.J.B.; Iversen, R.; Jeliazkov, J.R.; Gray, J.J.; Bergseng, E.; et al. Plasma Cells Are the Most Abundant Gluten Peptide MHC-expressing Cells in Inflamed Intestinal Tissues From Patients With Celiac Disease. *Gastroenterology* **2019**, *156*, 1428–1439.e10. [CrossRef]

19. Iversen, R.; Roy, B.; Stamnaes, J.; Høydahl, L.S.; Hnida, K.; Neumann, R.S.; Korponay-Szabó, I.R.; Lundin, K.E.A.; Sollid, L.M. Efficient T cell–B cell collaboration guides autoantibody epitope bias and onset of celiac disease. *Proc. Natl. Acad. Sci. USA* **2019**, *116*, 15134–15139. [CrossRef]

20. Bouziat, R.; Hinterleitner, R.; Brown, J.J.; Stencel-Baerenwald, J.E.; Ikizler, M.; Mayassi, T.; Meisel, M.; Kim, S.M.; Discepolo, V.; Pruijssers, A.J.; et al. Reovirus infection triggers inflammatory responses to dietary antigens and development of celiac disease. *Science* **2017**, *356*, 44–50. [CrossRef]

21. Bouziat, R.; Biering, S.B.; Kouame, E.; Sangani, K.A.; Kang, S.; Ernest, J.D.; Varma, M.; Brown, J.J.; Urbanek, K.; Dermody, T.S.; et al. Murine norovirus infection induces TH1 inflammatory responses to dietary antigens. *Cell Host Microbe* **2018**, *24*, 677–688.e5. [CrossRef] [PubMed]

22. Corouge, M.; Loridant, S.; Fradin, C.; Salleron, J.; Damiens, S.; Moragues, M.D.; Souplet, V.; Jouault, T.; Robert, R.; Dubucquoi, S.; et al. Humoral immunity links Candida albicans infection and celiac disease. *PLoS ONE* **2015**, *10*, e0121776. [CrossRef] [PubMed]

23. Caminero, A.; Galipeau, H.J.; McCarville, J.L.; Johnston, C.W.; Bernier, S.P.; Russell, A.K.; Jury, J.; Herran, A.R.; Casqueiro, J.; Tye-Din, J.A.; et al. Duodenal Bacteria From Patients With Celiac Disease and Healthy Subjects Distinctly Affect Gluten Breakdown and Immunogenicity. *Gastroenterology* **2016**, *151*, 670–683. [CrossRef] [PubMed]

24. Francavilla, R.; Cristofori, F.; Vacca, M.; Barone, M.; De Angelis, M. Advances in understanding the potential therapeutic applications of gut microbiota and probiotic mediated therapies in celiac disease. *Expert Rev. Gastroenterol. Hepatol.* **2020**, *14*, 323–333. [CrossRef]

25. Petersen, J.; Ciacchi, L.; Tran, M.T.; Loh, K.L.; Kooy-Winkelaar, Y.; Croft, N.P.; Hardy, M.Y.; Chen, Z.; McCluskey, J.; Anderson, R.P.; et al. T cell receptor cross-reactivity between gliadin and bacterial peptides in celiac disease. *Nat. Struct. Mol. Biol.* **2020**, *27*, 49–61. [CrossRef]

26. Liu, E.; Rewers, M.; Eisenbarth, G.S. Genetic testing: Who should do the testing and what is the role of genetic testing in the setting of celiac disease? *Gastroenterology* **2005**, *128*, 33–37. [CrossRef]

27. Withoff, S.; Li, Y.; Jonkers, I.; Wijmenga, C. Understanding Celiac Disease by Genomics. *Trends Genet.* **2016**, *32*, 295–308. [CrossRef]

28. Ricaño-Ponce, I.; Gutierrez-Achury, J.; Costa, A.F.; Deelen, P.; Kurilshikov, A.; Zorro, M.M.; Platteel, M.; van der Graaf, A.; Sugai, E.; Moreno, M.L.; et al. Immunochip meta-analysis in European and Argentinian populations identifies two novel genetic loci associated with celiac disease. *Eur. J. Hum. Genet.* **2020**, *28*, 313–323. [CrossRef]

29. Trynka, G.; Hunt, K.A.; Bockett, N.A.; Romanos, J.; Mistry, V.; Szperl, A.; Bakker, S.F.; Bardella, M.T.; Bhaw-Rosun, L.; Castillejo, G.; et al. Dense genotyping identifies and localizes multiple common and rare variant association signals in celiac disease. *Nat. Genet.* **2011**, *43*, 1193–1201. [CrossRef]

30. Kuja-Halkola, R.; Lebwohl, B.; Halfvarson, J.; Wijmenga, C.; Magnusson, P.K.E.; Ludvigsson, J.F. Heritability of non-HLA genetics in coeliac disease: A population-based study in 107 000 twins. *Gut* **2016**, *65*, 1793–1798. [CrossRef]

31. Van der Graaf, A.; Zorro, M.; Claringbould, A.; Vosa, U.; Aguirre-Gamboa, R.; Li, C.; Mooiweer, J.; Ricano-Ponce, I.; Borek, Z.; Koning, F.; et al. Systematic prioritization of candidate genes in disease loci identifies TRAFD1 as a master regulator of IFNγ signalling in celiac disease. *bioRxiv* **2020**, 1–40. [CrossRef]

32. Van der Wijst, M.G.P.; De Vries, D.H.; Brugge, H.; Westra, H.J.; Franke, L. An integrative approach for building personalized gene regulatory networks for precision medicine. *Genome Med.* **2018**, *10*. [CrossRef] [PubMed]

33. Abraham, G.; Rohmer, A.; Tye-Din, J.A.; Inouye, M. Genomic prediction of celiac disease targeting HLA-positive individuals. *Genome Med.* **2015**, *7*, 1–11. [CrossRef] [PubMed]

34. Sharp, S.A.; Jones, S.E.; Kimmitt, R.A.; Weedon, M.N.; Halpin, A.M.; Wood, A.R.; Beaumont, R.N.; King, S.; van Heel, D.A.; Campbell, P.M.; et al. A single nucleotide polymorphism genetic risk score to aid diagnosis of coeliac disease: A pilot study in clinical care. *Aliment. Pharmacol. Ther.* **2020**, *52*, 1165–1173. [CrossRef] [PubMed]

35. Moerkens, R.; Mooiweer, J.; Withoff, S.; Wijmenga, C. Celiac disease-on-chip: Modeling a multifactorial disease in vitro. *United Eur. Gastroenterol. J.* **2019**, *7*, 467–476. [CrossRef]

36. Vriezinga, S.L.; Schweizer, J.J.; Koning, F.; Mearin, M.L. Coeliac disease and gluten-related disorders in childhood. *Nat. Rev. Gastroenterol. Hepatol.* **2015**, *12*, 527–536. [CrossRef]

37. Korponay-Szabó, I.R.; Szabados, K.; Pusztai, J.; Uhrin, K.; Ludmány, É.; Nemes, É.; Kaukinen, K.; Kapitány, A.; Koskinen, L.; Sipka, S.; et al. Population screening for coeliac disease in primary care by district nurses using a rapid antibody test: Diagnostic accuracy and feasibility study. *Br. Med. J.* **2007**, *335*, 1244–1247. [CrossRef]

38. Singh, P.; Arora, A.; Strand, T.A.; Leffler, D.A.; Mäki, M.; Kelly, C.P.; Ahuja, V.; Makharia, G.K. Diagnostic Accuracy of Point of Care Tests for Diagnosing Celiac Disease: A Systematic Review and Meta-Analysis. *J. Clin. Gastroenterol.* **2019**, *53*, 535–542. [CrossRef]

39. Mooney, P.D.; Kurien, M.; Evans, K.E.; Chalkiadakis, I.; Hale, M.F.; Kannan, M.Z.; Courtice, V.; Johnston, A.J.;
     Irvine, A.J.; Hadjivassiliou, M.; et al. Point-of-care testing for celiac disease has a low sensitivity in endoscopy.
     Gastrointest. Endosc. **2014**, *80*, 456–462. [CrossRef]

40. Kurppa, K.; Taavela, J.; Saavalainen, P.; Kaukinen, K.; Lindfors, K. Novel diagnostic techniques for celiac
     disease. *Expert Rev. Gastroenterol. Hepatol.* **2016**, *10*, 795–805. [CrossRef]

41. Yazdani, R.; Azizi, G.; Abolhassani, H.; Aghamohammadi, A. Selective IgA Deficiency: Epidemiology,
     Pathogenesis, Clinical Phenotype, Diagnosis, Prognosis and Management. *Scand. J. Immunol.* **2017**, *85*, 3–12.
     [CrossRef] [PubMed]

42. Bizzaro, N.; Villalta, D.; Tonutti, E.; Doria, A.; Tampoia, M.; Bassetti, D.; Tozzoli, R. IgA and IgG Tissue
     Transglutaminase Antibody Prevalence and Clinical Significance in Connective Tissue Diseases, Inflammatory
     Bowel Disease, and Primary Biliary Cirrhosis. *Dig. Dis. Sci.* **2003**, *48*, 2360–2365. [CrossRef] [PubMed]

43. Ferrara, F.; Quaglia, S.; Caputo, I.; Esposito, C.; Lepretti, M.; Pastore, S.; Giorgi, R.; Martelossi, S.; Dal Molin, G.;
     Di Toro, N.; et al. Anti-transglutaminase antibodies in non-coeliac children suffering from infectious diseases.
     Clin. Exp. Immunol. **2010**, *159*, 217–223. [CrossRef] [PubMed]

44. Trovato, C.M.; Montuori, M.; Valitutti, F.; Leter, B.; Cucchiara, S.; Oliva, S. The Challenge of Treatment in
     Potential Celiac Disease. *Gastroenterol. Res. Pract.* **2019**, *2019*. [CrossRef]

45. Auricchio, R.; Mandile, R.; Del Vecchio, M.R.; Scapaticci, S.; Galatola, M.; Maglio, M.; Discepolo, V.; Miele, E.;
     Cielo, D.; Troncone, R.; et al. Progression of Celiac Disease in Children With Antibodies Against Tissue
     Transglutaminase and Normal Duodenal Architecture. *Gastroenterology* **2019**, *157*, 413–420.e3. [CrossRef]

46. See, J.A.; Kaukinen, K.; Makharia, G.K.; Gibson, P.R.; Murray, J.A. Practical insights into gluten-free diets.
     Nat. Rev. Gastroenterol. Hepatol. **2015**, *12*, 580–591. [CrossRef]

47. Leonard, M.M.; Weir, D.C.; Degroote, M.; Mitchell, P.D.; Singh, P.; Silvester, J.A.; Leichtner, A.M.; Fasano, A.
     Value of IgA tTG in Predicting Mucosal Recovery in Children with Celiac Disease on a Gluten-Free Diet.
     J. Pediatr. Gastroenterol. Nutr. **2017**, *64*, 286–291. [CrossRef]

48. Silvester, J.A.; Kurada, S.; Szwajcer, A.; Kelly, C.P.; Leffler, D.A.; Duerksen, D.R. Tests for Serum Transglutaminase
     and Endomysial Antibodies Do Not Detect Most Patients With Celiac Disease and Persistent Villous Atrophy
     on Gluten-free Diets: A Meta-analysis. *Gastroenterology* **2017**, *153*, 689–701.e1. [CrossRef]

49. Hollon, J.R.; Cureton, P.A.; Martin, M.L.; Puppa, E.L.L.; Fasano, A. Trace gluten contamination may play
     a role in mucosal and clinical recovery in a subgroup of diet-adherent non-responsive celiac disease patients.
     BMC Gastroenterol. **2013**, *13*, 40. [CrossRef]

50. Hære, P.; Høie, O.; Schulz, T.; Schönhardt, I.; Raki, M.; Lundin, K.E.A. Long-term mucosal recovery and
     healing in celiac disease is the rule—not the exception. *Scand. J. Gastroenterol.* **2016**, *51*, 1439–1446. [CrossRef]

51. Szakács, Z.; Mátrai, P.; Hegyi, P.; Szabó, I.; Vincze, Á.; Balaskó, M.; Mosdósi, B.; Sarlós, P.; Simon, M.;
     Márta, K.; et al. Younger age at diagnosis predisposes to mucosal recovery in celiac disease on a gluten-free
     diet: A meta-analysis. *PLoS ONE* **2017**, *12*, e0187526. [CrossRef] [PubMed]

52. Ludvigsson, J.F.; Ciacci, C.; Green, P.H.R.; Kaukinen, K.; Korponay-Szabo, I.R.; Kurppa, K.; Murray, J.A.;
     Lundin, K.E.A.; Maki, M.J.; Popp, A.; et al. Outcome measures in coeliac disease trials: The Tampere
     recommendations. *Gut* **2018**, *67*, 1410–1424. [CrossRef] [PubMed]

53. Manavalan, J.S.; Hernandez, L.; Shah, J.G.; Konikkara, J.; Naiyer, A.J.; Lee, A.R.; Ciaccio, E.; Minaya, M.T.;
     Green, P.H.R.; Bhagat, G. Serum cytokine elevations in celiac disease: Association with disease presentation.
     Hum. Immunol. **2010**, *71*, 50–57. [CrossRef] [PubMed]

54. Iervasi, E.; Auricchio, R.; Strangio, A.; Greco, L.; Saverino, D. Serum IL-21 levels from celiac disease patients
     correlates with anti-tTG IgA autoantibodies and mucosal damage. *Autoimmunity* **2020**, *53*, 225–230. [CrossRef]

55. Assarsson, E.; Lundberg, M.; Holmquist, G.; Björkesten, J.; Thorsen, S.B.; Ekman, D.; Eriksson, A.; Dickens, E.R.;
     Ohlsson, S.; Edfeldt, G.; et al. Homogenous 96-plex PEA immunoassay exhibiting high sensitivity, specificity,
     and excellent scalability. *PLoS ONE* **2014**, *9*, e95192. [CrossRef]

56. Goel, G.; Daveson, A.J.M.; Hooi, C.E.; Tye-Din, J.A.; Wang, S.; Szymczak, E.; Williams, L.J.; Dzuris, J.L.;
     Neff, K.M.; Truitt, K.E.; et al. Serum cytokines elevated during gluten-mediated cytokine release in coeliac
     disease. *Clin. Exp. Immunol.* **2020**, *199*, 68–78. [CrossRef]

57. Goel, G.; Tye-Din, J.A.; Qiao, S.W.; Russell, A.K.; Mayassi, T.; Ciszewski, C.; Sarna, V.K.; Wang, S.; Goldstein, K.E.;
     Dzuris, J.L.; et al. Cytokine release and gastrointestinal symptoms after gluten challenge in celiac disease.
     Sci. Adv. **2019**, *5*, eaaw7756. [CrossRef]

58. Tye-Din, J.A.; Skodje, G.I.; Sarna, V.K.; Dzuris, J.L.; Russell, A.K.; Goel, G.; Wang, S.; Goldstein, K.E.; Williams, L.J.; Sollid, L.M.; et al. Cytokine release after gluten ingestion differentiates coeliac disease from self-reported gluten sensitivity. *United Eur. Gastroenterol. J.* **2020**, *8*, 108–118. [CrossRef]

59. Sarna, V.K.; Skodje, G.I.; Reims, H.M.; Risnes, L.F.; Dahal-Koirala, S.; Sollid, L.M.; Lundin, K.E.A. HLA-DQ:gluten tetramer test in blood gives better detection of coeliac patients than biopsy after 14-day gluten challenge. *Gut* **2018**, *67*, 1606–1613. [CrossRef]

60. Christophersen, A.; Ráki, M.; Bergseng, E.; Lundin, K.E.; Jahnsen, J.; Sollid, L.M.; Qiao, S.W. Tetramer-visualized gluten-specific CD4+ t cells in blood as a potential diagnostic marker for coeliac disease without oral gluten challenge. *United Eur. Gastroenterol. J.* **2014**, *2*, 268. [CrossRef]

61. López-Palacios, N.; Pascual, V.; Castaño, M.; Bodas, A.; Fernández-Prieto, M.; Espino-Paisán, L.; Martínez-Ojinaga, E.; Salazar, I.; Martínez-Curiel, R.; Rey, E.; et al. Evaluation of T cells in blood after a short gluten challenge for coeliac disease diagnosis. *Dig. Liver Dis.* **2018**, *50*, 1183–1188. [CrossRef] [PubMed]

62. Zühlke, S.; Risnes, L.F.; Dahal-Koirala, S.; Christophersen, A.; Sollid, L.M.; Lundin, K.E.A. CD38 expression on gluten-specific T cells is a robust marker of gluten re-exposure in coeliac disease. *United Eur. Gastroenterol. J.* **2019**, *7*, 1337–1344. [CrossRef] [PubMed]

63. Bragde, H.; Jansson, U.; Fredrikson, M.; Grodzinsky, E.; Söderman, J. Potential blood-based markers of celiac disease. *BMC Gastroenterol.* **2014**, *14*, 176. [CrossRef] [PubMed]

64. Galatola, M.; Cielo, D.; Panico, C.; Stellato, P.; Malamisura, B.; Carbone, L.; Gianfrani, C.; Troncone, R.; Greco, L.; Auricchio, R. Presymptomatic Diagnosis of Celiac Disease in Predisposed Children: The Role of Gene Expression Profile. *J. Pediatr. Gastroenterol. Nutr.* **2017**, *65*, 314–320. [CrossRef] [PubMed]

65. Gebert, L.F.R.; MacRae, I.J. Regulation of microRNA function in animals. *Nat. Rev. Mol. Cell Biol.* **2019**, *20*, 21–37. [CrossRef] [PubMed]

66. Guo, J.; Meng, R.; Yin, Z.; Li, P.; Zhou, R.; Zhang, S.; Dong, X.; Liu, L.; Wu, G. A serum microRNA signature as a prognostic factor for patients with advanced NSCLC and its association with tissue microRNA expression profiles. *Mol. Med. Rep.* **2016**, *13*, 4643–4653. [CrossRef]

67. Iborra, M.; Bernuzzi, F.; Correale, C.; Vetrano, S.; Fiorino, G.; Beltrán, B.; Marabita, F.; Locati, M.; Spinelli, A.; Nos, P.; et al. Identification of serum and tissue micro-RNA expression profiles in different stages of inflammatory bowel disease. *Clin. Exp. Immunol.* **2013**, *173*, 250–258. [CrossRef]

68. Stachurska, A.; Zorro, M.M.; van der Sijde, M.R.; Withoff, S. Small and long regulatory RNAs in the immune system and immune diseases. *Front. Immunol.* **2014**, *5*, 513. [CrossRef]

69. Capuano, M.; Iaffaldano, L.; Tinto, N.; Montanaro, D.; Capobianco, V.; Izzo, V.; Tucci, F.; Troncone, G.; Greco, L.; Sacchetti, L. MicroRNA-449a overexpression, reduced NOTCH1 signals and scarce goblet cells characterize the small intestine of celiac patients. *PLoS ONE* **2011**, *6*, e29094. [CrossRef]

70. Magni, S.; Comani, G.B.; Elli, L.; Vanessi, S.; Ballarini, E.; Nicolini, G.; Rusconi, M.; Castoldi, M.; Meneveri, R.; Muckenthaler, M.U.; et al. MIRNAs affect the expression of innate and adaptive immunity proteins in celiac disease. *Am. J. Gastroenterol.* **2014**, *109*, 1662. [CrossRef]

71. Buoli Comani, G.; Panceri, R.; Dinelli, M.; Biondi, A.; Mancuso, C.; Meneveri, R.; Barisani, D. miRNA-regulated gene expression differs in celiac disease patients according to the age of presentation. *Genes Nutr.* **2015**, *10*, 482. [CrossRef] [PubMed]

72. Vaira, V.; Roncoroni, L.; Barisani, D.; Gaudioso, G.; Bosari, S.; Bulfamante, G.; Doneda, L.; Conte, D.; Tomba, C.; Bardella, M.T.; et al. microRNA profiles in coeliac patients distinguish different clinical phenotypes and are modulated by gliadin peptides in primary duodenal fibroblasts. *Clin. Sci.* **2014**, *126*, 417–423. [CrossRef] [PubMed]

73. Comincini, S.; Manai, F.; Meazza, C.; Pagani, S.; Martinelli, C.; Pasqua, N.; Pelizzo, G.; Biggiogera, M.; Bozzola, M. Identification of autophagy-related genes and their regulatory miRNAs associated with celiac disease in children. *Int. J. Mol. Sci.* **2017**, *18*, 391. [CrossRef] [PubMed]

74. Amr, K.S.; Bayoumi, F.S.; Eissa, E.; Abu-Zekry, M. Circulating microRNAs as potential non-invasive biomarkers in pediatric patients with celiac disease. *Eur. Ann. Allergy Clin. Immunol.* **2019**, *51*, 159–164. [CrossRef]

75. Bascuñán, K.A.; Pérez-Bravo, F.; Gaudioso, G.; Vaira, V.; Roncoroni, L.; Elli, L.; Monguzzi, E.; Araya, M. A miRNA-Based Blood and Mucosal Approach for Detecting and Monitoring Celiac Disease. *Dig. Dis. Sci.* **2020**, *65*, 1982–1991. [CrossRef]

76. Zahm, A.M.; Thayu, M.; Hand, N.J.; Horner, A.; Leonard, M.B.; Friedman, J.R. Circulating microRNA is a biomarker of pediatric crohn disease. *J. Pediatr. Gastroenterol. Nutr.* **2011**, *53*, 26–33. [CrossRef]

77. Cortez, M.A.; Bueso-Ramos, C.; Ferdin, J.; Lopez-Berestein, G.; Sood, A.K.; Calin, G.A. MicroRNAs in body fluids-the mix of hormones and biomarkers. *Nat. Rev. Clin. Oncol.* **2011**, *8*, 467–477. [CrossRef]

78. Robbins, P.D.; Morelli, A.E. Regulation of immune responses by extracellular vesicles. *Nat. Rev. Immunol.* **2014**, *14*, 195–208. [CrossRef]

79. Villarroya-Beltri, C.; Gutiérrez-Vázquez, C.; Sánchez-Cabo, F.; Pérez-Hernández, D.; Vázquez, J.; Martin-Cofreces, N.; Martinez-Herrera, D.J.; Pascual-Montano, A.; Mittelbrunn, M.; Sánchez-Madrid, F. Sumoylated hnRNPA2B1 controls the sorting of miRNAs into exosomes through binding to specific motifs. *Nat. Commun.* **2013**, *4*, 1–10. [CrossRef]

80. Mittelbrunn, M.; Gutiérrez-Vázquez, C.; Villarroya-Beltri, C.; González, S.; Sánchez-Cabo, F.; González, M.Á.; Bernad, A.; Sánchez-Madrid, F. Unidirectional transfer of microRNA-loaded exosomes from T cells to antigen-presenting cells. *Nat. Commun.* **2011**, *2*, 282. [CrossRef]

81. Montecalvo, A.; Larregina, A.T.; Shufesky, W.J.; Stolz, D.B.; Sullivan, M.L.G.; Karlsson, J.M.; Baty, C.J.; Gibson, G.A.; Erdos, G.; Wang, Z.; et al. Mechanism of transfer of functional microRNAs between mouse dendritic cells via exosomes. *Blood* **2012**, *119*, 756–766. [CrossRef] [PubMed]

82. Marasco, G.; Di Biase, A.R.; Schiumerini, R.; Eusebi, L.H.; Iughetti, L.; Ravaioli, F.; Scaioli, E.; Colecchia, A.; Festi, D. Gut Microbiota and Celiac Disease. *Dig. Dis. Sci.* **2016**, *61*, 1461–1472. [CrossRef] [PubMed]

83. Olivares, M.; Neef, A.; Castillejo, G.; De Palma, G.; Varea, V.; Capilla, A.; Palau, F.; Nova, E.; Marcos, A.; Polanco, I.; et al. The HLA-DQ2 genotype selects for early intestinal microbiota composition in infants at high risk of developing coeliac disease. *Gut* **2015**, *64*, 406–417. [CrossRef] [PubMed]

84. Olivares, M.; Walker, A.W.; Capilla, A.; Benítez-Páez, A.; Palau, F.; Parkhill, J.; Castillejo, G.; Sanz, Y. Gut microbiota trajectory in early life may predict development of celiac disease. *Microbiome* **2018**, *6*. [CrossRef]

85. Lerner, A.; Arleevskaya, M.; Schmiedl, A.; Matthias, T. Microbes and viruses are bugging the gut in celiac disease. Are they friends or foes? *Front. Microbiol.* **2017**, *8*. [CrossRef]

86. Plot, L.; Amital, H. Infectious associations of Celiac disease. *Autoimmun. Rev.* **2009**, *8*, 316–319. [CrossRef]

87. Lerner, A.; Aminov, R.; Matthias, T. Dysbiosis may trigger autoimmune diseases via inappropriate post-translational modification of host proteins. *Front. Microbiol.* **2016**, *7*. [CrossRef]

88. Stene, L.C.; Honeyman, M.C.; Hoffenberg, E.J.; Haas, J.E.; Sokol, R.J.; Emery, L.; Taki, I.; Norris, J.M.; Erlich, H.A.; Eisenbarth, G.S.; et al. Rotavirus infection frequency and risk of celiac disease autoimmunity in early childhood: A longitudinal study. *Am. J. Gastroenterol.* **2006**, *101*, 2333–2340. [CrossRef]

89. Lindfors, K.; Lin, J.; Lee, H.S.; Hyöty, H.; Nykter, M.; Kurppa, K.; Liu, E.; Koletzko, S.; Rewers, M.; Hagopian, W.; et al. Metagenomics of the faecal virome indicate a cumulative effect of enterovirus and gluten amount on the risk of coeliac disease autoimmunity in genetically at risk children: The TEDDY study. *Gut* **2020**, *69*, 1416–1422. [CrossRef]

90. Pabst, O.; Mowat, A.M. Oral tolerance to food protein. *Mucosal Immunol.* **2012**, *5*, 232–239. [CrossRef]

91. Ko, C.W.; Qu, J.; Black, D.D.; Tso, P. Regulation of intestinal lipid metabolism: Current concepts and relevance to disease. *Nat. Rev. Gastroenterol. Hepatol.* **2020**, *17*, 169–183. [CrossRef] [PubMed]

92. Sen, P.; Carlsson, C.; Virtanen, S.M.; Simell, S.; Hyöty, H.; Ilonen, J.; Toppari, J.; Veijola, R.; Hyötyläinen, T.; Knip, M.; et al. Persistent alterations in plasma lipid profiles before introduction of gluten in the diet associated with progression to celiac disease. *Clin. Transl. Gastroenterol.* **2019**, *10*. [CrossRef] [PubMed]

93. Auricchio, R.; Galatola, M.; Cielo, D.; Amoresano, A.; Caterino, M.; De Vita, E.; Illiano, A.; Troncone, R.; Greco, L.; Ruoppolo, M. A Phospholipid Profile at 4 Months Predicts the Onset of Celiac Disease in at-Risk Infants. *Sci. Rep.* **2019**, *9*, 1–12. [CrossRef] [PubMed]

94. Kirchberg, F.F.; Werkstetter, K.J.; Uhl, O.; Auricchio, R.; Castillejo, G.; Korponay-Szabo, I.R.; Polanco, I.; Ribes-Koninckx, C.; Vriezinga, S.L.; Koletzko, B.; et al. Investigating the early metabolic fingerprint of celiac disease—A prospective approach. *J. Autoimmun.* **2016**, *72*, 95–101. [CrossRef] [PubMed]

95. Loberman-Nachum, N.; Sosnovski, K.; Di Segni, A.; Efroni, G.; Braun, T.; BenShoshan, M.; Anafi, L.; Avivi, C.; Barshack, I.; Shouval, D.S.; et al. Defining the Celiac Disease Transcriptome using Clinical Pathology Specimens Reveals Biologic Pathways and Supports Diagnosis. *Sci. Rep.* **2019**, *9*, 1–10. [CrossRef] [PubMed]

96. Bragde, H.; Jansson, U.; Jarlsfelt, I.; Söderman, J. Gene expression profiling of duodenal biopsies discriminates celiac disease mucosa from normal mucosa. *Pediatr. Res.* **2011**, *69*, 530–537. [CrossRef]

97. Leonard, M.M.; Bai, Y.; Serena, G.; Nickerson, K.P.; Camhi, S.; Sturgeon, C.; Yan, S.; Fiorentino, M.R.; Katz, A.; Nath, B.; et al. RNA sequencing of intestinal mucosa reveals novel pathways functionally linked to celiac disease pathogenesis. *PLoS ONE* **2019**, *14*, 1–19. [CrossRef]

98.   Adriaanse, M.P.M.; Mubarak, A.; Riedl, R.G.; Ten Kate, F.J.W.; Damoiseaux, J.G.M.C.; Buurman, W.A.;
      Houwen, R.H.J.; Vreugdenhil, A.C.E.; Beeren, M.C.G.; Van Dael, C.M.L.; et al. Progress towards non-invasive
      diagnosis and follow-up of celiac disease in children; A prospective multicentre study to the usefulness of
      plasma I-FABP. *Sci. Rep.* **2017**, *7*, 1–10. [CrossRef]
99.   Singh, A.; Verma, A.K.; Das, P.; Prakash, S.; Pramanik, R.; Nayak, B.; Datta Gupta, S.; Sreenivas, V.; Kumar, L.;
      Ahuja, V.; et al. Non-immunological biomarkers for assessment of villous abnormalities in patients with
      celiac disease. *J. Gastroenterol. Hepatol.* **2020**, *35*, 438–445. [CrossRef]
100. Adriaanse, M.P.M.; Leffler, D.A.; Kelly, C.P.; Schuppan, D.; Najarian, R.M.; Goldsmith, J.D.; Buurman, W.A.;
      Vreugdenhil, A.C.E. Serum I-FABP Detects Gluten Responsiveness in Adult Celiac Disease Patients on
      a Short-Term Gluten Challenge. *Am. J. Gastroenterol.* **2016**, *111*, 1014–1022. [CrossRef]
101. Fragkos, K.C.; Forbes, A. Citrulline as a marker of intestinal function and absorption in clinical settings:
      A systematic review and meta-analysis. *United Eur. Gastroenterol. J.* **2018**, *6*, 181–191. [CrossRef] [PubMed]
102. Chretien, M.L.; Bailey, D.G.; Asher, L.; Parfitt, J.; Driman, D.; Gregor, J.; Dresser, G.K. Severity of coeliac disease
      and clinical management study when using a CYP3A4 metabolised medication: A phase i pharmacokinetic
      study. *BMJ Open* **2020**, *10*, 1–7. [CrossRef] [PubMed]
103. Morón, B.; Verma, A.K.; Das, P.; Taavela, J.; Dafik, L.; Diraimondo, T.R.; Albertelli, M.A.; Kraemer, T.;
      Mäki, M.; Khosla, C.; et al. CYP3A4-catalyzed simvastatin metabolism as a non-invasive marker of small
      intestinal health in celiac disease. *Am. J. Gastroenterol.* **2013**, *108*, 1344–1351. [CrossRef] [PubMed]
104. Bragde, H.; Jansson, U.; Fredrikson, M.; Grodzinsky, E.; Söderman, J. Celiac disease biomarkers identified by
      transcriptome analysis of small intestinal biopsies. *Cell. Mol. Life Sci.* **2018**, *75*, 4385–4401. [CrossRef] [PubMed]
105. Lang, C.C.; Brown, R.M.; Kinirons, M.T.; Deathridge, M.A.; Guengerich, F.P.; Kelleher, D.; O'Briain, D.S.;
      Ghishan, F.K.; Wood, A.J.J. Decreased intestinal CYP3A in celiac disease: Reversal after successful gluten-free
      diet: A potential source of interindividual variability in first-pass drug metabolism. *Clin. Pharmacol. Ther.*
      1996, *59*, 41–46. [CrossRef]
106. Heyman, M.; Abed, J.; Lebreton, C.; Cerf-Bensussan, N. Intestinal permeability in coeliac disease: Insight into
      mechanisms and relevance to pathogenesis. *Gut* **2012**, *61*, 1355–1364. [CrossRef]
107. Fasano, A.; Not, T.; Wang, W.; Uzzau, S.; Berti, I.; Tommasini, A.; Goldblum, S.E. Zonulin, a newly discovered
      modulator of intestinal permeability, and its expression in coeliac disease. *Lancet* **2000**, *355*, 1518–1519. [CrossRef]
108. Duerksen, D.R.; Wilhelm-Boyles, C.; Veitch, R.; Kryszak, D.; Parry, D.M. A comparison of antibody testing,
      permeability testing, and zonulin levels with small-bowel biopsy in celiac disease patients on a gluten-free diet.
      Dig. Dis. Sci. **2010**, *55*, 1026–1031. [CrossRef]
109. Kelly, C.P.; Green, P.H.R.; Murray, J.A.; Dimarino, A.; Colatrella, A.; Leffler, D.A.; Alexander, T.; Arsenescu, R.;
      Leon, F.; Jiang, J.G.; et al. Larazotide acetate in patients with coeliac disease undergoing a gluten challenge:
      A randomised placebo-controlled study. *Aliment. Pharmacol. Ther.* **2013**, *37*, 252–262. [CrossRef]
110. Leffler, D.A.; Kelly, C.P.; Green, P.H.R.; Fedorak, R.N.; Dimarino, A.; Perrow, W.; Rasmussen, H.; Wang, C.;
      Bercik, P.; Bachir, N.M.; et al. Larazotide acetate for persistent symptoms of celiac disease despite a gluten-free
      diet: A randomized controlled trial. *Gastroenterology* **2015**, *148*, 1311–1319.e6. [CrossRef]
111. Linsalata, M.; Riezzo, G.; D'Attoma, B.; Clemente, C.; Orlando, A.; Russo, F. Noninvasive biomarkers of gut
      barrier function identify two subtypes of patients suffering from diarrhoea predominant-IBS: A case-control
      study. *BMC Gastroenterol.* **2018**, *18*, 1–14. [CrossRef] [PubMed]
112. Vojdani, A.; Vojdani, E.; Kharrazian, D. Fluctuation of zonulin levels in blood vs stability of antibodies.
      World J. Gastroenterol. **2017**, *23*, 5669–5679. [CrossRef] [PubMed]
113. Ajamian, M.; Steer, D.; Rosella, G.; Gibson, P.R. Serum zonulin as a marker of intestinal mucosal barrier
      function: May not be what it seems. *PLoS ONE* **2019**, *14*, 1–14. [CrossRef] [PubMed]
114. Valitutti, F.; Fasano, A. Breaking Down Barriers: How Understanding Celiac Disease Pathogenesis Informed
      the Development of Novel Treatments. *Dig. Dis. Sci.* **2019**, *64*, 1748–1758. [CrossRef]
115. Leffler, D.; Schuppan, D.; Pallav, K.; Najarian, R.; Goldsmith, J.D.; Hansen, J.; Kabbani, T.; Dennis, M.;
      Kelly, C.P. Kinetics of the histological, serological and symptomatic responses to gluten challenge in adults
      with coeliac disease. *Gut* **2013**, *62*, 996–1004. [CrossRef]
116. Rajani, S.; Huynh, H.Q.; Shirton, L.; Kluthe, C.; Spady, D.; Prosser, C.; Meddings, J.; Rempel, G.R.; Persad, R.;
      Turner, J.M. A Canadian Study toward Changing Local Practice in the Diagnosis of Pediatric Celiac Disease.
      Can. J. Gastroenterol. Hepatol. **2016**, *2016*. [CrossRef]

117. Comino, I.; Fernández-Bañares, F.; Esteve, M.; Ortigosa, L.; Castillejo, G.; Fambuena, B.; Ribes-Koninckx, C.; Sierra, C.; Rodríguez-Herrera, A.; Salazar, J.C.; et al. Fecal Gluten Peptides Reveal Limitations of Serological Tests and Food Questionnaires for Monitoring Gluten-Free Diet in Celiac Disease Patients. *Am. J. Gastroenterol.* **2016**, *111*, 1456–1465. [CrossRef]

118. Moreno, M.D.L.; Cebolla, Á.; Munõz-Suano, A.; Carrillo-Carrion, C.; Comino, I.; Pizarro, Á.; León, F.; Rodríguez-Herrera, A.; Sousa, C. Detection of gluten immunogenic peptides in the urine of patients with coeliac disease reveals transgressions in the gluten-free diet and incomplete mucosal healing. *Gut* **2017**, *66*, 250–257. [CrossRef]

119. Gerasimidis, K.; Zafeiropoulou, K.; Mackinder, M.; Ijaz, U.Z.; Duncan, H.; Buchanan, E.; Cardigan, T.; Edwards, C.A.; McGrogan, P.; Russell, R.K. Comparison of clinical methods with the faecal gluten immunogenic peptide to assess gluten intake in coeliac disease. *J. Pediatr. Gastroenterol. Nutr.* **2018**, *67*, 356–360. [CrossRef]

120. Stefanolo, J.P.; Tálamo, M.; Dodds, S.; de la Paz Temprano, M.; Costa, A.F.; Moreno, M.L.; Pinto-Sánchez, M.I.; Smecuol, E.; Vázquez, H.; Gonzalez, A.; et al. Real-World Gluten Exposure in Patients With Celiac Disease on Gluten-Free Diets, Determined From Gliadin Immunogenic Peptides in Urine and Fecal Samples. *Clin. Gastroenterol. Hepatol.* **2020**. [CrossRef]

121. Lindfors, K.; Koskinen, O.; Laurila, K.; Collin, P.; Saavalainen, P.; Haimila, K.; Partanen, J.; Mäki, M.; Kaukinen, K. IgA-class autoantibodies against neuronal transglutaminase, TG6 in celiac disease: No evidence for gluten dependency. *Clin. Chim. Acta* **2011**, *412*, 1187–1190. [CrossRef] [PubMed]

122. Hadjivassiliou, M.; Aeschlimann, P.; Sanders, D.S.; Mäki, M.; Kaukinen, K.; Grünewald, R.A.; Bandmann, O.; Woodroofe, N.; Haddock, G.; Aeschlimann, D.P. Transglutaminase 6 antibodies in the diagnosis of gluten ataxia. *Neurology* **2013**, *80*, 1740–1745. [CrossRef] [PubMed]

123. Borroni, G.; Biagi, F.; Ciocca, O.; Vassallo, C.; Carugno, A.; Cananzi, R.; Campanella, J.; Bianchi, P.I.; Brazzelli, V.; Corazza, G.R. IgA anti-epidermal transglutaminase autoantibodies: A sensible and sensitive marker for diagnosis of dermatitis herpetiformis in adult patients. *J. Eur. Acad. Dermatology Venereol.* **2013**, *27*, 836–841. [CrossRef] [PubMed]

124. Sárdy, M.; Kárpáti, S.; Merkl, B.; Paulsson, M.; Smyth, N. Epidermal transglutaminase (TGase 3) is the autoantigen of dermatitis herpetiformis. *J. Exp. Med.* **2002**, *195*, 747–757. [CrossRef] [PubMed]

125. Taavela, J.; Viiri, K.; Popp, A.; Oittinen, M.; Dotsenko, V.; Peräaho, M.; Staff, S.; Sarin, J.; Leon, F.; Mäki, M.; et al. Histological, immunohistochemical and mRNA gene expression responses in coeliac disease patients challenged with gluten using PAXgene fixed paraffin-embedded duodenal biopsies. *BMC Gastroenterol.* **2019**, *19*, 1–10. [CrossRef] [PubMed]

126. Dotsenko, V.; Oittinen, M.; Taavela, J.; Popp, A.; Peräaho, M.; Staff, S.; Sarin, J.; Leon, F.; Isola, J.; Mäki, M.; et al. Genome-Wide Transcriptomic Analysis of Intestinal Mucosa in Celiac Disease Patients on a Gluten-Free Diet and Postgluten Challenge. *Cell. Mol. Gastroenterol. Hepatol.* **2020**. [CrossRef]

127. Mohamed, B.M.; Feighery, C.; Coates, C.; O'Shea, U.; Delaney, D.; O'Briain, S.; Kelly, J.; Abuzakouk, M. The absence of a mucosal lesion on standard histological examination does not exclude diagnosis of celiac disease. *Dig. Dis. Sci.* **2008**, *53*, 52–61. [CrossRef]

128. Misselwitz, B.; Butter, M.; Verbeke, K.; Fox, M.R. Update on lactose malabsorption and intolerance: Pathogenesis, diagnosis and clinical management. *Gut* **2019**, *68*, 2080–2091. [CrossRef]

129. Ojetti, V.; Gabrielli, M.; Migneco, A.; Lauritano, C.; Zocco, M.A.; Scarpellini, E.; Nista, E.C.; Gasbarrini, G.; Gasbarrini, A. Regression of lactose malabsorption in coeliac patients after receiving a gluten-free diet. *Scand. J. Gastroenterol.* **2008**, *43*, 174–177. [CrossRef]

130. Lamb, C.A.; Kennedy, N.A.; Raine, T.; Hendy, P.A.; Smith, P.J.; Limdi, J.K.; Hayee, B.; Lomer, M.C.E.; Parkes, G.C.; Selinger, C.; et al. British Society of Gastroenterology consensus guidelines on the management of inflammatory bowel disease in adults. *Gut* **2019**, *68*, s1–s106. [CrossRef]

131. Thorsvik, S.; Damås, J.K.; Granlund, A.B.; Flo, T.H.; Bergh, K.; Østvik, A.E.; Sandvik, A.K. Fecal neutrophil gelatinase-associated lipocalin as a biomarker for inflammatory bowel disease. *J. Gastroenterol. Hepatol.* **2017**, *32*, 128–135. [CrossRef] [PubMed]

132. Buisson, A.; Vazeille, E.; Minet-Quinard, R.; Goutte, M.; Bouvier, D.; Goutorbe, F.; Pereira, B.; Barnich, N.; Bommelaer, G. Fecal Matrix Metalloprotease-9 and Lipocalin-2 as Biomarkers in Detecting Endoscopic Activity in Patients with Inflammatory Bowel Diseases. *J. Clin. Gastroenterol.* **2018**, *52*, e53–e62. [CrossRef] [PubMed]

133. Ornatsky, O.; Bandura, D.; Baranov, V.; Nitz, M.; Winnik, M.A.; Tanner, S. Highly multiparametric analysis by mass cytometry. *J. Immunol. Methods* **2010**, *361*, 1–20. [CrossRef] [PubMed]
134. Van Unen, V.; Li, N.; Molendijk, I.; Temurhan, M.; Höllt, T.; van der Meulen-de Jong, A.E.; Verspaget, H.W.; Mearin, M.L.; Mulder, C.J.; van Bergen, J.; et al. Mass Cytometry of the Human Mucosal Immune System Identifies Tissue- and Disease-Associated Immune Subsets. *Immunity* **2016**, *44*, 1227–1239. [CrossRef]
135. Svensson, V.; Vento-Tormo, R.; Teichmann, S.A. Exponential scaling of single-cell RNA-seq in the past decade. *Nat. Protoc.* **2018**, *13*, 599–604. [CrossRef]
136. Atlasy, N.; Bujko, A.; Brazda, P.; Janssen-Megens, E.; Bækkevold, E.; Jahnsen, J.; Jahnsen, F.; Stunnenberg, H. Single cell transcriptome atlas of immune cells in human small intestine and in celiac disease. *bioRxiv Prepr.* **2019**, 6–8. [CrossRef]
137. Stoeckius, M.; Hafemeister, C.; Stephenson, W.; Houck-Loomis, B.; Chattopadhyay, P.K.; Swerdlow, H.; Satija, R.; Smibert, P. Simultaneous epitope and transcriptome measurement in single cells. *Nat. Methods* **2017**, *14*, 865–868. [CrossRef]
138. Reyes, M.; Billman, K.; Hacohen, N.; Blainey, P.C. Simultaneous Profiling of Gene Expression and Chromatin Accessibility in Single Cells. *Adv. Biosyst.* **2019**, *3*. [CrossRef]
139. Satija, R.; Farrell, J.A.; Gennert, D.; Schier, A.F.; Regev, A. Spatial reconstruction of single-cell gene expression data. *Nat. Biotechnol.* **2015**, *33*, 495–502. [CrossRef]
140. Achim, K.; Pettit, J.B.; Saraiva, L.R.; Gavriouchkina, D.; Larsson, T.; Arendt, D.; Marioni, J.C. High-throughput spatial mapping of single-cell RNA-seq data to tissue of origin. *Nat. Biotechnol.* **2015**, *33*, 503–509. [CrossRef]
141. Chang, Q.; Ornatsky, O.I.; Siddiqui, I.; Loboda, A.; Baranov, V.I.; Hedley, D.W. Imaging Mass Cytometry. *Cytom. Part A* **2017**, *91*, 160–169. [CrossRef] [PubMed]

4

Psychiatric Comorbidity in Children and Adults with Gluten-Related Disorders

Mahmoud Slim [1], Fernando Rico-Villademoros [2] and Elena P. Calandre [2,*]

[1] Division of Neurology, The Hospital for Sick Children, The Peter Gilgan Centre for Research and Learning, 686 Bay St., Toronto, ON M5G 0A4, Canada; mahmoud.slim@gmail.com
[2] Instituto de Neurociencias, Universidad de Granada, Avenida del Conocimiento s/n, 18100 Armilla, Granada, Spain; fernando.ricovillademoros@gmail.com
* Correspondence: calandre@gmail.com

Abstract: Gluten-related disorders are characterized by both intestinal and extraintestinal manifestations. Previous studies have suggested an association between gluten-related disorder and psychiatric comorbidities. The objective of our current review is to provide a comprehensive review of this association in children and adults. A systematic literature search using MEDLINE, Embase and PsycINFO from inception to 2018 using terms of 'celiac disease' or 'gluten-sensitivity-related disorders' combined with terms of 'mental disorders' was conducted. A total of 47 articles were included in our review, of which 28 studies were conducted in adults, 11 studies in children and eight studies included both children and adults. The majority of studies were conducted in celiac disease, two studies in non-celiac gluten sensitivity and none in wheat allergy. Enough evidence is currently available supporting the association of celiac disease with depression and, to a lesser extent, with eating disorders. Further investigation is warranted to evaluate the association suggested with other psychiatric disorders. In conclusion, routine surveillance of potential psychiatric manifestations in children and adults with gluten-related disorders should be carried out by the attending physician.

Keywords: celiac disease; non-celiac gluten sensitivity; psychiatric disorders; depression; anxiety disorders; eating disorders; ADHD; autism; psychosis

1. Introduction

Gluten-related disorders include three pathologies caused by the ingestion of gluten-containing cereals grains, namely celiac disease (CD), non-celiac gluten sensitivity (NCGS) and wheat allergy (WA) [1]. Although all of them are due to the toxicity of gluten proteins in the sensitive subject, their respective pathogenetic mechanisms differ.

Celiac disease is a systemic autoimmune disease due to a permanent intolerance to gluten which causes villous atrophy of the intestinal mucosa. It involves both innate and adaptive immune responses that appear in genetically predisposed subjects exposed to gluten and, unlike food allergies, it is not mediated by an immediate hypersensitivity reaction. It is a polygenic multifactorial disorder whose development depends on the genetic constitution of the subject, on his/her exposure to gluten intake, and on different environmental factors [2,3]. To date, the only effective treatment for the disease is to observe a life-long strict gluten-free diet although other therapeutic approaches are being explored [4].

In relation to the genetic background of the disease, two HLA class II genes, the HLA-DQ2 and the HLA-DQ8 heterodimers are present in almost all CD patients and their simultaneous absence in a subject usually rules out a diagnosis of CD. However, these genes are also common in the general population and the implication of other non-HLA genes is being investigated by genome wide association studies [5]. Environmental factors that facilitate or, conversely, protect against the development of CD are defectively known although they are considered important given that the genetic background is not enough to explain the increasing incidence and prevalence of CD [2]. Infant feeding practices such as the timing of the first gluten introduction in the diet and the presumed protective role of maternal breastfeeding that were once considered important, have been recently shown to be irrelevant in relation to the development of CD [6]. In contrast, gastrointestinal infections and antibiotics use during the first year of life seem to be associated with a higher risk of developing CD [7]; these latter factors could be related with the composition of gut microbiota that seems to be different between children with and without CD [8].

As both the two most relevant genes associated with the development of CD as well as the consumption gluten-containing foods are fairly prevalent in most of the world, it is not surprising that there is high worldwide prevalence of CD [9]. The global worldwide prevalence of CD has been shown to be higher when diagnosed only by serological tests, i.e., anti-tissue transglutaminase and/or antiendomysial antibodies (1.4%, 95% confidence interval [CI] 1.1–1.7%) than when diagnosed with intestinal biopsy (0.7%, 95% CI 0.5–0.9%) [10]. Some striking differences have been found among different geographic areas; differences that are probably due to different genetic haplotypes, different patterns of gluten-containing foods intake, and environmental differences. CD has been found to be more frequent in females than in males and in children than in adults [10]. A fact worthy of mention is that the CD prevalence has been increasing during the last decades [2,10]. This increase must be partially attributed to an augmented awareness about the disease and more accurate diagnosis, but environmental factors are also responsible for being the most relevant the increase to gluten exposure in countries where nutrition traditionally relied on the intake of gluten-free grains such as rice or corn [3].

The clinical manifestations of CD can be both gastrointestinal and extraintestinal. Gastrointestinal symptoms include diarrhea, steatorrhea, abdominal pain, abdominal bloating, vomiting and failure to thrive due to the malabsorption process. This kind of symptomatology is more frequent in children and was formerly called "typical CD", a term that has currently been replaced by "classic" CD [3]. Among the extraintestinal manifestations, some of them such as ferropenic anemia, osteopenia and osteoporosis, short stature or dental enamel hypoplasia, are a consequence of the intestinal malabsorption process. Others, however, seem to be due to the noxious effect of gluten in the affected organs; dermatitis herpetiformis, gluten ataxia, gluten encephalopathy, epileptic seizures or elevation of liver enzymes are examples of the latter. Extraintestinal symptoms, which are more frequently found among adolescents and adults, were initially known as "atypical" CD, a term that has now been replaced by "symptomatic" CD [3].

CD is frequently comorbid with mainly other autoimmune disorders, although non-exclusively, type1 diabetes, Graves' disease and inflammatory bowel diseases [11,12]. It has also been found to be associated with a higher risk of non-Hodgkin lymphoma [13,14] and with Down [15,16] and Turner syndromes [15,17].

Unlike CD, NCGS has not been shown to be associated with underlying autoimmune mechanisms. Similar to patients with CD, subjects that experience NCGS may, after gluten intake, suffer a wide variety of intestinal and/or extraintestinal symptoms that improve after following a gluten-free diet. Contrarily to CD, the presence of anti-tissue transglutaminase and/or antiendomysial antibodies is always negative, the HLA-DQ2/HLA-DQ8 combination in these patients is only slightly more frequent than in the general population, and there is no atrophy of the small intestine mucosa although a rise in intraepithelial intestinal lymphocytes has been observed [18]. Its prevalence is not yet well-known although it does not seem to be an uncommon disease [19]. The pathogenetic mechanisms of NCGS are, at present, poorly understood. Patients with NCGS benefit from a gluten-free diet but they have been also shown to improve following a low FODMAPs (fermentable, oligo-, di-, monosaccharides and polyols) diet, a fact that suggests that other constituents of grains may be responsible for the symptoms of the disease [20].

Wheat allergy is an IgE-mediated reaction to the proteins contained in wheat and in particular, although not exclusively, the omega-5-gliadin. WA can be developed by inhalation of wheat flour, the so-called baker's asthma and baker's rhinitis which are considered occupational diseases, or by wheat ingestion [21]. The latter case, which is the most frequent, may cause urticaria, angioedema and/or gastrointestinal symptoms such as nausea, vomiting, abdominal bloating, abdominal pain and diarrhea; in the most severe cases it can induce systemic anaphylaxis [18]. WA is especially frequent in children, being less commonly seen in adolescents and adults. The treatment is based on the avoidance of wheat-containing foods, being less restrictive compared to gluten-free diet in CD, as it does not require the restriction of rye and barley-containing foods [22].

Psychiatric disturbances have frequently been reported in patients with CD. Several narrative reviews of the literature undertaken in the last five years indicate that CD could be associated with a wide spectrum of psychiatric disorders, including anxiety disorders, dysthymia, major depression, bipolar disorders, schizophrenia, eating disorders, autism spectrum disorders, and attention-deficit hyperactive disorders [23–27]. However, these otherwise important reviews have several limitations. Several of them were focused on specific psychiatric disorders such as anxiety and depression [24], mood disorders and schizophrenia [25], or severe psychiatric disorders [27]. Some others, according to their objectives comprised the whole spectrum of psychiatric disorders, but they do not specify their search strategies and/or the biomedical literature database used for the review [23,26]. Finally, when specified, literature searches were almost restricted to PubMed, thus providing a limited review of the literature on this topic. Moreover, none of the previous have evaluated the association of psychiatric disorders in children and adults with gluten-related disorders separately. The aim of this manuscript is presenting a comprehensive review of the literature on the potential association of gluten-related disorders with the whole spectrum of psychiatric disorders using the most common literature databases for this kind of evaluation (namely, Medline, EMBASE and PyscINFO).

2. Methodology

2.1. Search Strategy

We searched the medical literature for published studies indexed in the Medline (1966 to January 2018), EMBASE (1947 to January 2018), and PsycINFO (1967 to January 2018). The search strategy included terms of 'celiac disease' or 'gluten-sensitivity related disorders' combined with terms of 'mental disorders' as described in Supplementary Table S1. No limits or restrictions were applied. Retrieved references were pooled and managed using EndNote X8 (Clarivate Analytics, Philadelphia, PA, USA).

2.2. Inclusion Criteria

We included studies that investigated the prevalence, incidence or the likelihood of presenting mental or psychiatric disorders in patients with CD or gluten-sensitivity related disorders. For that purpose, comparative observational or interventional studies, including meta-analysis, assessing the aforementioned objectives as part of their primary or secondary objectives were included. Only studies published in English, Spanish, French, Portuguese, or Italian were included. Case-reports, case-series, abstracts and editorials were excluded. The relationship between CD and psychiatric disorders may be bidirectional. Our purpose was to assess the comorbidity between gluten-related disorders and psychiatric manifestations; thus, those studies assessing the prevalence, incidence or likelihood of presenting CD or gluten-related disorders in patients with diagnosed psychiatric disorders were excluded.

Study eligibility was independently evaluated by the three investigators (MS, EPC, FRV). Discrepancies in the evaluation were resolved by consensus among study investigators.

2.3. Data Extraction

Standardized data collection forms were used to extract data that included: (1) name of the first author; (2) year of publication; (3) country where the study was conducted; (4) study objective(s);

(5) study design; (6) assessment tools used in psychiatric comorbidities evaluation; (7) Disease diagnostic criteria; (8) sample size and demographic characteristics; and (9) summary of outcomes. Data extraction was independently completed by two investigators (MS and FRV). Discrepancies in data extraction were solved by consensus.

3. Results

3.1. Study Selection

Our systematic search strategy identified 1375 potentially relevant articles (730 articles from EMBASE, 453 articles from MEDLINE and 192 articles from PsycINFO). After removing 461 duplicate articles, 914 articles underwent title and abstract screening. Seven hundred and eighty-eight articles were excluded as they were case-reports, editorials, animal studies, basic science studies, did not include comparator group, or were published in a language other than those specified in the inclusion criteria, leaving 126 articles for a full-text screening. Two studies were excluded because we were unable to obtain their full text [28,29]. A total of 77 were excluded following full-text review because they were either published in abstract form, did not meet the specific objectives set for our current review or did not report outcomes of interest, leaving a total of 47 articles that were included in our review, of which 28 studies were conducted in the adult population, 11 studies were conducted in the pediatric population and eight studies included both adults and children. Mixed studies (including children and adults, $n = 8$) were classified under the corresponding population group with a larger sample size (pediatrics ($n = 4$), adults ($n = 4$)) (Figure 1).

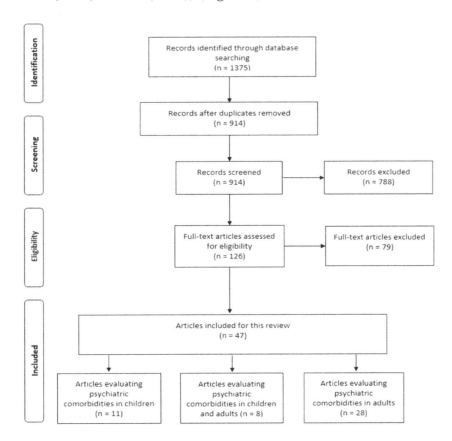

Figure 1. PRISMA flow chart.

3.2. Studies Conducted in Children with CD

We found 15 studies that evaluated psychiatric disorders in children or young adults with CD, 11 of which were conducted in clinical-based settings and four were conducted in community-based settings (Table 1). Studies were published between 1997 and 2018 [30–44]. Most studies ($n = 12$) were cross-sectional, although one of them included a subsequent longitudinal phase [41]. Three studies used a population-based cohort design and were conducted in Sweden using the same data source for patients with CD [31,34,44]. Finally, one study used a cohort design [38]. With the exception of this later study which was conducted in several countries [38], the remaining studies were conducted in European countries or Turkey.

According to a population-based cohort study, children with CD have a 70% increased likelihood of presenting a psychiatric disorder with intellectual disability being the most likely disorder (HR 1.7, 95% CI 1.4 to 2.1) [44]. A summary of results of studies evaluating the association between CD and the occurrence or presence of psychiatric disorders is presented in Table 2. Regarding specific conditions, cohort studies have shown that CD is associated with an increased likelihood of occurrence of depression (HR = 1.8, 95% CI 1.6 to 2.2) [34] or mood disorders (HR 1.2, 95% CI 1.0–1.4) [44], although this latter result did not reach statistical significance. In contrast, most cross-sectional studies have found that the point prevalence of depression or the severity of depressive symptoms did not differ in children with CD as compared with controls [33,35–37]. Pynnonen et al. [32], using a cross sectional study, found no differences between patients with CD and controls in the point prevalence of major depressive disorder, but the lifetime prevalence of major depressive disorder was significantly increased in patients with CD (31% vs. 7%; OR = 6.06, 95% CI 1.18–31.23). Although a population-based study found an increased likelihood of occurrence of anxiety disorder in patients with CD as compared with controls (HR 1.2, 95% CI 1.0 to 1.4, $p < 0.05$) [44], cross-sectional studies have not shown differences between patients with CD and controls in the prevalence or severity of symptom of anxiety [32,35,36]. In children, no association has been found between CD and the occurrence of bipolar disorder [34].

The association of CD with psychotic disorders in children has been scarcely investigated, showing no association with the occurrence of schizophrenia [31] or psychotic disorder [44]; an association has been reported between CD and non-schizophrenic non-affective psychosis (HR 1.61, 95% CI 1.19–2.20) [31].

A population-based study found a significant association between CD and the occurrence of an eating disorder (HR 1.4, 95% CI 1.1 to 1.8) [44], and the presence of the disorder seems to have a negative impact on some dimensions of quality of life (namely, ill-being and joy-in-life) [39]. A population-based cohort found an excess likelihood of occurrence of an autism spectrum disorder in patients with CD as compared to controls [44]; however, a cross-sectional study did not find an association between both disorders [30]. A slight, but significant, increase in the likelihood of occurrence of attention deficit and hyperactive disorder (ADHD) in patients with CD has been reported [44].

Several factors have been suggested to contribute to depressive symptomatology in the pediatric population including the presence of parental depressive disorders, low parental educational level, divorce of the parents, presence of functional comorbid conditions and female gender [32,33,43]. Older age, higher body mass index and history of dietary restrictions were linked to higher risk of eating disorders [39,40].

3.3. Studies Conducted in Adults with CD

We found 32 studies that evaluated psychiatric comorbidities in adult patients with CD or NCGS, 18 of which were conducted in clinical-based settings and nine were conducted in community-based settings (Table 3). Studies were published between 1982 and 2018 [45–76]. More than half of these studies were of cross-sectional design [45,48,51,53–57,59,60,63,67,68,71,72,74–76] and four of them were representative of the general population [47,70,73,76].

Table 1. Objectives and design of studies evaluating the association between gluten-related disorders and psychiatric disorders in children and young adults.

Author (Year)	Country	Primary Objective	Design ‡	Study Setting	Psychiatric Comorbidity Assessment	Celiac Disease Diagnostic Criteria
Autism spectrum disorders						
Pavone (1997) [30]	Italy	To evaluate behavioral problems and autistic features in children with CD	Cross-sectional	Clinical	DSM-III-R	Biopsy
Schizophrenia Spectrum						
Ludvigsson (2007) * [31]	Sweden	To determine the risk of non-affective psychosis in patients with CD in a national general population cohort	Population-based cohort	Community	ICD	ICD
Bipolar, depressive and anxiety disorders						
Pynnonen (2004) [32]	Finland	To compare the prevalence of current and lifetime mental disorders in adolescents with CD and controls	Cross-sectional	Clinical	K-SADS-PL Youth Self-Report BDI and BAI HDRS and HARS	Biopsy
Accomando (2005) * [33]	Italy	To investigate the relationship between CD and depression	Cross-sectional	Clinical	CDQ (adults) CDS (children)	NR
Ludvigsson (2007) * [34]	Sweden	To investigate the risk of subsequent depression and bipolar in patients with CD	Population-based cohort	Community	ICD	NR
Fidan (2013) [35]	Turkey	To investigate the depression and anxiety levels of children and adolescents with celiac disease and the impact of these on quality of life	Cross-sectional	Clinical	CDI STAIC	NR
Esenyel (2014) [36]	Turkey	To explore the diet compliance and depression and anxiety levels of pediatric celiac children and their families after a GFD	Cross-sectional	Clinical	CDI SCARED	ESPGHAN criteria
Simsek (2015) [37]	Turkey	To evaluate depressive symptoms at time of CD diagnosis and 6 months following GFD initiation	Phase 1: Cross-sectional Phase 2: Case-series	Clinical	CDI HRQOL (Kid-KINDL)	Biopsy
Smith (2017) [38]	USA, Finland, Germany, and Sweden	To assess mother's report of psychological functioning in children with CDA	Cohort	Community	CBCL	Serology and optional biopsy
Feeding and eating disorders						
Wagner (2015) [39]	Austria	To assess the determinants of eating disorders in female adolescents with CD	Cross-sectional	Clinical	EDI-2 EDE DSM-IV for subclinical eating disorders CDI (total score ≥ 18)	Both
Babio (2018) * [40]	Spain	To assess the risk of eating disorders in individuals between 10 and 23 years old diagnosed with CD	Cross-sectional	Clinical	CEAT EAT-26 SCFF BITE BSQ	Both

Table 1. *Cont.*

Author (Year)	Country	Primary Objective	Design ‡	Study Setting	Psychiatric Comorbidity Assessment	Celiac Disease Diagnostic Criteria
Overall psychological status						
Terrone (2013) [41]	Italy	To screen for neurological and behavioral disorders in children with CD	Phase 1: cross-sectional Phase 2: cohort	Clinical	PSC (total score $\geq$ 28)	ESPGHAN criteria
Various psychiatric conditions						
Ruggieri (2008) [42]	Italy	To determine the prevalence of neurologic symptoms in children with gluten sensitivity enteropathy	Cross-sectional	Clinical	NR	Both
Mazzone (2011) [43]	Italy	To identify psychological features in children with CD following strict GFD	Cross-sectional	Clinical	MASC CBCL CDI DSM-IV-TR criteria to assess autistic disorders	ESPGHAN criteria
Butwicka (2017) [44]	Sweden	To examine the risk of psychiatric disorders in children with a biopsy-verified diagnosis of CD and to examine the prevalence of psychiatric disorders before CD is diagnosed in children	Population-based cohort	Community	ICD	Biopsy

* Included patients of all age groups (pediatrics and adults); ‡ The design was determined by the authors of the current review which might not coincide with the design described in the original studies; for studies including multiple methodologies, the design that achieved the objectives of interest was selected; BAI: Beck Anxiety Inventory; BDI: Beck Depression Inventory; BITE: Bulimia Investigatory Test Edinburgh; BSQ: Body Shape Questionnaire; CBCL: Achenbach Child Behavior Checklist; CD: celiac disease; CDA: celiac disease autoimmunity; CDI: Child Depression Inventory; CDQ: Clinical Depression Questionnaire; CDS: Children Depression Scale; CEAT: Children Eating Attitudes Test; DSM: Diagnostic and Statistical Manual of Mental Disorders; EAT: Eating Attitudes Test; EDE: Eating Disorder Examination; EDI: Eating Disorder Inventory; ESPGHAN: The European Society for Pediatric Gastroenterology, Hepatology, and Nutrition; GFD: gluten-free diet; HARS: Hamilton Anxiety Rating Scale; HDRS: Hamilton Depression Rating Scale; HRQOL: Health-Related Quality of Life; ICD: International Classification of Disease; KINDL: German questionnaire for measuring quality of life in children and adolescents; K-SADS-PL: Schedule for Affective Disorders and Schizophrenia for school-Age Children-Present and Lifetime version; MASC: Multidimensional Anxiety Scale for Children; NR: not reported; PSC: Pediatric Symptom Checklist; SCARED: Childhood Anxiety Disorders Screening Measure; SCFF: Sick Control Fat Food;STAIC: State-Trait Anxiety Inventory for Children.

Table 2. Summary of outcomes evaluating the association between gluten-related disorders and psychiatric disorders in children and young adults.

Author (Year)	Design	Sample Size and Demographic Characteristics	Summary of Outcomes	Associated Factors with Psychiatric Comorbidities and Other Relevant Information
Autism spectrum disorders				
Pavone (1997) [30]	Cross-sectional	CD, n = 120 (mean age 9.6 years, 48% females) Recently-diagnosed CD, n = 27 CD on strict GFD, n = 70 GFD non-adherent CD, n = 23 Controls, n = 20 (mean age 9.6 years, 48% females)	- Autism diagnosis: none of the recently-diagnosed CD - Language delay: Two subjects in GFD-compliant, one subject in the non-adherent group - Differences were not statistically significant compared to controls	NR
Schizophrenia Spectrum				
Ludvigsson (2007) [31]	Population-based cohort study	CD, n = 14,003 (age at diagnosis, 0–15 years 66% & ≥16 years 34%, 59% females) Controls, n = 68,125 (matched age and gender)	- Likelihood of psychosis in CD vs. controls using a Cox regression model stratified for gender, age, year of study entry and county: Any non-affective psychosis (schizophrenia and other psychoses) HR = 1.55 (95% CI: 1.16–2.06) Non-schizophrenic non-affective psychosis HR = 1.61 (95% CI: 1.19–2.20) Schizophrenia HR = 1.43 (95% CI: 0.77–2.67)	NR
Bipolar, depressive and anxiety disorders				
Pynnonen (2004) [32]	Cross-sectional	CD, n = 29 (mean age 14.2 years, 55% females) Controls, n = 29 (mean age 14.4 years, 55% females)	- Lifetime prevalence of major depression disorder (CD vs. controls): 31% vs. 7%, p <0.05. OR = 6.06 (95% CI: 1.18–31.23). - Disruptive behavior disorders (CD vs. controls): 28% vs. 3%, p <0.05. OR = 10.67 (95% CI: 1.24–92). - Lifetime prevalence of anxiety disorders (CD vs. controls): 21% vs. 24%, p = NS - Differences in the prevalence of current depressive, anxiety, or disruptive behavior disorders between the two groups were non-significant	- History of parental depressive disorder was more common in CD patients with depressive symptomatology compared to CD without depressive symptomatology - Parental educational level, divorce of parents, poor weight or height gain, and somatic symptoms were not associated with mental disorders
Accomando (2005) [33]	Cross-sectional	CD, n = 42 (17 adults and 25 children) HC, n = 42	Prevalence of depression (CD vs. HC): 26.2% vs. 30.9%, p = NS	- Females predominated in CD patients with depression (not reaching statistical significance) - Depression was more common in CD with functional comorbid conditions (specific conditions not specified)
Ludvigsson (2007) [34]	Population-based cohort study	CD, n = 13,776 (median age at diagnosis 2 years, 58.6% females) Controls, n = 66,815 (median age at diagnosis 2 years, 58.7% females)	- CD was associated with an increased risk of subsequent depression (HR = 1.8, 95% CI: 1.6–2.2) - No significant association between CD and bipolar disorder was reported (HR = 1.1, 95% CI: 0.7–1.7)	- Socioeconomic index didn't have any confounding effect on the later schizophrenia diagnosis in CD
Fidan (2013) [35]	Cross-sectional	CD, n =30 (mean age 12.4 ± 3.1 years, 57% females). HC, n = 30 (mean age NR, 57% females)	- CD vs. HC: CDI: 10.8 ± 7.4 vs. 8.8 ± 6.8, p=0.28 STAIC-State Anxiety: 34.6 ± 6.1 vs. 32.8 ± 7.2, p = 0.30 STAIC-Trait Anxiety: 33.7 ± 6.5 vs. 33 ± 6.3, p =0.64	- Data on the impact of depression and anxiety on HRQOL NR

Table 2. *Cont.*

Author (Year)	Design	Sample Size and Demographic Characteristics	Summary of Outcomes	Associated Factors with Psychiatric Comorbidities and Other Relevant Information
Esenyel (2014) [36]	Cross-sectional	CD, $n = 30$ (mean age 11.9 ± 2 years, 70% females) HC, $n =20$ (mean age 12 ± 2 years, 55% females)	- CD vs. HC: CDI points: 8.73 ± 5.51 vs. 8.3 ± 4.02, $p = 0.921$ SCARED points: 24.5 ± 14.41 vs. 17.85 ± 9.12, $p = 0.120$ - There were no differences in depression and anxiety scores between patients with CD compliant or non-compliant with a GFD	NR
Simsek (2015) [37]	Phase 1: Cross-sectional Phase 2: Case-series	CD, $n = 25$ (mean age 11.8 years, 72% females) Controls, $n = 25$ (mean age 12.2 years, 64%)	- At the time of diagnosis (CD vs. controls): CDI scores: 9 vs. 6, p = NS - 6 months following GFD initiation: CDI scores in CD: 9 before diet vs. 9.5 after diet, p = NS	- Total scores of HRQOL were significantly lower in CD patients ($p <0.05$)
Smith (2017) [38]	Cohort	Aware-CDA, $n = 440$ (58% females) Unware-CDA, $n = 66$ (50% females) No CDA, $n = 3651$ (NR)	- At 3.5 years of age, unaware-CDA mothers reported more anxious/depressed symptoms, aggressive behavior, and externalizing composite score compared to aware-CDA group ($p <0.05$) or without CDA ($p <0.05$) - At 3.5 years of age, Aware-CDA mothers reported significantly fewer problems on the anxious/depressed subscale compared to No CDA group ($p = 0.03$) - At 4.5 years, there were no significant differences	NR

Feeding and eating disorders

Author (Year)	Design	Sample Size and Demographic Characteristics	Summary of Outcomes	Associated Factors with Psychiatric Comorbidities and Other Relevant Information
Wagner (2015) [39]	Cross-sectional	CD, $n = 206$ (mean age NR) CD with ED, $n = 32$ (mean age 16.4 yeas) CD without ED, $n = 174$ (mean age 14.5 years) Controls, $n = 53$ (mean age 14.7 years)	- Lifetime prevalence of EDs: 5.3% of girls with CD: anorexia nervosa ($n = 1$), bulimia nervosa ($n = 4$), and EDs not otherwise specified ($n = 6$); 3.9% suffered from current ED - Criteria for lifetime subclinical EDs: 21 girls (10.2%) with CD - Higher BMI and self-directedness were predictors of greater risk of ED - Higher BMI and lower joy in life were reported by patients with CD with ED compared with patients without EDs, even when controlling for age and depression levels	- No differences between patients (with CD) with and without EDs in coping strategies were found - Higher BMI and lower self-directedness were linked to higher risk of ED in CD
Babio (2018) [40]	Cross-sectional	CD, $n = 98$ (mean age 15 years, 60% females) Controls, $n = 98$ (mean age 15 years, 60% females)	- No significant differences in the median scores of the screening tools for EDs between CD and HC - CD vs. HC: β coefficient = 2.15 (1.04); $p = 0.04$ in a multiple linear regression model for EAT after adjusting for several factors	- Only significant results for one out of the 4 models (one for each screening test) - Age > 13 years old was positively associated with an increase in the score on the EAT

Overall psychological status

Author (Year)	Design	Sample Size and Demographic Characteristics	Summary of Outcomes	Associated Factors with Psychiatric Comorbidities and Other Relevant Information
Terrone (2013) [41]	Phase 1: cross-sectional Phase 2: cohort	CD, $n = 139$ (mean age 10 years, 64.7% females): Group A ($n =40$): newly diagnosed CD Group B ($n = 54$): CD in remission on GFD > 1 year Group C ($n = 45$): potential CD	- Comparison of mean PSC scores using ANOVA: Group A, 14.8 ± 4.2 (one pathological score) vs. Group B, 12.3 ± 6.4 (one pathological score) vs. Group C, 7.6 ± 6 ($p <0.0001$)	NR

Table 2. *Cont.*

Author (Year)	Design	Sample Size and Demographic Characteristics	Summary of Outcomes	Associated Factors with Psychiatric Comorbidities and Other Relevant Information
Various psychiatric conditions				
Ruggieri (2008) [42]	Cross-sectional	GS, n = 835 (demographic characteristics NR) Controls, n = 300 (demographic characteristics NR)	- 3 out of 835 children had bipolar disorders - None of the controls had psychiatric disorders	NR
Mazzone (2011) [43]	Cross-sectional	CD, n = 100 (mean age 10.4 years, 65% females) HC, n = 100 (mean age 11.5 years, 58% females)	- MASC scores: CD children showed significantly higher scores (50 ± 8.3 vs. 42.9 ± 6.6, p <0.01) - CDI scores: CD children showed significantly higher scores (8.1 ± 5.7 vs. 5.6 ± 3.4, p <0.01) - No significant differences were found in CBCL analysis - Two children in the CD group were classified within the spectrum of autistic disorders	- CD males showed significantly higher scores for total CBCL - CD females showed an increased rate of anxiety and depression symptoms, as indicated by significantly higher MASC and CDI scores
Butwicka (2017) [44]	Population-based cohort study	CD, n = 10,903 (median age 3 years, 62% females) Controls, n = 1,042,072 (age NR but matched, 61% females)	- HRs from a Multivariate Cox regression adjusted for maternal/paternal age at child's birth, maternal/paternal country of birth, level of education of higher-educated parent, gestational age, birth weight, birth cohort, Apgar score, and history of psychiatric disorders before recruitment: Any psychiatric disorder 1.4 (95% CI: 1.3–1.4) Psychotic disorders 1.9 (95% CI: 1.0–3.5) Mood disorders 1.2 (95% CI: 1.0–1.4) Anxiety disorders 1.2 (95% CI: 1.0–1.4) EDs 1.4 (95% CI: 1.1–1.8) Substance misuse 1.0 (95% CI: 0.9–1.3) Behavioral disorders 1.4 (95% CI: 1.2–1.6) ADHD 1.2 (95% CI: 1.0–1.4) Autism spectrum disorder 1.3 (95% CI: 1.1–1.7) Intellectual disability 1.7 (95% CI: 1.4–2.1)	NR

ADHD: Attention-Deficit Hyperactivity Disorder; ANOVA: analysis of variance; BMI: body mass index; CBCL: Achenbach Child Behavior Checklist; CD: celiac disease; CDA: celiac disease autoimmunity; CDI: Child Depression Inventory; CI: confidence interval; EAT: Eating Attitudes Test; ED: eating disorder; GFD: gluten free diet; GS: gluten sensitivity; HC: healthy controls; HR: hazard ratio; HRQOL: Health-Related Quality of Life; MASC: Multidimensional Anxiety Scale for Children; NR: not reported; NS: not significant; OR: odd ratio; PSC: Pediatric Symptom Checklist; SCARED: Childhood Anxiety Disorders Screening Measure; STAIC: State–Trait Anxiety Inventory for Children; *vs*: versus.

Table 3. Objectives and design of studies evaluating the association between gluten-related disorders and psychiatric disorders in adults.

Author (Year)	Country	Primary Objective	Design ‡	Study Setting	Psychiatric Comorbidity Assessment	Celiac Disease Diagnostic Criteria
Attention-Deficit/Hyperactivity Disorder						
Zelnik (2004) * [45]	Israel	To evaluate neurologic disorders including ADHD in CD	Cross-sectional	Clinical	DSM criteria for ADHD	Both
Autism spectrum disorders						
Ludvigsson (2013) * [46]	Sweden	To examine the association between autistic spectrum disorder and CD	Cohort study	Community	ICD	Group 1: villous atrophy, Marsh stage 3 Group 2: villous atrophy, Marsh stages 1–2 Group 3: normal mucosa and positive serologic findings
Schizophrenia Spectrum						
West (2006) [47]	UK	To compare the risk of schizophrenia in patients with CD, ulcerative colitis, Crohn's disease with the general population	Population-based cross-sectional	Community	NR	NR
Eaton (2006) [48]	Denmark	To estimate the association of schizophrenia with autoimmune disorders	Cross-sectional	Community	ICD	ICD
Benros (2011) [49]	Denmark	To investigate whether autoimmune diseases are associated with increased risk of schizophrenia	Population-based retrospective cohort	Community	ICD	NR
Wijampreecha (2018) [50]	USA	To evaluate the risk of developing schizophrenia among patients with CD	Meta-analysis	NA	NR	NR
Bipolar, depressive or anxiety disorders						
Hallert (1982) [51] Hallert (1983) [52]	Sweden	To compare the prevalence of psychiatric illness among patients with CD vs. controls and to assess the effects of gluten withdrawal and vitamin B6 supplement on depressive symptoms	Phase 1: cross-sectional Phase 2: case-series	Clinical	MMPI	Both (serological and biopsy) combined with morphological improvement with GFD
Addolorato (1996) [53]	Italy	To conduct psychometric evaluation in patients with CD or IBD compared to healthy controls	Cross-sectional	Clinical	STAI IDSQ	Both
Ciacci (1998) [54]	Italy	To explore the relevance of depressive symptoms in a large series of adult celiacs	Cross-sectional	Clinical	SRDS	Both
Addolorato (2001) [55]	Italy	To evaluate state and trait anxiety and depression in adult CD patients before and after 1 year of GFD	Phase 1: Cross-sectional Phase 2: Case-series	Clinical	STAI SRDS	Both
Cicarelli (2003) [56]	Italy	To evaluate the prevalence of headache, mood disorders, epilepsy, ataxia and peripheral neuropathy in adult celiac patients	Cross-sectional	Clinical	DSM-IV	Both
Carta (2002) [57] Carta (2003) [58]	Italy	To evaluate the association between celiac disease and specific anxiety and depressive disorders	Cross-sectional	Clinical	CIDI-DSM-IV	Both
Addolorato (2008) [59]	Italy	To evaluate social phobia in CD patients	Cross-sectional	Clinical	LSAS total > 30 SRDS > 49	Both

Table 3. *Cont.*

Author (Year)	Country	Primary Objective	Design ‡	Study Setting	Psychiatric Comorbidity Assessment	Celiac Disease Diagnostic Criteria
Garud (2009) [60]	US	To determine the prevalence of psychiatric and autoimmune disorders in patients with CD in the US compared with control groups	Cross-sectional	Community	Clinical charts	Biopsy
Smith (2012) [61]	Denmark	To investigate whether CD is reliably linked with anxiety and/or depression	Meta-analysis	NA	NA	NA
Peters (2014) [62]	Australia	To investigate the effect of gluten on mental state among patients with NCGS	Randomized, double-blind, cross-over trial	Clinical	STPI	Challenging with varying amounts of gluten
Carta (2015) [63]	Italy	To measure the association between CD and affective disorders	Cross-sectional	Clinical	DSM-IV	NR
Di Sabatino (2015) [64]	Italy	To assess the effects of gluten administration on intestinal and extraintestinal symptoms in subjects with NCGS	Randomized, double-blind, placebo-controlled cross-over trial	Clinical	Extraintestinal symptoms, including depression, were self-reported by patients as absent or present	Self-reported persistence of relevant intestinal and extraintestinal symptoms at low gluten doses
Tortora (2013) [65]	Italy	To evaluate the prevalence of post-partum depression in CD	Cross-sectional	Clinical	EPDS (Total score > 10 possible PPD)	Both
Sainsbury (2018) [66]	UK	To synthesize the evidence on the relationship between depression and degree of adherence to GFD in patients with CD	Meta-analysis	NA	NA	NA
Feeding and eating disorders						
Passananti (2013) [67]	Italy	To investigate the prevalence of eating disorders in patients with celiac disease	Cross-sectional	Clinical	Structured psychological assessment using: BES (Total score ≥ 17) EAT-26 (Total score ≥ 20) EDI-2 M-SDS (Total score > 44) SCL-90	Both
Satherley (2016) [68]	United Kingdom	To examine the prevalence of eating disorders in women with CD	Cross-sectional	Clinical	EAT-26 (Total score > 20) BES (Moderate bingeing, score > 17; severe bingeing, score > 27) DASS-21	Self-reported a biopsy-confirmed diagnosis
Märild (2017) * [69]	Sweden	To determine whether women with CD are at increased risk of diagnosis of anorexia nervosa	Register-based cohort study	Community	ICD	Group 1: villous atrophy, Marsh stage 3 Group 2: villous atrophy, Marsh stages 1–2 Group 3: normal mucosa and positive serologic findings
Sleep-Wake disorders						
Märild (2015) * [70]	Sweden	To estimate the risk of repeated use of hypnotics among individuals with CD as a proxy measure for poor sleep	Population-based cohort study	Community	Prescribed Drug Register in Sweden—Use of hypnotics	Biopsy

Table 3. *Cont.*

Author (Year)	Country	Primary Objective	Design ‡	Study Setting	Psychiatric Comorbidity Assessment	Celiac Disease Diagnostic Criteria
Substance-related and addictive disorders						
Roos (2006) [71]	Sweden	To assess psychological well-being in adults with CD with proven remission (treated for 10 years)	Cross-sectional	Clinical	PGWB	Remission was ascertained with a return of villous structure at repeat biopsy (82%) or negative serology (18%)
Gili (2013) [72]	Spain	To study the impact of alcohol disorders on length of hospital stays, over-expenditures during hospital stays, and excess mortality in CD patients	Cross-sectional	Clinical	ICD	ICD
Neurocognitive Disorders						
Lebwohl (2016) [73]	Sweden	To determine whether patients with CD have an increased risk of dementia	Population-based cohort	Community	ICD	Biopsy
Various psychiatric conditions						
Fera (2003) [74]	Italy	To estimate the incidence of psychiatric disorders in celiac disease patients on gluten withdrawal	Cross-sectional	Clinical	DSM-IV criteria	Biopsy & Clinical history
Sainsbury (2013) [75]	Australia	To compare the relevant impact of psychological symptoms to known negative impacts of gastrointestinal symptoms and adherence to the GFD on quality of life	Study 1: Cross-sectional Study 2: Cross-sectional	Clinical	DASS EDI-3 CISS	Biopsy
Zylberberg (2017) [76]	US	To assess the prevalence of depression and insomnia among patients with CD, both diagnosed and undiagnosed, and people without CD who avoid gluten	Population-based cross-sectional	Community	PHQ-9 (Total score on questions 1-9 $\geq$ 10) SDQ	Diagnosed CD: self-reported diagnosis Undiagnosed CD: serology

* Included patients of all age groups (pediatrics and adults); ‡ The design was determined by the authors of the current review which might not coincide with the design described in the original studies; for studies including multiple methodologies, the design that achieved the objectives of interest was selected; ADHD: Attention-deficit/hyperactivity disorder; BES: Binge Eating Scale; CD: celiac disease; CDS: Children Depression Scale; CIDI-DSM-IV: Composite International Diagnostic Interview for DSM-IV; CISS: Coping Inventory for Stressful Situations; DASS: Depression Anxiety Stress Scale; DSM: Diagnostic and Statistical Manual of Mental Disorders; EAT: Eating Attitudes Test; EDI: Eating Disorder Inventory; EDRS: Eating Disorder Risk Scale; EPDS: Edinburgh Postnatal Depression Scale; GFD: gluten-free diet; HADS: Hospital Anxiety and Depression Scale; IBD: inflammatory bowel disease; ICD: International Classification of Disease; IDSQ: Ipat Depression Scale Questionnaire; LSAS: Liebowitz Social Anxiety Scale; MMPI: Minnesota Multiphasic Personality Inventory; M-SDS: Modified Zung Self-Rating Depression Scale; NA: not applicable; NCGS: non-celiac gluten sensitivity; NR: not reported; PGWB: Psychological General Well-being; PHQ: Patient Health Questionnaire; PPD: post-partum depression; PSS: Perceived Stress Scale; SCL: Symptom Check List; SDQ: Sleep Disorder Questionnaire; SRDS: Zung Self-Rating Depression Scale; STAI: State and Trait Anxiety Inventory; STPI: Spielberger State Trait Personality Inventory.

A summary of results of studies evaluating the association between CD and the occurrence or presence of psychiatric disorders is presented in Table 4.

The prevalence rates of depression or depressive symptomatology were significantly higher in patients with CD compared to controls in the majority of the published studies except for two [56,60]. Nevertheless, significant variability in the point-prevalence of depression or depressive symptomatology exists, ranging from 14% to 68.7% [53,56,57,59,60,63]. In a meta-analysis conducted by Smith et al. [61], depression was shown to be more common and severe in CD than in healthy adults, but not compared to patients with other medical conditions. Comorbid illnesses, including type I diabetes mellitus or subclinical thyroid disease, and stress were associated with the presence of depressive symptomatology in CD [57,60]. Increased severity of gastrointestinal symptoms in CD was linked to worsened depressive symptoms [75] which, in turn, led to poorer QOL compared to controls [63]. Although gluten-free diet (GFD) did not lead to any improvement in depressive symptoms in two longitudinal studies [52,55], a meta-analysis conducted by Sainsbury et al. [66] found a moderate association between poor adherence to GFD and greater depressive symptoms. With respect to post-partum depression, it was assessed in a single study in which it turned out to be significantly more prevalent in women with CD compared to controls (41% vs. 11%, $p < 0.01$) [65].

Table 4. Summary of outcomes evaluating the association between gluten-related disorders and psychiatric disorders in adults.

Author (Year)	Design	Sample Size and Demographic Characteristics	Summary of Outcomes	Associated Factors with Psychiatric Comorbidities and other Relevant Information
Attention-Deficit/Hyperactivity Disorder				
Zelnik (2004) [45]	Cross-sectional	CD, $n = 111$ (mean age 20.1 years, 57.7% females) Controls, $n = 211$ (mean age 20.1 years, 59.7% females)	- ADHD diagnosis: 20.7% in CD vs. 10.5% in controls (p <0.01) CD, 20.3% of female patients and 21.2% of male patients Controls, 8.7% of females and 12.9% males	- No gender differences were found in the prevalence of ADHD in patients with CD - Differences in ADHD were not different among CD patients presenting with infantile form of CD or late-onset symptoms
Autism spectrum disorders				
Ludvigsson (2013) [46]	Cohort study	Group 1, $n = 26,995$ (age at diagnosis, 0–19 years 40.4%, >20 years 59.6%; 62.1% females); Controls, $n = 134,076$ (matched age and gender) Group 2, $n = 12,304$ (age at diagnosis, 0–19 years 8.9%, >20 years 91.1%; 56.9% females); Controls, $n = 60,654$ (matched age and gender) Group 3, $n = 3719$ (age at diagnosis, 0–19 years 25.3%, >20 years 74.7%; 62.1% females); Controls, $n = 18,478$ (matched age and gender)	- Risk of later ASD diagnosis: Group 1: HR = 1.39 (95% CI: 1.13–1.71) Group 2: HR =2.01 (95% CI: 1.29–3.13) Group 3: HR = 3.09 (95% CI: 1.99–4.8)	NR
Schizophrenia Spectrum				
West (2006) [47]	Population-based case-control	CD, $n = 4732$; matched controls, $n = 23,620$ Crohn's disease, $n = 5961$; matched controls, $n = 29,843$ Ulcerative colitis, $n = 8301$; matched controls, $n = 41,589$ Demographics NR	- Prevalence of schizophrenia 0.25% in CD, 0.27% in Crohn's disease and 0.24% in ulcerative colitis, 0.37% in general population - ORs for schizophrenia compared to controls adjusted for smoking status: 0.76 (95% CI: 0.4–1.4) in CD, 0.74 (95% CI: 0.4–1.3) in Crohn's disease, 0.71 (95% CI 0.4–1.1) in ulcerative colitis	NR
Eaton (2006) [48]	Cross-sectional	Schizophrenia, $n = 7704$, 25 controls for each case. Demographics NR	- Prior CD diagnosis in subjects with schizophrenia: Crude incidence rate: 3.8 (95% CI: 1.3–11) Adjusted incidence rate: 3.6 (95% CI: 1.2–10.6)	NR
Benros (2011) [49]	Population-based cohort	Schizophrenia, $n = 39,076$: Prior diagnosis of autoimmune disease, $n = 927$, autoimmune disease and infections, $n = 444$, without autoimmune disease, $n = 37,705$ Demographics NR	- The risk of schizophrenia among individuals with CD was increased: CD without infection: Incidence rate ratio = 2.11 (95% CI: 1.09–3.61) CD with infections: Incidence rate ratio = 2.47 (95% CI: 1.13–4.61)	NR
Wijarnpreecha (2018) [50]	Meta-analysis	Four studies were included	- Higher risk of schizophrenia among patients with CD was found; pooled OR = 2.03 (95% CI: 1.45–2.86)	NR

Table 4. *Cont.*

Author (Year)	Design	Sample Size and Demographic Characteristics	Summary of Outcomes	Associated Factors with Psychiatric Comorbidities and other Relevant Information
Bipolar, depressive and anxiety disorders				
Hallert (1982) [51] Hallert (1983) [52]	Phase 1: cross-sectional Phase 2: case-series	CD, $n = 12$ (mean age 47 years, 67% females) Controls undergoing cholecystectomy, $n = 12$ (mean age 47 years, 67% females)	- MMPI depression subscale: Significantly higher scores in CD vs. controls (70.3 ± 12.5 vs. 59.2 ± 9.3, p <0.01) - MMPI sores: Post-remission in small intestinal mucosa following GFD in CD: no improvement in mood (70 ± 12.5 at point 0 vs. 68 ± 14 at year 1, p = NS) - Post-cholecystectomy in controls: No change in MMPI scores - Supplementation with Vitamin B6 80 mg/day for 6 months: Significant decrease in depressive symptoms (68 ± 14.0 to 56 ± 8.5, p <0.01)	- In patients with CD, significant correlation was found between depression scores and degree of steatorrhea - No correlation was found between abdominal complaints (diarrhea and pain) and depression scores
Addolorato (1996) [53]	Case-control	CD, $n = 20$ (mean age 37 years, 56% females) IBD, $n = 16$ (mean age 32 years, 56% females) Controls, $n = 16$ (mean age 35 years, 56% females)	- Prevalence of State anxiety: 62.5% in CD, 50% in IBD, and 31.3% in controls (p = NS). - Prevalence of depression: 68.7% in CD, 37.5% in IBD, and 18.8% in controls (p <0.01 for CD vs. controls only)	NR
Ciacci (1998) [54]	Cross-sectional	CD, $n = 92$ (mean age 29.4 years, 70% females) CPH, $n = 48$ (mean age 31.8 years, 34% females) Controls, $n = 100$ (mean age 30 years, 71% females)	- Mean scores of the M-SDS: CD: 31.81 ± 7.84 CPH: 28.73 ± 7.09 (p = 0.038 vs. CD) Controls: 27.14 ± 5.26 (p <0.0001 vs. CD)	- Demographic characteristics did not influence M-SDS scores - Depressive symptoms are present to a similar extent in patients with childhood- and adulthood-diagnosed CD
Addolorato (2001) [55]	Phase 1: Cross-sectional Phase 2: Case-series	CD, $n = 35$ (mean age 29.8 years, 60% females) Controls, $n = 59$ (mean age 31.7 years, 54% females)	*Before diet:* - Prevalence of high levels of state anxiety: CD vs. control: 71.4% versus 23.7% (p <0.0001) - Prevalence of high levels of trait anxiety: CD vs. controls: 25.7% versus 15.2% (p = NS) - Prevalence of depression CD vs. controls: 57.1% versus 9.6% (p <0.0001) *After 1 year of GFD (T0 vs. T1)* - Prevalence of high levels of state anxiety: T0 71.4% versus T1: 25.7% (p <0.001) - Prevalence of high levels of trait anxiety: T0: 25.7% versus T1: 17.1% (p = NS) - Prevalence of depression T0: 57.1% versus T1:45.7 (p = NS)	NR
Cicarelli (2003) [56]	Cross-sectional	CD, $n = 176$ (mean age 30.9 years, 75% females) Controls, $n = 52$ (mean age 31.7 years, 65% females)	- Prevalence of mood disorders (CD vs. controls): Mood disorders 50 (29%) vs. 9 (17%), p = NS Depression episodes 24 (14%) vs. 7 (13%), p = NS Dysthymia 26 (15%) vs. 2 (4%), p <0.05	- Adherence to a strict gluten-free diet was associated with a significant reduction of dysthymia

Table 4. *Cont.*

Author (Year)	Design	Sample Size and Demographic Characteristics	Summary of Outcomes	Associated Factors with Psychiatric Comorbidities and other Relevant Information
Bipolar, depressive and anxiety disorders				
Carta (2002) [57] Carta (2003) [58]	Cross-sectional	CD, $n = 36$ (mean age 41.1 years, 75% females) Controls, $n = 144$ (mean age 41.3 years, 75% females)	- Lifetime prevalence of psychiatric disorders (cases vs. controls): Major depressive disorder 15 (41.7%) vs. 30 (20.8%), $p = 0.01$ Dysthymic disorder 3 (8.3%) vs. 2 (1.4%), $p = 0.05$ Adjustment disorders 11 (30.5%) vs. 11 (7.6%), $p = 0.001$ Generalized anxiety disorder 10 (27.7%) vs. 23 (16%), $p = NS$ Panic disorder 5 (13.9%) vs. 3 (2.1%), $p = 0.001$ Specific phobia 1 (2.7%) vs. 6 (4.2%), $p = NS$ Social phobia 3 (8.3%) vs. 10 (6.9%), $p = NS$ Recurrent brief depression 36.1% versus 6.9% (OR = 7.6; 95% CI: 3.2–17.8)	- Earlier onset of CD was linked to higher prevalence of major depressive disorder - Subclinical thyroid disease appears to represent a significant risk factor for these psychiatric disorders
Addolorato (2008) [59]	Cross-sectional	CD, $n = 40$ (mean age 38 years, 86% females) HC, $n = 50$ (mean age 36 years, 80% females)	- Prevalence of social phobia: 70% in CD vs. 16% in HC ($p < 0.0001$) - Prevalence of depression: 53% in CD vs. 8% in HC ($p < 0.0001$)	- The prevalence of social phobia or depression in patients with CD did not differ among subjects newly diagnosed with CD and those already on GFD
Garud (2009) [60]	Cross-sectional	CD, $n = 600$ (mean age 54 males & 49 females, 75% females) IBS, $n = 200$ (mean age 48 males & 45 females, 75% females) Controls, $n = 200$ (mean age 52 males & 47 females, 75% females)	Prevalence of depression: 17.2% in CD vs. 18.5% in IBS ($p = 0.74$ vs. CD) and 16% in controls ($p = 0.79$ vs. CD)	- Among CD patients, type 1 diabetes mellitus was identified as a significant risk factor for depression ($p < 0.01$) with 37% of patients with both CD and type 1 DM having clinical depression
Smith (2012) [61]	Meta-analysis	Eleven studies on depression and eight studies on anxiety were included	- Depression is more common and severe in CD than in healthy adults with an overall effect size of 0.97 - Anxiety did not differ significantly between CD and healthy adults - No differences in depression or anxiety in CD vs. other medical disorders	- Other medical conditions included: Crohn's disease, DM, IBD, lactose intolerance, surgery patients, CPH
Peters (2014) [62]	Randomized, double-blind, cross-over trial	NCGS, $n = 22$ (median age 48 years, 77% females)	- Gluten ingestion effect on STPI depression scores: Significantly higher scores in CD vs. controls (mean difference = 2.03, 95% CI: 0.55–3.51, $p = 0.01$) - No differences in other STPI state indices or for any STPI trait measures	NR
Carta (2015) [63]	Cross-sectional	CD, $n = 46$ (mean age 41 years, 83% females) Controls, $n = 240$ (mean age 41 years, 83% females)	- Prevalence of depression: 30.0% in CD vs. 8.3% in controls, $p < 0.0001$ - Prevalence of panic disorder: 18.3% in CD vs. 5.4% in controls, $p < 0.001$ - Prevalence of bipolar disorder: 4.3% in CD vs. 0.4% in controls, $p < 0.005$	- Patients with CD but without comorbidity with major depression, panic disorder, or bipolar disorder do not show worse QOL than controls
Di Sabatino (2015) [64]	Randomized, double-blind, placebo-controlled cross-over trial	NCGS, $n = 61$ (mean age 39 years, 87% females) randomly assigned to: Gluten 4.375 mg/day for 1 week Placebo 4.375 g/day rice starch for 1 week Wash-out period: 1 week	- Depression was significantly worsened by gluten ingestion ($p = 0.02$)	NR

Table 4. *Cont.*

Author (Year)	Design	Sample Size and Demographic Characteristics	Summary of Outcomes	Associated Factors with Psychiatric Comorbidities and other Relevant Information
Bipolar, depressive and anxiety disorders				
Tortora (2013) [65]	Cross-sectional	CD, $n = 70$ (mean age 33 years) Controls, $n = 70$ (mean age 32 years)	- EPDS scores in CD women vs. controls: 9.9 ± 5.9 vs. 6.7 ± 3.7, $p < 0.01$ - EPDS >10: 47% in CD vs. 14% in controls (OR = 3.3, $p < 0.01$) - PPD diagnosis: 41% of CD women with vs. 11% in controls ($p < 0.01$)	- A significant association was observed between the onset of PPD and a previous menstrual disorder in women suffering from CD - QOL scores were significantly higher in women with CD
Sainsbury (2018) [66]	Meta-analysis	Eight studies were included in quantitative analysis (total $n = 1644$, mean age ranged from 39 to 57 years, % of females ranged from 76.6% to 100%)	- Moderate association between poor adherence to GFD and greater depressive symptoms ($r = 0.398$, 95% CI: 0.32–0.47) with marked heterogeneity in effects ($I^2 = 66.8\%$) - Exclusion of studies with high or unclear risk of bias did not alter the results	- Poorer QOL was correlated with a higher incidence of psychological and gastrointestinal symptoms, greater reliance on maladaptive coping strategies, and poorer GFD adherence
Feeding and eating disorders				
Passananti (2013) [67]	Cross-sectional	CD, $n = 100$ (mean age 29 years, 72% females) HC, $n = 100$ (mean age 30 years, 68% females)	- BES ≥ 17: 6% in CD vs. 0% controls (p = NS) - Women with CD had significantly higher scores in pulse thinness, social insecurity, perfectionism, inadequacy, ascetisim, and interpersonal diffidence compared to HC women of the Eating Disorder Inventory - EAT-26 ≥ 20: 16% in CD vs. 4% in HC ($p = 0.01$) - SRDS > 44: 39% in CD vs. 6% in controls ($p < 0.001$) - SCL-90 pathological scores: 42% in CD vs. 6% in HC ($p < 0.0001$)	- EAT-26 demonstrated association between indices of diet-related disorders in both CD and the female gender after controlling for anxiety and depression
Satherley (2016) [68]	Cross-sectional	CD, $n = 157$ (mean age 38 years, sex NR) IBD, $n = 116$ (mean age 36 years, sex NR) DM-type 2, $n = 88$ (mean age 47 years, sex NR) HC, $n = 142$ (mean age 33 years, sex NR)	- EAT-26 > 20: 15.7% in CD vs. 8.8% in DM and 3.8% in HC ($p < 0.05$) - BES > 17: 19.4% in CD vs. 2.3% in controls ($p < 0.05$) - Mean EAT-26 and BES scores: 11.1 in CD vs. 7.7 in controls ($p < 0.05$) and 11.2 in CD vs. 3.9 in controls ($p < 0.05$), respectively - Significant associations between EAT-26 and BES scores with DASS-21 scores were reported ($p < 0.008$)	- Dietary-management and gastrointestinal symptoms were significantly associated with EAT scores in CD
Mårild (2017) [69]	Population-based cohort study	Group 1, $n = 17{,}959$ (median age 28 years); Matched controls, $n = 89{,}379$ Group 2, $n = 7455$ (median age 46 years); Matched controls, $n = 36{,}940$ Group 3, $n = 2307$ (median age 38 years); Matched controls, $n = 11{,}499$	- Risk of developing anorexia nervosa: Group 1: HR=1.46 (95% CI: 1.08–1.98) Group 2: HR=2.12 (95% CI: 0.97–4.67) Group 3: HR=2.45 (95% CI: 1.10–5.45) - Adjustment for education level, socioeconomic status, and type 1 DM didn't affect conclusions in all groups	- There was no significantly increased risk for subsequent anorexia nervosa among males with CD

Table 4. *Cont.*

Author (Year)	Design	Sample Size and Demographic Characteristics	Summary of Outcomes	Associated Factors with Psychiatric Comorbidities and other Relevant Information
Sleep-Wake disorders				
Mårild (2015) [70]	Population-based cohort study	CD, n = 2933 (median age 28 years, 61.2% females) Controls, n = 14,571 (median age 28 years, 61.3 females)	- Poor sleep in CD vs. controls: 12.5% vs. 9.8% (HR = 1.36, 95% CI: 1.30–1.41) - Individuals with CD had a similar increased risk irrespective of age at CD diagnosis, sex and type of hypnotic used	- Overall, poor sleep was more prevalent in females than in males. However, differences in risk estimates for poor sleep were small between females and males with CD - Adjustment for sleep apnea and restless leg syndrome did not influence the risk of poor sleep in CD
Substance-related and addictive disorders				
Roos (2006) [71]	Cross-sectional	CD, n = 51 (age 45–64 years, 59% females) Controls, n = 182 (age 45–64 years, 57% females)	- PGWB index scores: 103 (95% CI: 99–107) in CD vs. 103 (95% CI: 100–106) in controls (p = NS)	- Males with CD tended to score higher on the PGWB domains than the male controls - CD women scored somewhat lower in the PGWB domains than the female controls - CD men tended to score higher than the CD women in all six domains of the PGWB
Gili 2013 [72]	Cross-sectional	CD, n = 3327 (mean age 49 years and 70% females). Controls, n = 5,471,988) (mean age 58 years and 54% females).	- Prevalence of alcohol disorders: 4.9% in CD vs. 6.3% in controls (p = 0.0009)	- The presence of alcohol disorders in CD increased the length of stay, costs and had an excess of mortality
Neurocognitive Disorders				
Lebwohl (2016) [73]	Population-based cohort	CD, n = 8846 (mean age 64 years and 56% females). Control, n = 43,474 (mean age 64 years and 56% females).	- In a median follow-up period of 8.4 years: 4.3% of CD patients and 4.4% of controls had a diagnosis of dementia (HR 1.07; 95% CI 0.95–1.20) - A subgroup analysis showed an increased risk of vascular dementia (HR 1.28; 95% CI 1.00–1.64)	- A significant association between CD and dementia among the age group 60–69 was found, which was not present in the younger or older age groups - Increased risk of dementia was found in the first year following CD diagnosis
Various psychiatric conditions				
Fera (2003) [74]	Cross-sectional	CD, n = 100 (mean age 40 years, 75% females) DM, n = 100 (mean age 53 years, 74% females) HC, n = 100 (mean age 41 years, 68% females)	- CD, prevalence of OCD 28%, depressive disorder/dysthymia 19% - DM, prevalence of OCD 0%, depressive disorder/dysthymia 10% HC, anxiety and depression in 10% of subjects	- QOL was poorer in both CD and diabetic patients than in healthy controls and significantly correlated with anxiety
Sainsbury (2013) [75]	Study 1: cross-sectional	n = 390 (mean age 44 years, 82.8% females)	- Severe gastrointestinal symptoms at CD diagnosis were associated with: increased depression (r = 0.28, p <0.001), anxiety (r = 0.29, p <0.001), stress (r = 0.28, p <0.001), eating disorder (r = 0.15, p <0.01), and emotion-oriented coping (r = 0.17, p <0.01)	- Poorer QOL was significantly associated with a greater number and longer duration of CD symptoms prior to diagnosis - Higher number of symptoms was associated with poorer QOL - There were no gender differences in QOL, although females reported a greater number of symptoms - More severe gastrointestinal symptoms at diagnosis were also associated with increased psychological manifestations

Table 4. Cont.

Various psychiatric conditions

Author (Year)	Design	Sample Size and Demographic Characteristics	Summary of Outcomes	Associated Factors with Psychiatric Comorbidities and other Relevant Information
Sainsbury (2013) [75]	Study 2: cross-sectional	$n = 189$ (mean age 46.5 years, 87.3% females)	- Hierarchical regression analyses: Current psychological distress significantly contributed to poor QOL (accounting for 23.8% of the variance in QOL)	
Zylberberg (2017) [76]	Population-based cross-sectional	Diagnosed CD, $n = 27$ (age NR, 78% females) Undiagnosed CD, $n = 79$ (age NR, 58% females) PWAG; $n = 213$ (age NR, 55% females) Controls; $n = 14,769$ (demographic characteristics NR)	- Prevalence of depression: 8.2% of controls vs. 3.9% in CD ($p = 0.18$) and 2.9% in PWAGs (0.002) - Prevalence of sleep difficulty: 37.3% in CD, 34.1% in PWAGs vs. 27.4% in controls ($p = $ NS) - Multivariate analysis adjusted for race/ethnicity, annual household income, number of healthcare visits: PWAGS, significantly lower odds of depression (OR = 0.25, 95% CI: 0.12–0.5, $p = 0.0001$) CD, OR = 0.30; 95% CI: 0.08–1.19, $p = 0.09$	-QOL: The presence of physical, mental, and emotional limitations was reported in 2.9% of controls vs. 13.8% diagnosed CD ($p = 0.004$), 9.6% with undiagnosed CD ($p = 0.02$), and 5.1% in PWAGs ($p = 0.18$)

ADHD: Attention-Deficit Hyperactivity Disorder; ASD: Autistic Spectrum Disorders; BES: Binge Eating Scale; CD: celiac disease; CI: confidence interval; CPH: Chronic persistent hepatitis; DASS: Depression Anxiety Stress Scale; DM: Diabetes Mellitus; EAT: Eating Attitudes Test; EPDS: Edinburgh Postnatal Depression Scale; GFD: gluten-free diet; HC: healthy controls; HR: hazard ratio; IBD: Inflammatory Bowel Disease; IBS: Irritable Bowel Disease; MMPI: Minnesota Multiphasic Personality Inventory; M-SDS: Modified Zung Self-Rating Depression Scale; NCGS: non-celiac gluten sensitivity; NR: not reported; NS: not significant; OCD: Obsessive-Compulsive Disorder; OR: odd ratio; PGWB: Psychological General Well-being; PWAG: people who avoid gluten; QOL: quality of life; RR: relative risk; SCL: Symptom Check List; SRDS: Zung Self-Rating Depression Scale; vs: versus.

In two studies conducted by the same research group, the prevalence of state anxiety in patients with CD was substantially higher than in controls (62.5% vs. 31.3%, and 71.4% vs. 23.7%), although the difference was statistically significant in only one study [53,55]. Generalized anxiety disorder diagnosis in CD was not shown to be prevalent in CD compared to controls [57] and the overall prevalence of anxiety was not significantly higher compared to healthy adults in the meta-analysis conducted by Smith et al. [61]. The prevalence of social phobia in CD reached 70% in one cross-sectional study [59]; however, its lifetime prevalence in another study was only 8.3% [57]. Bipolar disorder and panic disorders were significantly more prevalent in patients with CD [57,58,63].

Three studies assessed the prevalence and risk of eating disorders in CD. Their prevalence was significantly higher in adults with CD compared to healthy controls as demonstrated via the elevated scores on the different assessment scales employed in two cross-sectional studies [67,68]. Elevated Eating Attitudes Test scores were seen in around 16% of patients with CD in both studies, whereas elevated Binge Eating Scale scores were only elevated in one study with 19.7% of adults with CD reporting high scores [68]. Moreover, severe gastrointestinal symptoms were linked to greater risk of eating disorders [75]. In the register-based cohort and case-control study conducted by Marild et al. [69], the likelihood of developing anorexia nervosa was significantly higher in women with CD (HR = 1.46, 95% CI: 1.08–1.98) and the likelihood was highest in women with normal mucosa and positive serology (HR = 2.45, 95% CI: 1.1–5.45).

While patients with CD were less likely to experience alcohol-related disorders [72], their risk of developing dementia was significantly higher as shown in a population-based cohort study [70,73]. The likelihood of developing poor sleep in CD based on the use of hypnotics was significantly elevated compared to controls HR = 1.36, 95% CI: 1.3–1.41) in the population-based case-control study conducted by Marild et al. [70]. On the other hand, sleep difficulty as measured with the Patient Health Questionnaire did not differ significantly between adults with CD and controls (37.3% vs. 27.4%, $p = 0.15$) in a population-based cross-sectional study [76].

While gender did not seem to affect the prevalence rates of ADHD in CD patients [45], males with CD were less likely to experience poor sleep problems [70] or subsequent anorexia nervosa [69] and they tended to score higher on the different Psychological General Well-being Index domains [71]. Conflicting results concerning the effect of the CD onset time on psychological symptomatology were obtained; on one hand, earlier onset of CD symptoms was linked to higher prevalence of major depressive disorder in one study [57] and on the other hand, depressive symptomatology scores did not differentiate between childhood or adulthood diagnosis of CD [54]. Finally, severe gastrointestinal symptomatology significantly correlated with increased psychological manifestations [68,75].

The risk of schizophrenia in patients with CD was assessed in three studies [47–49]. While one population-based case-control study showed no increased risk of schizophrenia in CD (OR = 0.75, 95% CI: 0.4–1.4) [47], its risk was shown to be significantly elevated in a population-based cohort study (Incidence rate ratio = 2.11, 95% CI: 1.1–3.6) and a cross-sectional study (adjusted incidence rate = 3.6, 95% CI: 1.2–10.6) [48,49]. In a meta-analysis including four studies, an increased risk of schizophrenia among patients with CD was found (OR = 2.03, 95% CI: 1.45–2.86) [50]. With respect to autistic spectrum disorders, its risk in a population-based cohort of CD appeared to be increased with the highest risk being present in patients with normal mucosa and positive serologic findings (HR = 3.09, 95% CI: 1.99–4.8) [46].

ADHD was assessed in one cross-sectional study that reported an increased prevalence of this disorder in adults with CD compared to controls (20.7% vs. 10.5%, $p <0.01$) [45]. The overall psychological status in adults with CD was evaluated in one study whereby no difference in the total Psychological General Well-Being Index was found between CD and controls [71].

In the two studies that evaluated the effects of gluten ingestion in adults with NCGS [62,64], significant worsening of depressive symptomatology [64] and increase in the depression subscale scores of Spielberger State Trait Personality Inventory [62] were reported.

4. Discussion

Our current review of the literature revealed the existence of an association between CD and other gluten-related disorders with psychiatric disorders across different age groups. CD is primarily an autoimmune disorder that is characterized by villous atrophy of the intestinal mucosa along with intraepithelial lymphocytosis and crypt hyperplasia [77]. Nevertheless, a major shift in clinical presentation with extraintestinal manifestations becoming more prevalent than classical gastrointestinal symptoms has been suggested [78]. The reviewed data demonstrate that a wide range of psychiatric disorders have been investigated in CD and NCGS including autism spectrum disorders, schizophrenia, attention-deficit disorder, depression and mood disorders, anxiety disorders, bipolar disorder, feeding and eating disorders, sleep disorders, substance-related and addictive disorders and neurocognitive disorders.

Most of the cross-sectional studies in the pediatric population did not find any significant differences in the point prevalence of depression or anxiety disorders [32,33,35–37], however, these studies had several methodological limitations which mainly included small sample size (ranging between 29 and 42 children with CD), the lack of specialized psychiatric clinical assessment, and the absence of adequate blinding measures to limit assessment bias. On the other hand, two population-based cohort studies including >9000 children each provided evidence for an increased likelihood of occurrence of depression and anxiety disorders in patients with CD [34,44]. In the cohort study conducted by Ludvigsson et al. [34], it was shown that adults and children with CD are at increased risk of being diagnosed with depression but not bipolar disorder later in life (i.e., during adulthood for children diagnosed with CD), whereas in the study conducted by Butwicka et al. [44], CD was identified as a risk factor for mood disorders, anxiety disorders, eating disorders, behavioral disorders, ADHD, ASD, and intellectual disability diagnosed prior to 18 years of age. Although the analyses in the two previous cohort studies were controlled for children's age, stratified analyses to identify the likelihood of occurrence of specific psychiatric disorders across the different age groups are worth evaluation taking into consideration the variation in clinical presentation across the developmental span between 0 and 15 years of age [79].

In adults, the point-prevalence of depression was significantly higher in patients with CD in the majority of published studies. These findings were ascertained by a population-based cohort study in which the HR of depression (in participants ≥16 years at diagnosis) was two folds higher than controls [34] and by a meta-analysis in which depression was shown to be more common and severe in CD than in healthy adults with an overall effect size of 0.97 [61]. A comprehensive review, evaluating the comorbidity of depression and anxiety in CD, concluded that these disorders are common disorders among patients with CD and contribute to a poorer quality of life [24]. Nevertheless, the lack of differences in the prevalence of depression when compared to patients with other physical disorders [61] raises a question about the existence of a specific underlying pathophysiological mechanism in patients with CD or whether depression represents a non-specific disorder affected by physical and psychosocial distress. The association between chronic medical diseases and depression is well-known and many different causes, including both genetic predisposition and environmental factors have been shown to be involved [80–82]. This association is frequently bidirectional, as the presence of physical illness often worsens the affective disorder and vice versa [81]. The current information relative to depression in patients with CD does not allow, at the present time, to ascertain the exact relationship and the predisposing factors involved between CD or NCGS and depressive symptomatology.

The association between CD and eating disorders has been investigated in a limited number of studies. Current findings reveal an elevated prevalence of eating disorders in CD among both children and adults with CD [39,40,44,67–69]. These disorders encompassed anorexia nervosa, bulimia nervosa and binge eating. Poor dietary management can occur as a result of physical dissatisfaction, which is not uncommon in patients with CD [83]. Moreover, evidence from the current literature suggests that young adults with chronic illnesses that require dietary modification are at higher risk of developing pathological eating practices [39]. The elevated lifetime comorbidity between depression and eating disorders [84] could be another explanatory mechanism of increased prevalence of eating disorders in CD patients who are more prone to developing depressive symptomatology.

Concerning psychotic disorders, the current evidence provided by solely two population-based cohort studies does not support the presence of an association between these disorders and CD in children [31,44]. However, children and young adults ($\geq$16 years of age) with CD were 1.8-fold more likely to experience non-schizophrenic non-affective psychosis [31]. The authors of the latter cohort study yet did not rule out the presence of a potential association between CD and schizophrenia as the risk of the latter disorder was high despite the low number of individuals with schizophrenia. These findings were similar to another population-based case-control study conducted in adults in which no evidence of an increased risk of schizophrenia in CD was found [47]. In contrast, Benros et al. [49] demonstrated an increased incidence of schizophrenia in patients with prior CD in their population-based cohort study. Furthermore, Eaton et al. [48] showed also 3.8-fold increase in incidence rates of prior CD diagnosis in subjects with schizophrenia. However, in the latter study, data on parents' celiac status were also included in their analysis which might have led to biased findings. A meta-analysis including four studies demonstrated the presence of an increased risk of schizophrenia among patients with CD [50]. We believe that the pooled-effect estimate in the previous meta-analysis could be biased because their pooled analysis on one hand missed the negative findings reported by West et al. [47] and on the other hand included the findings of a study in which the prevalence of CD in patients with schizophrenia was investigated [85]. The objectives and outcome measures of the latter study [85] did not match the principal objective of the meta-analysis whereby the authors investigated the prevalence of autoimmune diseases (including CD) in patients with schizophrenia and not the other way around [85]. The association between CD and gluten-related disorders with schizophrenia has been under investigation for more than five decades but most studies evaluated the prevalence or risk of gluten-related disorders in patients already diagnosed with schizophrenia [86]. Current evidence suggests a two-fold increase in the prevalence of CD in schizophrenia patients [87] and an association between gluten ingestion and exacerbation of schizophrenia symptoms [88]; nonetheless, these findings are highly inconsistent across different clinical, immunological, and epidemiological studies [86] and have not been replicated in patients presenting with CD.

The underlying mechanisms behind the association between CD and psychiatric disorders are not well-known. Nevertheless, several potential biological and psychosocial explanations have been suggested: (i) Several psychiatric disorders such as depression, anxiety, and ADHD, among others have been linked to certain nutritional and vitamin deficiencies [89] and it is well-known that patients with CD often suffer from malnutrition prior to diagnosis or as a result of dietary non-compliance [90]; (ii) The immune-mediated processes underlying CD have been postulated as potential causative factors of the different psychiatric manifestations taking into consideration the involvement of chronic immune system activation in the etiology of various psychiatric conditions [91]; (iii) The bidirectional communication between the gastrointestinal tract [92] and the brain may suggest that alterations in the intestinal permeability, which is cardinal manifestation in CD [93], could be eventually involved in the pathophysiology of psychiatric manifestations in patients with CD; (iv) Finally, psychosocial aspects commonly seen in CD could place this population at an increased risk of developing psychiatric disorders, for instance, the introduction of GFD is associated with radical changes in daily life activities, eating habits and lifestyle which could be particularly stressful and difficult to accept [43,94]. In addition, effective adherence to GFD entails greater burden manifested via increased daily expenditure on more expensive products, social isolation and constant fear about dietary mistakes [95].

The studies included in this review provided limited data on potential factors associated with psychiatric comorbidity in patients with CD. Bearing in mind this limitation, none of the demographic factors has been consistently associated with the presence or occurrence of psychiatric comorbidities and the role of ethnicity in this context has not been studied. Regarding clinical factors, only severity of CD symptoms appears to be associated with the presence and/or severity of psychiatric disorders [33,51,52,68,75]. In this regard, the significant positive association between increased severity of gastrointestinal symptoms and worsening of psychiatric manifestations [75] and QOL [63] in CD indirectly demonstrates the importance of adherence to GFD. Nevertheless, few studies have documented the beneficial effects of GFD on psychiatric manifestations in patients with CD [27,66], with the majority of these studies suffering from several methodological flaws limiting our capacity of reaching definitive conclusions supporting the role of GFD in this context.

Only two studies in patients with NCGS supported the association between this relatively new entity and depressive symptomology [62,64]. It has not been until recently that standardized diagnostic criteria for NCGS were established [19], which might explain the limited number of studies investigating psychiatric comorbidities in NCGS. In our current review search, we could not find any study that investigated psychiatric comorbidities in patients with WA.

Limitations of our current review are essentially derived from the limited quality of the majority of the studies that have investigated psychiatric disorders in CD. Most of these studies are of cross-sectional design which does not allow establishing causal relationships and are of small sample size, whereas very few population-based studies have been published.

Evaluating psychiatric comorbidities in different age groups adds strength to our current review since up to the current date, none of the previous reviews had evaluated the evidence of psychiatric disorders in children and adults with CD separately. Interestingly, according to our review, the presence of CD in childhood seems to be associated with an increased risk of developing psychiatric disorders later during adulthood, but not with an increased prevalence of these disorders during childhood.

5. Conclusions

Our current comprehensive review ascertains the presence of an association between CD and psychiatric disorders with varying grades of evidence from one condition to another. In our view, there is enough evidence supporting an association of CD with depression and, to a lesser extent, with eating disorders. Some studies also point out to an association between CD and panic disorder, autism and ADHD, but the evidence is limited, and these potential associations should be further investigated. Finally, the data regarding the association of CD with schizophrenia or other anxiety disorders is conflicting. Overall, psychiatric symptomatology which could be perceived as part of the atypical manifestations of this chronic condition are linked to significant distortion in quality of life and moderately increased risk of suicide [96] and thus warrants further attention. Therefore, gastroenterologists and other healthcare professionals involved in the management of patients with CD should be aware of the increased risk of psychiatric disorders in these patients. Thus, routine surveillance of potential psychiatric manifestations, especially anxiety and/or depressive symptomatology that seem to be the most common forms of disturbances, should be carried out by the attending physician in order to refer the patient to the mental health services if necessary.

Author Contributions: Conceptualization, E.P.C; Methodology, M.S., F.R.-V. and E.P.C.; Data extraction, F.R.-V. and M.S.; Writing—Original Draft Preparation, M.S., F.R.-V. and E.P.C.; Writing—Review and Editing, M.S., F.R.-V. and E.P.C.

References

1. Sapone, A.; Bai, J.C.; Ciacci, C.; Dolinsek, J.; Green, P.H.; Hadjivassiliou, M.; Kaukinen, K.; Rostami, K.; Sanders, D.S.; Schumann, M.; et al. Spectrum of gluten-related disorders: Consensus on new nomenclature and classification. *BMC Med.* **2012**, *10*, 13. [CrossRef] [PubMed]
2. Guandalini, S.; Assiri, A. Celiac disease: A review. *JAMA Pediatr.* **2014**, *168*, 272–278. [CrossRef] [PubMed]
3. Green, P.H.; Lebwohl, B.; Greywoode, R. Celiac disease. *J. Allergy Clin. Immunol.* **2015**, *135*, 1099–1106, quiz 1107. [CrossRef] [PubMed]

4.   Ludvigsson, J.F.; Bai, J.C.; Biagi, F.; Card, T.R.; Ciacci, C.; Ciclitira, P.J.; Green, P.H.; Hadjivassiliou, M.; Holdoway, A.; van Heel, D.A.; et al. Diagnosis and management of adult coeliac disease: Guidelines from the british society of gastroenterology. *Gut* **2014**, *63*, 1210–1228. [CrossRef] [PubMed]

5.   Uibo, R.; Tian, Z.; Gershwin, M.E. Celiac disease: A model disease for gene-environment interaction. *Cell. Mol. Immunol.* **2011**, *8*, 93–95. [CrossRef] [PubMed]

6.   Szajewska, H.; Shamir, R.; Chmielewska, A.; Piescik-Lech, M.; Auricchio, R.; Ivarsson, A.; Kolacek, S.; Koletzko, S.; Korponay-Szabo, I.; Mearin, M.L.; et al. Systematic review with meta-analysis: Early infant feeding and coeliac disease—Update 2015. *Aliment. Pharmacol. Ther.* **2015**, *41*, 1038–1054. [CrossRef] [PubMed]

7.   Canova, C.; Zabeo, V.; Pitter, G.; Romor, P.; Baldovin, T.; Zanotti, R.; Simonato, L. Association of maternal education, early infections, and antibiotic use with celiac disease: A population-based birth cohort study in northeastern italy. *Am. J. Epidemiol.* **2014**, *180*, 76–85. [CrossRef] [PubMed]

8.   Olivares, M.; Neef, A.; Castillejo, G.; Palma, G.D.; Varea, V.; Capilla, A.; Palau, F.; Nova, E.; Marcos, A.; Polanco, I.; et al. The hla-dq2 genotype selects for early intestinal microbiota composition in infants at high risk of developing coeliac disease. *Gut* **2015**, *64*, 406–417. [CrossRef] [PubMed]

9.   Catassi, C.; Gatti, S.; Lionetti, E. World perspective and celiac disease epidemiology. *Dig. Dis.* **2015**, *33*, 141–146. [CrossRef] [PubMed]

10. Singh, P.; Arora, A.; Strand, T.A.; Leffler, D.A.; Catassi, C.; Green, P.H.; Kelly, C.P.; Ahuja, V.; Makharia, G.K. Global prevalence of celiac disease: Systematic review and meta-analysis. *Clin. Gastroenterol. Hepatol.* **2018**, *16*, 823–836.e2. [CrossRef] [PubMed]

11. Lauret, E.; Rodrigo, L. Celiac disease and autoimmune-associated conditions. *BioMed Res. Int.* **2013**, *2013*, 127589. [CrossRef] [PubMed]

12. Assa, A.; Frenkel-Nir, Y.; Tzur, D.; Katz, L.H.; Shamir, R. Large population study shows that adolescents with celiac disease have an increased risk of multiple autoimmune and nonautoimmune comorbidities. *Acta Paediatr.* **2017**, *106*, 967–972. [CrossRef] [PubMed]

13. Viljamaa, M.; Kaukinen, K.; Pukkala, E.; Hervonen, K.; Reunala, T.; Collin, P. Malignancies and mortality in patients with coeliac disease and dermatitis herpetiformis: 30-year population-based study. *Dig. Liver Dis.* **2006**, *38*, 374–380. [CrossRef] [PubMed]

14. Ilus, T.; Kaukinen, K.; Virta, L.J.; Pukkala, E.; Collin, P. Incidence of malignancies in diagnosed celiac patients: A population-based estimate. *Am. J. Gastroenterol.* **2014**, *109*, 1471–1477. [CrossRef] [PubMed]

15. Bai, J.C.; Fried, M.; Corazza, G.R.; Schuppan, D.; Farthing, M.; Catassi, C.; Greco, L.; Cohen, H.; Ciacci, C.; Eliakim, R.; et al. World gastroenterology organisation global guidelines on celiac disease. *J. Clin. Gastroenterol.* **2013**, *47*, 121–126. [CrossRef] [PubMed]

16. Pavlovic, M.; Berenji, K.; Bukurov, M. Screening of celiac disease in down syndrome—Old and new dilemmas. *World J. Clin. Cases* **2017**, *5*, 264–269. [CrossRef] [PubMed]

17. Jenkins, H.R.; Murch, S.H.; Beattie, R.M.; Coeliac Disease Working Group of British Society of Paediatric Gastroenterology, Hepatology and Nutrition. Diagnosing coeliac disease. *Arch. Dis. Child.* **2012**, *97*, 393–394. [CrossRef] [PubMed]

18. Elli, L.; Branchi, F.; Tomba, C.; Villalta, D.; Norsa, L.; Ferretti, F.; Roncoroni, L.; Bardella, M.T. Diagnosis of gluten related disorders: Celiac disease, wheat allergy and non-celiac gluten sensitivity. *World J. Gastroenterol.* **2015**, *21*, 7110–7119. [CrossRef] [PubMed]

19. Catassi, C.; Elli, L.; Bonaz, B.; Bouma, G.; Carroccio, A.; Castillejo, G.; Cellier, C.; Cristofori, F.; de Magistris, L.; Dolinsek, J.; et al. Diagnosis of non-celiac gluten sensitivity (ncgs): The salerno experts' criteria. *Nutrients* **2015**, *7*, 4966–4977. [CrossRef] [PubMed]

20. Nijeboer, P.; Bontkes, H.J.; Mulder, C.J.; Bouma, G. Non-celiac gluten sensitivity. Is it in the gluten or the grain? *J. Gastrointest. Liver Dis.* **2013**, *22*, 435–440.

21. Cianferoni, A. Wheat allergy: Diagnosis and management. *J. Asthma Allergy* **2016**, *9*, 13–25. [CrossRef] [PubMed]

22. Pietzak, M. Celiac disease, wheat allergy, and gluten sensitivity: When gluten free is not a fad. *JPEN J. Parenter. Enter. Nutr.* **2012**, *36*, 68s–75s. [CrossRef] [PubMed]

23. Jackson, J.R.; Eaton, W.W.; Cascella, N.G.; Fasano, A.; Kelly, D.L. Neurologic and psychiatric manifestations of celiac disease and gluten sensitivity. *Psychiatr. Q.* **2012**, *83*, 91–102. [CrossRef] [PubMed]

24. Zingone, F.; Swift, G.L.; Card, T.R.; Sanders, D.S.; Ludvigsson, J.F.; Bai, J.C. Psychological morbidity of celiac disease: A review of the literature. *United Eur. Gastroenterol. J.* **2015**, *3*, 136–145. [CrossRef] [PubMed]

25. Porcelli, B.; Verdino, V.; Bossini, L.; Terzuoli, L.; Fagiolini, A. Celiac and non-celiac gluten sensitivity: A review on the association with schizophrenia and mood disorders. *Auto Immun. Highlights* **2014**, *5*, 55–61. [CrossRef] [PubMed]

26. Cossu, G.; Carta, M.G.; Contu, F.; Mela, Q.; Demelia, L.; Elli, L.; Dell'Osso, B. Coeliac disease and psychiatric comorbidity: Epidemiology, pathophysiological mechanisms, quality-of-life, and gluten-free diet effects. *Int. Rev. Psychiatry* **2017**, *29*, 489–503. [CrossRef] [PubMed]

27. Brietzke, E.; Cerqueira, R.O.; Mansur, R.B.; McIntyre, R.S. Gluten related illnesses and severe mental disorders: A comprehensive review. *Neurosci. Biobehav. Rev.* **2018**, *84*, 368–375. [CrossRef] [PubMed]

28. Da Silva Kotze, L.M.; David Paiva, A.D.; Roberto Kotze, L. Emotional disturbances in children and adolescents with celiac disease. *Rev. Bras. Med. Psicossom.* **2000**, *4*, 9–15.

29. Horvath-Stolarczyk, A.; Sidor, K.; Dziechciarz, P.; Siemińska, J. Assessment of emotional status, selected personality traits and depression in young adults with celiac disease. *Pediatr. Wspolcz.* **2002**, *4*, 241–246.

30. Pavone, L.; Fiumara, A.; Bottaro, G.; Mazzone, D.; Coleman, M. Autism and celiac disease: Failure to validate the hypothesis that a link might exist. *Biol. Psychiatry* **1997**, *42*, 72–75. [CrossRef]

31. Ludvigsson, J.F.; Osby, U.; Ekbom, A.; Montgomery, S.M. Coeliac disease and risk of schizophrenia and other psychosis: A general population cohort study. *Scand. J. Gastroenterol.* **2007**, *42*, 179–185. [CrossRef] [PubMed]

32. Pynnönen, P.A.; Isometsä, E.T.; Aronen, E.T.; Verkasalo, M.A.; Savilahti, E.; Aalberg, V.A. Mental disorders in adolescents with celiac disease. *Psychosomatics* **2004**, *45*, 325–335. [CrossRef] [PubMed]

33. Accomando, S.; Fragapane, M.L.; Montaperto, D.; Trizzino, A.; Amato, G.M.; Calderone, F.; Accomando, I. Coeliac disease and depression: Two related entities? *Dig. Liver Dis.* **2005**, *37*, 298–299. [CrossRef] [PubMed]

34. Ludvigsson, J.F.; Reutfors, J.; Osby, U.; Ekbom, A.; Montgomery, S.M. Coeliac disease and risk of mood disorders—A general population-based cohort study. *J. Affect. Disord.* **2007**, *99*, 117–126. [CrossRef] [PubMed]

35. Fidan, T.; Ertekin, V.; Karabag, K. Depression-anxiety levels and the quality of life among children and adolescents with coeliac disease. *Dusunen Adam* **2013**, *26*, 232–238. [CrossRef]

36. Esenyel, S.; Unal, F.; Vural, P. Depression and anxiety in child and adolescents with follow-up celiac disease and in their families. *Turk. J. Gastroenterol.* **2014**, *25*, 381–385. [CrossRef] [PubMed]

37. Simsek, S.; Baysoy, G.; Gencoglan, S.; Uluca, U. Effects of gluten-free diet on quality of life and depression in children with celiac disease. *J. Pediatr. Gastroenterol. Nutr.* **2015**, *61*, 303–306. [CrossRef] [PubMed]

38. Smith, L.B.; Lynch, K.F.; Kurppa, K.; Koletzko, S.; Krischer, J.; Liu, E.; Johnson, S.B.; Agardh, D.; Rewers, M.; Bautista, K.; et al. Psychological manifestations of celiac disease autoimmunity in young children. *Pediatrics* **2017**, *139*, e20162848. [CrossRef] [PubMed]

39. Wagner, G.; Zeiler, M.; Berger, G.; Huber, W.D.; Favaro, A.; Santonastaso, P.; Karwautz, A. Eating disorders in adolescents with celiac disease: Influence of personality characteristics and coping. *Eur. Eat. Disord. Rev.* **2015**, *23*, 361–370. [CrossRef] [PubMed]

40. Babio, N.; Alcázar, M.; Castillejo, G.; Recasens, M.; Martínez-Cerezo, F.; Gutiérrez-Pensado, V.; Vaqué, C.; Vila-Martí, A.; Torres-Moreno, M.; Sánchez, E.; et al. Risk of eating disorders in patients with celiac disease. *J. Pediatr. Gastroenterol. Nutr.* **2018**, *66*, 53–57. [CrossRef] [PubMed]

41. Terrone, G.; Parente, I.; Romano, A.; Auricchio, R.; Greco, L.; Del Giudice, E. The pediatric symptom checklist as screening tool for neurological and psychosocial problems in a paediatric cohort of patients with coeliac disease. *Acta Paediatr. Int. J. Paediatr.* **2013**, *102*, e325–e328. [CrossRef] [PubMed]

42. Ruggieri, M.; Incorpora, G.; Polizzi, A.; Parano, E.; Spina, M.; Pavone, P. Low prevalence of neurologic and psychiatric manifestations in children with gluten sensitivity. *J. Pediatr.* **2008**, *152*, 244–249. [CrossRef] [PubMed]

43. Mazzone, L.; Reale, L.; Spina, M.; Guarnera, M.; Lionetti, E.; Martorana, S.; Mazzone, D. Compliant gluten-free children with celiac disease: An evaluation of psychological distress. *BMC Pediatr.* **2011**, *11*, 46. [CrossRef] [PubMed]

44. Butwicka, A.; Lichtenstein, P.; Frisen, L.; Almqvist, C.; Larsson, H.; Ludvigsson, J.F. Celiac disease is associated with childhood psychiatric disorders: A population-based study. *J. Pediatr.* **2017**, *184*, 87–93.e81. [CrossRef] [PubMed]

45. Zelnik, N.; Pacht, A.; Obeid, R.; Lerner, A. Range of neurologic disorders in patients with celiac disease. *Pediatrics* **2004**, *113*, 1672–1676. [CrossRef] [PubMed]

46. Ludvigsson, J.F.; Reichenberg, A.; Hultman, C.M.; Murray, J.A. A nationwide study of the association between celiac disease and the risk of autistic spectrum disorders. *JAMA Psychiatry* **2013**, *70*, 1224–1230. [CrossRef] [PubMed]

47. West, J.; Logan, R.F.; Hubbard, R.B.; Card, T.R. Risk of schizophrenia in people with coeliac disease, ulcerative colitis and crohn's disease: A general population-based study. *Aliment. Pharmacol. Ther.* **2006**, *23*, 71–74. [CrossRef] [PubMed]

48. Eaton, W.W.; Byrne, M.; Ewald, H.; Mors, O.; Chen, C.Y.; Agerbo, E.; Mortensen, P.B. Association of schizophrenia and autoimmune diseases: Linkage of danish national registers. *Am. J. Psychiatry* **2006**, *163*, 521–528. [CrossRef] [PubMed]

49. Benros, M.E.; Nielsen, P.R.; Nordentoft, M.; Eaton, W.W.; Dalton, S.O.; Mortensen, P.B. Autoimmune diseases and severe infections as risk factors for schizophrenia: A 30-year population-based register study. *Am. J. Psychiatry* **2011**, *168*, 1303–1310. [CrossRef] [PubMed]

50. Wijarnpreecha, K.; Jaruvongvanich, V.; Cheungpasitporn, W.; Ungprasert, P. Association between celiac disease and schizophrenia: A meta-analysis. *Eur. J. Gastroenterol. Hepatol.* **2018**, *30*, 442–446. [CrossRef] [PubMed]

51. Hallert, C.; Aström, J. Psychic disturbances in adult coeliac disease. II. Psychological findings. *Scand. J. Gastroenterol.* **1982**, *17*, 21–24. [CrossRef] [PubMed]

52. Hallert, C.; Aström, J.; Walan, A. Reversal of psychopathology in adult coeliac disease with the aid of pyridoxine (vitamin b6). *Scand. J. Gastroenterol.* **1983**, *18*, 299–304. [CrossRef] [PubMed]

53. Addolorato, G.; Stefanini, G.F.; Capristo, E.; Caputo, F.; Gasbarrini, A.; Gasbarrini, G. Anxiety and depression in adult untreated celiac subjects and in patients affected by inflammatory bowel disease: A personality "trait" or a reactive illness? *Hepato-Gastroenterology* **1996**, *43*, 1513–1517. [PubMed]

54. Ciacci, C.; Iavarone, A.; Mazzacca, G.; De Rosa, A. Depressive symptoms in adult coeliac disease. *Scand. J. Gastroenterol.* **1998**, *33*, 247–250. [CrossRef] [PubMed]

55. Addolorato, G.; Capristo, E.; Ghittoni, G.; Valeri, C.; Masciana, R.; Ancona, C.; Gasbarrini, G. Anxiety but not depression decreases in celiac patients after one-year gluten-free diet: A longitudinal study. *Scand. J. Gastroenterol.* **2001**, *36*, 502–506. [CrossRef] [PubMed]

56. Cicarelli, G.; Della Rocca, G.; Amboni, M.; Ciacci, C.; Mazzacca, G.; Filla, A.; Barone, P. Clinical and neurological abnormalities in adult celiac disease. *Neurol. Sci.* **2003**, *24*, 311–317. [CrossRef] [PubMed]

57. Carta, M.G.; Hardoy, M.C.; Boi, M.F.; Mariotti, S.; Carpiniello, B.; Usai, P. Association between panic disorder, major depressive disorder and celiac disease: A possible role of thyroid autoimmunity. *J. Psychosom. Res.* **2002**, *53*, 789–793. [CrossRef]

58. Carta, M.G.; Hardoy, M.C.; Usai, P.; Carpiniello, B.; Angst, J. Recurrent brief depression in celiac disease. *J. Psychosom. Res.* **2003**, *55*, 573–574. [CrossRef]

59. Addolorato, G.; Mirijello, A.; D'Angelo, C.; Leggio, L.; Ferrulli, A.; Vonghia, L.; Cardone, S.; Leso, V.; Miceli, A.; Gasbarrini, G. Social phobia in celiac disease. *Scand. J. Gastroenterol.* **2008**, *43*, 410–415. [CrossRef] [PubMed]

60. Garud, S.; Leffler, D.; Dennis, M.; Edwards-George, J.; Saryan, D.; Sheth, S.; Schuppan, D.; Jamma, S.; Kelly, C.P. Interaction between psychiatric and autoimmune disorders in coeliac disease patients in the northeastern united states. *Aliment. Pharmacol. Ther.* **2009**, *29*, 898–905. [CrossRef] [PubMed]

61. Smith, D.F.; Gerdes, L.U. Meta-analysis on anxiety and depression in adult celiac disease. *Acta Psychiatr. Scand.* **2012**, *125*, 189–193. [CrossRef] [PubMed]

62. Peters, S.L.; Biesiekierski, J.R.; Yelland, G.W.; Muir, J.G.; Gibson, P.R. Randomised clinical trial: Gluten may cause depression in subjects with non-coeliac gluten sensitivity—An exploratory clinical study. *Aliment. Pharmacol. Ther.* **2014**, *39*, 1104–1112. [CrossRef] [PubMed]

63. Carta, M.G.; Conti, A.; Lecca, F.; Sancassiani, F.; Cossu, G.; Carruxi, R.; Boccone, A.; Cadoni, M.; Pisanu, A.; Moro, M.F.; et al. The burden of depressive and bipolar disorders in celiac disease. *Clin. Pract. Epidemiol. Ment. Health* **2015**, *11*, 180–185. [CrossRef] [PubMed]

64. Di Sabatino, A.; Volta, U.; Salvatore, C.; Biancheri, P.; Caio, G.; De Giorgio, R.; Di Stefano, M.; Corazza, G.R. Small amounts of gluten in subjects with suspected nonceliac gluten sensitivity: A randomized, double-blind, placebo-controlled, cross-over trial. *Clin. Gastroenterol. Hepatol.* **2015**, *13*, 1604–1612.e1603. [CrossRef] [PubMed]

65. Tortora, R.; Imperatore, N.; Ciacci, C.; Zingone, F.; Capone, P.; Leo, M.; Pellegrini, L.; De Stefano, G.; Caporaso, N.; Rispo, A. High prevalence of post-partum depression in coeliac women. *Dig. Liver Dis.* **2013**, *45*, S120. [CrossRef]

66. Sainsbury, K.; Marques, M.M. The relationship between gluten free diet adherence and depressive symptoms in adults with coeliac disease: A systematic review with meta-analysis. *Appetite* **2018**, *120*, 578–588. [CrossRef] [PubMed]

67. Passananti, V.; Siniscalchi, M.; Zingone, F.; Bucci, C.; Tortora, R.; Iovino, P.; Ciacci, C. Prevalence of eating disorders in adults with celiac disease. *Gastroenterol. Res. Pract.* **2013**, *2013*, 491657. [CrossRef] [PubMed]

68. Satherley, R.M.; Howard, R.; Higgs, S. The prevalence and predictors of disordered eating in women with coeliac disease. *Appetite* **2016**, *107*, 260–267. [CrossRef] [PubMed]

69. Marild, K.; Størdal, K.; Bulik, C.M.; Rewers, M.; Ekbom, A.; Liu, E.; Ludvigsson, J.F. Celiac disease and anorexia nervosa: A nationwide study. *Pediatrics* **2017**, *139*, e20164367. [CrossRef] [PubMed]

70. Marild, K.; Morgenthaler, T.I.; Somers, V.K.; Kotagal, S.; Murray, J.A.; Ludvigsson, J.F. Increased use of hypnotics in individuals with celiac disease: A nationwide case-control study. *BMC Gastroenterol.* **2015**, *15*, 10. [CrossRef] [PubMed]

71. Roos, S.; Karner, A.; Hallert, C. Psychological well-being of adult coeliac patients treated for 10 years. *Dig. Liver Dis.* **2006**, *38*, 177–180. [CrossRef] [PubMed]

72. Gili, M.; Béjar, L.; Ramirez, G.; Lopez, J.; Cabanillas, J.L.; Sharp, B. Celiac disease and alcohol use disorders: Increased length of hospital stay, overexpenditures and attributable mortality. *Rev. Esp. Enferm. Dig.* **2013**, *105*, 537–543. [CrossRef] [PubMed]

73. Lebwohl, B.; Luchsinger, J.A.; Freedberg, D.E.; Green, P.H.; Ludvigsson, J.F. Risk of dementia in patients with celiac disease: A population-based cohort study. *J. Alzheimer's Dis.* **2016**, *49*, 179–185. [CrossRef] [PubMed]

74. Fera, T.; Cascio, B.; Angelini, G.; Martini, S.; Guidetti, C.S. Affective disorders and quality of life in adult coeliac disease patients on a gluten-free diet. *Eur. J. Gastroenterol. Hepatol.* **2003**, *15*, 1287–1292. [CrossRef] [PubMed]

75. Sainsbury, K.; Mullan, B.; Sharpe, L. Reduced quality of life in coeliac disease is more strongly associated with depression than gastrointestinal symptoms. *J. Psychosom. Res.* **2013**, *75*, 135–141. [CrossRef] [PubMed]

76. Zylberberg, H.M.; Demmer, R.T.; Murray, J.A.; Green, P.H.R.; Lebwohl, B. Depression and insomnia among individuals with celiac disease or on a gluten-free diet in the United States: Results from the national health and nutrition examination survey (nhanes) 2009–2014. *Gastroenterology* **2017**, *152*, S482–S483. [CrossRef]

77. Dickson, B.C.; Streutker, C.J.; Chetty, R. Coeliac disease: An update for pathologists. *J. Clin. Pathol.* **2006**, *59*, 1008–1016. [CrossRef] [PubMed]

78. Leffler, D.A.; Green, P.H.; Fasano, A. Extraintestinal manifestations of coeliac disease. *Nat. Rev. Gastroenterol. Hepatol.* **2015**, *12*, 561–571. [CrossRef] [PubMed]

79. Scott, J.G.; Mihalopoulos, C.; Erskine, H.E.; Roberts, J.; Rahman, A. Childhood mental and developmental disorders. In *Mental, Neurological, and Substance Use Disorders: Disease Control Priorities*, 3rd ed.; Patel, V., Chisholm, D., Dua, T., Laxminarayan, R., Medina-Mora, M.E., Eds.; The World Bank: Washington, DC, USA, 2016; Volume 4.

80. Egede, L.E. Major depression in individuals with chronic medical disorders: Prevalence, correlates and association with health resource utilization, lost productivity and functional disability. *Gen. Hosp. Psychiatry* **2007**, *29*, 409–416. [CrossRef] [PubMed]

81. Katon, W.J. Epidemiology and treatment of depression in patients with chronic medical illness. *Dialog. Clin. Neurosci.* **2011**, *13*, 7–23.

82. Kang, H.J.; Kim, S.Y.; Bae, K.Y.; Kim, S.W.; Shin, I.S.; Yoon, J.S.; Kim, J.M. Comorbidity of depression with physical disorders: Research and clinical implications. *Chonnam Med. J.* **2015**, *51*, 8–18. [CrossRef] [PubMed]

83. Karwautz, A.; Wagner, G.; Berger, G.; Sinnreich, U.; Grylli, V.; Huber, W.D. Eating pathology in adolescents with celiac disease. *Psychosomatics* **2008**, *49*, 399–406. [CrossRef] [PubMed]

84. Hudson, J.I.; Hiripi, E.; Pope, H.G., Jr.; Kessler, R.C. The prevalence and correlates of eating disorders in the national comorbidity survey replication. *Biol. Psychiatry* **2007**, *61*, 348–358. [CrossRef] [PubMed]

85. Chen, S.J.; Chao, Y.L.; Chen, C.Y.; Chang, C.M.; Wu, E.C.; Wu, C.S.; Yeh, H.H.; Chen, C.H.; Tsai, H.J. Prevalence of autoimmune diseases in in-patients with schizophrenia: Nationwide population-based study. *Br. J. Psychiatry* **2012**, *200*, 374–380. [CrossRef] [PubMed]

86. Ergun, C.; Urhan, M.; Ayer, A. A review on the relationship between gluten and schizophrenia: Is gluten the cause? *Nutr. Neurosci.* **2017**. [CrossRef] [PubMed]

87. Cascella, N.G.; Kryszak, D.; Bhatti, B.; Gregory, P.; Kelly, D.L.; Mc Evoy, J.P.; Fasano, A.; Eaton, W.W. Prevalence of celiac disease and gluten sensitivity in the united states clinical antipsychotic trials of intervention effectiveness study population. *Schizophr. Bull.* **2011**, *37*, 94–100. [CrossRef] [PubMed]

88. Kalaydjian, A.E.; Eaton, W.; Cascella, N.; Fasano, A. The gluten connection: The association between schizophrenia and celiac disease. *Acta Psychiatr. Scand.* **2006**, *113*, 82–90. [CrossRef] [PubMed]

89. Kaplan, B.J.; Crawford, S.G.; Field, C.J.; Simpson, J.S. Vitamins, minerals, and mood. *Psychol. Bull.* **2007**, *133*, 747–760. [CrossRef] [PubMed]

90. Wierdsma, N.J.; van Bokhorst-de van der Schueren, M.A.; Berkenpas, M.; Mulder, C.J.; van Bodegraven, A.A. Vitamin and mineral deficiencies are highly prevalent in newly diagnosed celiac disease patients. *Nutrients* **2013**, *5*, 3975–3992. [CrossRef] [PubMed]

91. Najjar, S.; Pearlman, D.M.; Alper, K.; Najjar, A.; Devinsky, O. Neuroinflammation and psychiatric illness. *J. Neuroinflam.* **2013**, *10*, 43. [CrossRef] [PubMed]

92. Grenham, S.; Clarke, G.; Cryan, J.F.; Dinan, T.G. Brain-gut-microbe communication in health and disease. *Front. Physiol.* **2011**, *2*, 94. [CrossRef] [PubMed]

93. Heyman, M.; Abed, J.; Lebreton, C.; Cerf-Bensussan, N. Intestinal permeability in coeliac disease: Insight into mechanisms and relevance to pathogenesis. *Gut* **2012**, *61*, 1355–1364. [CrossRef] [PubMed]

94. Leffler, D.A.; Edwards-George, J.; Dennis, M.; Schuppan, D.; Cook, F.; Franko, D.L.; Blom-Hoffman, J.; Kelly, C.P. Factors that influence adherence to a gluten-free diet in adults with celiac disease. *Dig. Dis. Sci.* **2008**, *53*, 1573–1581. [CrossRef] [PubMed]

95. Lebwohl, B.; Ludvigsson, J.F.; Green, P.H. Celiac disease and non-celiac gluten sensitivity. *BMJ* **2015**, *351*, h4347. [CrossRef] [PubMed]

96. Ludvigsson, J.F.; Sellgren, C.; Runeson, B.; Langstrom, N.; Lichtenstein, P. Increased suicide risk in coeliac disease—A Swedish nationwide cohort study. *Dig. Liver Dis.* **2011**, *43*, 616–622. [CrossRef] [PubMed]

5

Relevance of HLA-DQB1*02 Allele in the Genetic Predisposition of Children with Celiac Disease: Additional Cues from a Meta-Analysis

Cristina Capittini [1], Annalisa De Silvestri [1], Chiara Rebuffi [2], Carmine Tinelli [1] and Dimitri Poddighe [3,*]

[1] Scientific Direction, Clinical Epidemiology and Biometric Unit, Fondazione IRCCS Policlinico San Matteo, 27100 Pavia, Italy; C.Capittini@smatteo.pv.it (C.C.); a.desilvestri@smatteo.pv.it (A.D.S.); ctinelli@smatteo.pv.it (C.T.)

[2] Grant Office and Scientific Documentation Center, Fondazione IRCCS Policlinico San Matteo, 27100 Pavia, Italy; C.Rebuffi@smatteo.pv.it

[3] Department of Medicine, Nazarbayev University School of Medicine, Nur-Sultan City 010000, Kazakhstan

[*] Correspondence: dimitri.poddighe@nu.edu.kz

Abstract: *Background and Objectives:* Celiac disease (CD) is a multifactorial immune-mediated disorder, triggered by the ingestion of gluten in genetically-predisposed subjects carrying MHC-DQ2 and -DQ8 heterodimers, which are encoded by four HLA-DQ allelic variants, overall. This meta-analysis aims at providing further epidemiological support to the predominant relevance of one specific allele, namely HLA-DQB1*02, in the predisposition and genetic risk of CD. *Materials and Methods:* We performed a search of MEDLINE/PubMed, Embase, Web of Science, and Scopus, retrieving all publications (case–control study, cross-sectional, and retrospective cohort study) on the association between HLA class II polymorphisms and first-degree relatives (FDRs) of children with CD. After a critical reading of the articles, two investigators independently performed data extraction according to the following inclusion criteria: HLA class II genes, any DQ and DR molecules, and CD diagnosed following the current clinical guidelines. A third participant was consulted for discussion to reach an agreement concerning discrepancies. *Results:* Our search strategy selected 14 studies as being eligible for inclusion, and those were submitted for data extraction and analysis. These studies were published between 1999 and 2016 and, collectively, enrolled 3063 FDRs. Positive and negative likelihood ratios (LR+ and LR−, respectively) for CD diagnosis, according to the presence of the HLA-DQ genotype coding a complete MHC-DQ2 and/or MHC-DQ8 molecules, were 1.449 (CI 1.279–1.642) and 0.187 (CI 0.096–0.362), respectively. If only the isolated presence of HLA-DQB1*02 allele is considered, the pooled estimation of LR+ was 1.659 (CI 1.302–2.155) and, importantly, the LR− still showed a very good discriminatory power of 0.195 (CI 0.068–0.558). *Conclusions:* Through our differential meta-analysis, comparing the presence of the genotype coding the full MHC-DQ2 and/or DQ8 molecules with the isolated presence of HLA-DQB1*02 allelic variant, we found that the LR− of the latter analysis maintained the same value. This observation, along with previous evidences, might be useful to consider potential cost-effective widened screening strategies for CD in children.

Keywords: celiac disease; children; HLA-DQB1*02; screening; first-degree relatives

1. Introduction

Celiac disease (CD) is a multifactorial immune-mediated disorder, triggered by the ingestion of gluten and other gluten-related proteins in genetically predisposed subjects. Importantly, the HLA-DQ alleles, coding α and β chains of the MHC-DQ2 and -DQ8 heterodimers, have been shown to be a necessary, but not sufficient, immunogenetic background for the development of CD. These HLA-DQ haplotypes have been estimated to contribute up to 25%–40% of the genetic risk for CD and have been reported to be present in around 35–40% of the general population in North America and Europe, where the prevalence of CD is close to 1% and, probably, even more if only the pediatric population is considered [1,2].

In particular, children are a vulnerable population with respect to the complications and long-term consequences of untreated CD, taking into account also their longer life-expectancy. Moreover, in addition to gastrointestinal symptoms, a considerable number of patients with CD present extra-gastrointestinal manifestations only (leading to under-diagnosis and/or significant diagnostic delays), and some patients may be completely asymptomatic, although they often report a subjective improvement after starting a gluten-free diet. Long-term complications of untreated CD are plausible, but there are still few studies addressing this specific issue [2–6].

All these epidemiological and clinical aspects have stimulated the scientific debate about the possibility to implement a wider screening strategy to identify CD patients, especially in children. Indeed, the screening approach by active case-finding, limited to the first-degree relatives (FDRs) of CD patients and children affected with other autoimmune diseases or chromosomal aberrations (known to be statistically associated with CD), was only partially effective as most asymptomatic or mildly symptomatic patients have no clear risk factors and, thus, cannot be detected [7,8]. However, extending the serological screening to all children and repeating it at several ages in childhood, is not a sustainable approach and, therefore, alternative strategies must be sought.

It is well known that HLA-DQ genotyping is useful to ascertain the susceptibility to CD with very high—if not absolute—discriminatory power. Indeed, it is very unlikely that individuals who do not carry any specific HLA-DQ alleles, coding MHC-DQ2 (HLA-DQA1*05 + HLA-DQB1*02) and MHC-DQ8 (HLA-DQA1*03 + HLA-DQB1*03:02) heterodimers, can develop CD [1,8]. Such a knowledge resulted to be very useful in the diagnostic approach to some complex cases (e.g. patients with antibody deficiencies) and, importantly, was able to avoid the duodenal biopsies in those children fulfilling some specific clinical and serological criteria, according to the ESPGHAN (European Society for Pediatric Gastroenterology, Hepatology and Nutrition) guidelines, published in 2012 [9]. Recently, several groups started to investigate the possibility to take advantage of specific HLA-DQ genetic analyses for a potential multi-step approach to extend the screening for CD to children who are not considered to be at higher risk, as defined above. That may be feasible through a reduction of the costs for the genetic analysis, compared to the high-resolution HLA genotyping. For this purpose, one contributing factor may be limiting the genetic analysis to specific CD-predisposed HLA-DQ alleles and, in particular, to the HLA-DQB1*02 allele, which plays a relevant role in CD genetic predisposition, according to the risk gradient showed in Figure 1 [8,10–12]. Through this meta-analysis, we aim at providing further epidemiological support to this potential approach.

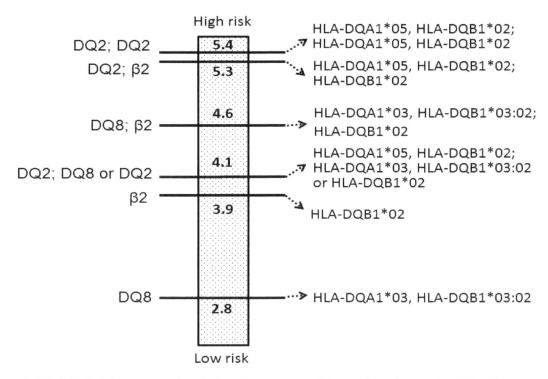

Figure 1. HLA-DQ risk gradient for Celiac Disease according to the odds-ratio (OR) values from our previous meta-analysis (modified from De Silvestri et al.).

2. Materials and Methods

2.1. Protocol

This work was written according to PRISMA guidelines [13], as described in Figure 2. Through this meta-analysis, we aimed at quantitatively evaluating the association between HLA-DQ polymorphisms and the susceptibility to CD in FDRs of pediatric CD patients.

2.2. Search Strategy

We performed a search of PubMed, EMBASE, Web of Science, and Scopus, retrieving all publications (case-control study, cross-sectional, and retrospective cohort study) on the association between HLA class II polymorphisms and first-degree relatives (FDRs) of CD children. We searched all articles published up to September 2018 in several languages (English, French, German, Italian, Portuguese, and Spanish).

We performed the search strategy using a free-text search (keywords) and thesaurus descriptors search (MeSH and Emtree) for each concept, adapted by a trained librarian for all the selected databases. In detail, an expert librarian performed the search by using the following terms: ("celiac disease" [MeSH] OR "celiac disease" [tiab] OR "coeliac disease" [tiab]) AND ("Histocompatibility Antigens Class II" [Mesh] OR "Histocompatibility Antigens Class II" [tiab]) AND ("nuclear family" [mesh] OR relative* [tiab] OR sibling* [tiab] OR parent* [tiab]) AND ("mass screening" [mesh] OR screening [tiab] OR prevalence[tiab] OR "Prevalence" [Mesh] OR "Predictive Value of Tests" [Mesh] OR "predictive value" [tiab]). In Embase, the search used the following terms: ('celiac disease'/exp OR 'celiac disease':ti,ab OR 'coeliac disease':ti,ab) AND ('HLA antigen class 2'/exp OR "Histocompatibility Antigens Class II":ti,ab) AND ('nuclear family'/exp OR relative*:ti,ab OR sibling*:ti,ab OR parent*:ti,ab) AND ('screening'/exp OR screening:ti,ab OR 'Prevalence'/exp OR prevalence:ti,ab OR 'predictive value'/exp OR 'predictive value':ti,ab). In Web of Science, the search used the following terms: ("celiac disease" OR "coeliac disease") AND HLA AND (relative* OR sibling* OR parent*) AND (screening OR prevalence OR "predictive value"). In Scopus, the search used the following terms: "celiac disease" OR "coeliac disease" AND HLA AND (relative* OR sibling* OR parent*) AND (screening OR prevalence OR "predictive value").

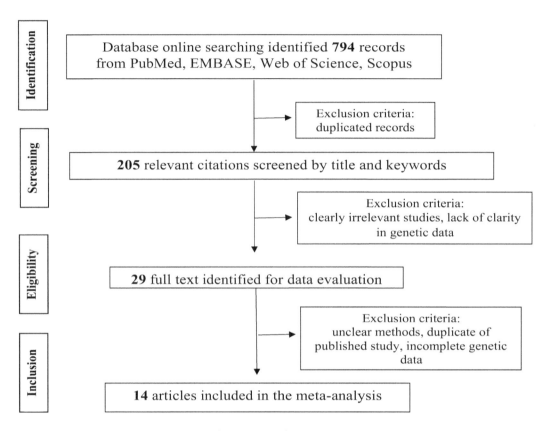

Figure 2. Flow diagram of the study following the PRISMA guidelines.

2.3. Data Extraction

After a critical reading of the articles, two investigators independently performed data extraction according to the following inclusion criteria: HLA class II genes, any DQ and DR molecules, and celiac disease diagnosed following the clinical criteria set by Meeuwisse (1969–1970), Walker-Smith et al. (1990–2012), and Husby et al. (2012 ESPGHAN guidelines) [9,14,15]. The third participant was consulted for discussion to reach an agreement concerning discrepancies.

2.4. Data Synthesis and Meta-Analysis

STATA 14.2 (StataCorp., College Station, TX, USA) and METADISC 1.4 were used for statistical analysis to perform meta-analysis the [16]. Heterogeneity was checked through the χ^2-test and the I-squared statistics [17]. The criteria for identification of heterogeneity were p values less than 0.10 for the χ^2-test and an I-squared value greater than 50%. When there was no statistical evidence for heterogeneity in effect sizes, we used the fixed-effect model to analyze odds ratios (ORs) or relative risks in FDRs. When significant heterogeneity was identified, we used the random-effects model (REM) and explored sources of significant heterogeneity [18,19].

We considered all studies including subjects analyzed for both the HLA-DQA1*05 and HLA-DQB1*02 alleles (coding the DQ2 molecule) and/or for the HLA-DQA1*03 and HLA-DQB1*03:02 alleles (coding the DQ8 molecule). For each selected study, we calculated sensitivity, specificity, positive likelihood ratio (LR+), and negative likelihood ratio (LR−) to develop CD. In order to produce clinically useful statistics, we calculated the pooled LR+ and LR− values. For all estimated values, we provided the 95% confidence interval (CI).

3. Results

3.1. Study Selection

Our search strategy yielded 794 papers for consideration. Following elimination of duplicates, 205 titles and/or abstracts were reviewed. Of these, 176 were excluded and, among the remaining 29 full-text manuscripts, 14 studies were deemed eligible for inclusion and were submitted to data extraction and analysis (refer to Figure 2). These studies were published between 1999 and 2016 and, collectively, enrolled 3063 FDRs. In detail, our analysis included three studies from India, two studies each from Chile, Italy, and Spain, and 1 study each from Brazil, Cuba, Jordan, Finland, and the USA [20–33].

Among the 3063 FDRs, 1720 patients were MHC-DQ2 or -DQ8 carriers, but only 352 were diagnosed with CD; among these, 337 patients were MHC-DQ2 or -DQ8 carriers. Thus, the prevalence of CD among FDRs was around 11.5% (CI 10–12).

3.2. Study Quality

The quality of selected studies, in terms of laboratory methods, methods description, statistical methodology and clinical features, was assessed according to PRISMA standards and resulted to be appropriate.

3.3. Meta-Analysis According to the Complete MHC-DQ2 and/or DQ8 Genotype

In our meta-analysis, we expressed these parameters as positive and negative likelihood ratios (LR+ and LR−, respectively) for CD, according to the presence of the HLA-DQ genotype coding complete MHC-DQ2 and/or MHC-DQ8 molecules. The pooled estimation of LR+ was 1.449 (CI 1.279–1.642), whereas LR− was 0.187 (0.096–0.362). While this HLA-DQ background is known to provide a low specificity (Table 1), its presence is actually characterized with very high sensitivity for CD, showing a good discriminatory power between genetically predisposed CD (not necessarily affected) patients and those who will not develop CD, as shown in Table 2.

Table 1. Positive likelihood ratio (LR+) of MHC-DQ2 and/or -DQ8 genotype in first-degree relatives (FDRs) of pediatric celiac disease (CD) patients (Heterogeneity χ^2 = 132.54 (d.f. = 13), p < 0.001; Inconsistency (I-squared) = 90.2%; and estimate of between-study variance (Tau-squared) = 0.0455).

Summary—Positive Likelihood Ratio (Random Effects Model)				
Study (Year)	Country	LR+	95% Conf. Interval	% Weight
Araya et al. (2015)	Chile	1.008	0.749–1.357	5.92
Araya et al. (2000)	Chile	7.557	4.475–12.762	3.47
Bonamico et al. (2006)	Italy	1.779	1.572–2.014	8.20
Cintado et al. (2006)	Cuba	1.054	0.809–1.372	6.38
Elakawi et al. (2010)	Jordan	1.487	1.061–2.084	5.40
Farre et al. (1999)	Spain	1.563	1.317–1.854	7.64
Karinen et al. (2006)	Finland		1.008–1.255	8.35
Martins et al. (2010)	Brazil	1.691	1.393–2.052	7.35
Megiorni et al. (2009)	Italy	1.707	1.590–1.832	8.67
Mishra et al. (2016)	India	1.304	1.126–1.511	7.94
Rubio-Tapia et al. (2010)	USA	1.413	1.302–1.533	8.59
Singla et al. (2016)	India	1.148	1.040–1.268	8.45
Srivastava et al. (2010)	India	1.063	0.783–1.443	5.82
Vaquero et al. (2014)	Spain	1.530	1.309–1.789	7.83
(REM) pooled LR+		1.449	1.279–1.642	

Table 2. Negative likelihood ratio (LR−) of MHC-DQ2 and/or -DQ8 genotype in FDRs of pediatric CD patients (Heterogeneity χ^2 = 20.34 (d.f. = 13), p = 0.087; inconsistency (I-squared) = 36.1%; and estimate of between-study variance (Tau-squared) = 0.4949).

Summary—Negative Likelihood Ratio (Random Effects Model)				
Study (Year)	Country	LR−	95% Conf. Interval	% Weight
Araya et al. (2015)	Chile	0.933	0.065–13.461	4.86
Araya et al. (2000)	Chile	0.081	0.006–1.178	4.86
Bonamico et al. (2006)	Italy	0.107	0.028–0.416	11.74
Cintado et al. (2006)	Cuba	0.641	0.041–10.017	4.64
Elakawi et al. (2010)	Jordan	0.217	0.015–3.170	4.83
Farre et al. (1999)	Spain	0.108	0.007–1.636	4.72
Karinen et al. (2006)	Finland	0.526	0.265–1.044	18.52
Martins et al. (2010)	Brazil	0.158	0.024–1.054	7.99
Megiorni et al. (2009)	Italy	0.044	0.006–0.310	7.73
Mishra et al. (2016)	India	0.188	0.047–0.757	11.43
Rubio-Tapia et al. (2010)	USA	0.042	0.003–0.656	4.61
Singla et al. (2016)	India	0.173	0.011–2.730	4.61
Srivastava et al. (2010)	India	0.652	0.045–9.460	4.85
Vaquero et al. (2014)	Spain	0.043	0.003–0.674	4.60
(REM) pooled LR−		0.187	0.096–0.362	

3.4. Meta-Analysis According to the Isolated Presence of HLA-DQB1*02 Allele

DQB1*02 sensitivity was 0.938 (CI 0.891–0.968) and specificity was 0.425 (CI 0.400–0.451). We meta-analyzed the LR+ and LR− of FDRs according to the presence of the DQB1*02 allele. The pooled estimate of LR+ was 1.659 (CI 1.302–2.155) (Table 3), whereas LR− showed a good discriminatory power of 0.195 (CI 0.068–0.558) (Table 4).

Table 3. Positive likelihood ratio (LR+) related to the DQB1*02 allele in FDRs of pediatric CD patients (Heterogeneity χ^2 = 89.02 (d.f. = 6), p < 0.001; inconsistency (I-squared) = 93.3%; and estimate of between-study variance (Tau-squared) = 0.0906).

Summary—Positive Likelihood Ratio (Random Effects Model)			
Study (Year)	LR+	95% Conf. Interval	% Weight
Araya et al. (2015)	7.557	4.475–12.762	9.44
Cintado et al. (2006)	1.054	0.809–1.372	14.07
Elakawi et al. (2010)	1.487	1.061–2.084	12.72
Farre et al. (1999)	1.563	1.317–1.854	15.58
Karinen et al. (2006)	1.125	1.008–1.255	16.32
Martins et al. (2010)	1.691	1.393–2.052	15.24
Megiorni et al. (2009)	1.707	1.590–1.832	16.64
(REM) pooled LR+	1.659	1.302–2.115	

Table 4. Negative likelihood ratio (LR−) related to the DQB1*02 allele in FDRs of pediatric CD patients (Heterogeneity χ^2 = 12.06 (d.f. = 6), p = 0.061; inconsistency (I-squared) = 50.2%; and estimate of between-study variance (Tau-squared) = 0.9053).

Summary—Negative Likelihood Ratio (Random Effects Model)			
Study (year)	LR−	95% Conf. Interval	% Weight
Araya et al. (2015)	0.081	0.006–1.178	10.43
Cintado et al. (2006)	0.641	0.041–10.017	10.03
Elakawi et al. (2010)	0.217	0.015–3.170	10.38
Farre et al. (1999)	0.108	0.007–1.636	10.18
Karinen et al. (2006)	0.526	0.265–1.044	28.05
Martins et al. (2010)	0.158	0.024–1.054	15.66
Megiorni et al. (2009)	0.044	0.006–0.310	15.26
(REM) pooled LR−	0.195	0.068–0.558	

4. Discussion

This meta-analysis confirmed the very high negative predictive value associated with the absence of the HLA-DQ genotype, coding MHC-DQ2 and/or -DQ8, as regards the risk to developing CD. This long-established knowledge has been exploited to complete and/or refine the diagnostic work-up of patients suspected to be affected with CD, but having doubtful histopathological findings or concomitant diseases that can impair the reliability of the serological screening (e.g., IgA deficiency, common variable immunodeficiency) [22,34]. More recently, this genetic analysis has been included in the ESPGHAN guidelines to diagnose CD without performing any duodenal biopsy in children with consistent symptoms, high-titer of anti-tTG IgA, and EMA positivity [9]. However, beyond these practical conditions, the poor positive predictive value of being carrier of MHC-DQ2 and/or -DQ8 heterodimers, cannot provide any additional usefulness to the diagnosis of CD, in addition to confirming the necessary genetic predisposition.

Additionally, in this meta-analysis we separately analyzed the positive and negative predictive values (expressed as positive and negative LRs, respectively) related to the presence and absence of the HLA-DQB1*02 allele. Recently, Megiorni et al. reviewed the role of HLA-DQA1 and HLA-DQB1 in the predisposition to CD. They described a risk gradient whereby patients who are DQ2/DQ8 heterozygous and DQ2 homozygous showed a very high risk and, to follow, there were patients who were DQ8 homozygous, DQ8 heterozygous, along with DQ2 heterozygous, and, then, people carrying a double dose of DQB1*02 only [35]. Importantly, these latter patients showed a similar risk of CD as the previous categories, although they did not carry the complete MHC-DQ2 or MHC-DQ8 heterodimer.

Recently, a previous meta-analysis by our group supported this observation: we showed that a double dose of HLA-DQB1*02 was associated with the highest risk to develop pediatric CD (OR > 5), regardless of other HLA-DQ alleles. Moreover, even a single "dose" of HLA-DQB1*02 was associated with a relatively high risk (OR around 4) for pediatric CD. Basically, our statistical analysis suggested that children carrying only one HLA-DQB1*02 copy (without any other allele related to MHC-DQ2 or MHC-DQ8 molecules) have a similar predisposition/risk to become celiac as children expressing the full MHC-DQ2 and/or MHC-DQ8 molecules [8]. Accordingly, the original research by Megiorni et al., including 437 Italian children with CD and 551 controls, described a disease risk of 1:26 for children being homozygous for HLA-DQB1*02 (despite the absence of the other genes coding for DQ2 or DQ8); children being double heterozygous DQ2/DQ8, heterozygous DQ2 with double dose HLA-DQB1*02, and DQ8 heterozygous along with one HLA-DQB1*02 allele, showed a disease risk of 1:7, 1:10, and 1:24, respectively [28]. Therefore, all these studies suggested a major relevance of HLA-DQB1*02 allele in conferring the risk to develop pediatric CD, rather than the expression of the full MHC-DQ2 and/or -DQ8 heterodimers. Moreover, a risk gradient according to the dose ("single" or "double" copy of HLA-DQB1*02) has been evidenced.

Through our differential meta-analysis, comparing the presence of the full MHC-DQ2 and/or DQ8 genotypes and the isolated presence of HLA-DQB1*02 allelic variant, we found that the negative LR (namely the negative predictive value) was basically the same (0.187 vs. 0.195). Unfortunately, we could not obtain enough data to perform the same statistical analysis considering the HLA-DQB1*03:02 solely, as its frequency in the general population and CD patients is much lower compared to the HLA-DQB1*02 allele.

However, some molecular studies supported this concept that HLA-DQB1*02 may play a major role in the interaction between class II MHC molecule and the gliadin-derived peptide to be presented to T-lymphocytes, in order to trigger all immunological events involved in the pathogenesis of CD [36]. Indeed, the high content of proline and glutamine residues of MHC-DQ2-restricted gliadin epitopes resulted to be fundamental for the interaction and binding to the class II MHC molecules. One research showed that some specific DQ2 β chain residues, participating in the formation of the peptide-binding cleft (particularly Arg-β70 and Lys-β71 of β chain encoded by HLA-DQB1*02), are mainly responsible for the interaction with several residues of the gliadin epitope and, thus, may be critical to the CD predisposition [37].

Previously, we showed that 90–95% of CD children seem to carry at least a single copy of HLA-DQB1*02, regardless of the remaining HLA-DQ genotype [8]. Moreover, we supported this finding in our monocentric case series, including 269 children with CD, where >97% of all these CD children possessed at least one copy of HLA-DQB1*02 allele in their individual genotype [38]. Here, we looked at the HLA-DQ asset in the FDRs of pediatric CD patients and we found that the almost absolute negative LR was maintained, even when we considered only HLA-DQB1*02 in our analysis. This comparison suggests that the absence of this allele from the individual HLA-DQ genotype might rule out any individual predisposition to develop CD, as well as the analysis of the full genotype coding complete MHC-DQ2/DQ8 heterodimer(s) can do, without any significant decrease in the negative predictive value for CD.

These observations may contribute to the debate about the potential and cost-effective implementation of wider or mass-screening strategies for CD in children. Indeed, a low-cost HLA-DQ analysis, specific for CD predisposition, may allow to select those 30–40% of children who really deserve the serological screening [39–41].

The qualitative analysis to screen the presence of HLA-DQB1*02 in order to establish the genetic predisposition in the general population, may be one potential approach, and the complete HLA-DQ genotyping might be reserved to children with clinical suspicion, if needed [8,10,12]. Of course, further epidemiological, clinical and genetic researches are required in order to establish if this approach may be appropriate, feasible and cost-effective. However, other researchers considered a potential multi-step approach to screen CD, starting from the analysis of the specific genetic predisposition to CD through low-cost molecular methods. Recently, Verma et al. proposed a rapid HLA-DQ typing method to identify subjects genetically susceptible to CD. Basically, they performed a PCR through a kit containing the primers for the HLA-DQ target alleles only, on blood samples from CD patients, FDRs and controls. They could show an excellent concordance with the results obtained through conventional high-resolution HLA-DQ typing, in terms of presence or absence of HLA-DQ2 and HLA-DQ8 alleles [11]. The implementation of cost-effective screening strategies may be very helpful, not only in Western countries (where CD has been widely studied and described), but also in developing countries, where a number of health system-related barriers have not permitted an evidence-based approach to the diagnosis of CD, yet [42–44].

Therefore, if our observations will be supported by further and independent studies, those may represent an additional contribution to reduce the cost of a targeted genetic analysis for CD.

5. Conclusions

Through a differential meta-analysis, comparing the presence of the genotype coding the full MHC-DQ2 and/or DQ8 molecules and the isolated presence of HLA-DQB1*02 allelic variant, we found that the LR− of the latter analysis maintained the same value. This observation, along with the previous evidences, might be useful to consider potential cost-effective widened screening strategies for CD in children.

Author Contributions: D.P. and C.C. conceived and wrote this manuscript; A.D.S. and C.T. analyzed data; C.R. made the systematic search; A.D.S. collected data and made the tables; C.C. made the figures; D.P. and C.T. provided substantial intellectual contribution; C.C., A.D.S., C.R., C.T., D.P. approved the manuscript.

References

1. Lindfors, K.; Ciacci, C.; Kurppa, K.; Lundin, K.E.A.; Makharia, G.K.; Mearin, M.L.; Murray, J.A.; Verdu, E.F.; Kaukinen, K. Coeliac disease. *Nat. Rev. Dis. Primers* **2019**, *5*, 3. [CrossRef] [PubMed]
2. Lebwohl, B.; Sanders, D.S.; Green, P.H.R. Coeliac disease. *Lancet* **2018**, *391*, 70–81. [CrossRef]
3. Ludvigsson, J.F. Mortality and malignancy in celiac disease. *Gastrointest. Endosc. Clin. N. Am.* **2012**, *22*, 705–722. [CrossRef]
4. Abdul Sultan, A.; Crooks, C.J.; Card, T.; Tata, L.J.; Fleming, K.M.; West, J. Causes of death in people with coeliac disease in England compared with the general population: A competing risk analysis. *Gut* **2015**, *64*, 1220–1226. [CrossRef] [PubMed]
5. Paarlahti, P.; Kurppa, K.; Ukkola, A.; Collin, P.; Huhtala, H.; Mäki, M.; Kaukinen, K. Predictors of persistent symptoms and reduced quality of life in treated coeliac disease patients: A large cross-sectional study. *BMC Gastroenterol.* **2013**, *13*, 75. [CrossRef]
6. Stordal, K.; Bakken, I.J.; Suren, P. Epidemiology of coeliac disease and comorbidity in Norwegian children. *J. Pediatr. Gastroenterol. Nutr.* **2013**, *57*, 467–471. [CrossRef] [PubMed]
7. Bjorck, S.; Brundin, C.; Lorinc, E.; Lynch, K.F.; Agardh, D. Screening detects a high proportion of celiac disease in young HLA-genotyped children. *J. Pediatr. Gastroenterol. Nutr.* **2010**, *50*, 49–53. [CrossRef]
8. De Silvestri, A.; Capittini, C.; Poddighe, D.; Valsecchi, C.; Marseglia, G.; Tagliacarne, S.C.; Scotti, V.; Rebuffi, C.; Pasi, A.; Martinetti, M.; Tinelli, C. HLA-DQ genetics in children with celiac disease: A meta-analysis suggesting a two-step genetic screening procedure starting with HLA-DQ β chains. *Pediatr. Res.* **2018**, *83*, 564–572. [CrossRef]
9. Husby, S.; Koletzko, S.; Korponay-Szabó, I.R.; Mearin, M.L.; Phillips, A.; Shamir, R.; Troncone, R.; Giersiepen, K.; Branski, D.; Catassi, C.; et al. ESPGHAN Working Group on Coeliac Disease Diagnosis; ESPGHAN Gastroenterology Committee; European Society for Pediatric Gastroenterology, Hepatology, and Nutrition. European Society for Pediatric Gastroenterology, Hepatology, and Nutrition guidelines for the diagnosis of coeliac disease. *J. Pediatr. Gastroenterol. Nutr.* **2012**, *54*, 136–160. [PubMed]
10. Poddighe, D. Individual screening strategy for pediatric celiac disease. *Eur. J. Pediatr.* **2018**, *177*, 1871. [CrossRef] [PubMed]
11. Verma, A.K.; Singh, A.; Gatti, S.; Lionetti, E.; Galeazzi, T.; Monachesi, C.; Franceschini, E.; Ahuja, V.; Catassi, C.; Makharia, G.K. Validation of a novel single-drop rapid human leukocyte antigen-DQ2/-DQ8 typing method to identify subjects susceptible to celiac disease. *JGH Open* **2018**, *2*, 311–316. [CrossRef]
12. Poddighe, D. Relevance of HLA-DQB1*02 allele in predisposing to Coeliac Disease. *Int. J. Immunogenet.* **2019**, in press. [CrossRef]
13. Moher, D.; Liberati, A.; Tetzlaff, J.; Altman, D.G.; PRISMA Group. Preferred reporting items for systematic reviews and meta-analyses: The PRISMA statement. *J. Clin. Epidemiol.* **2009**, *62*, 1006–1012. [CrossRef]
14. Meeuwisse, G.W. Round table discussion. Diagnostic criteria in coeliac disease. *Acta Paediatr. Scand.* **1970**, *59*, 461–463.
15. Walker-Smith, J.A.; Guandalini, S.; Schmitz, J. Revised criteria for diagnosis of coeliac disease. *Arch. Dis. Child.* **1990**, *65*, 909–911.
16. Zamora, J.; Abraira, V.; Muriel, A.; Khan, K.; Coomarasamy, A. Meta-DiSc: A software for metaanalysis of test accuracy data. *BMC Med. Res. Methodol.* **2006**, *6*, 31. [CrossRef] [PubMed]
17. Higgins, J.P.; Thompson, S.G. Quantifying heterogeneity in a meta-analysis. *Stat. Med.* **2002**, *21*, 1539–1558. [CrossRef] [PubMed]

18.   Der Simonian, R.; Laird, N. Meta-analysis in clinical trials. *Control. Clin. Trials* **1986**, *7*, 177–188. [CrossRef]
19.   Higgins, J.P.T.; Green, S. Cochrane Handbook for Systematic Reviews of Interventions, Version 5.1.0 (updated March 2011). The Cochrane Collaboration. Available online: http://www.cochrane-handbook.org (accessed on 1 March 2015).
20.   Araya, M.; Oyarzun, A.; Lucero, Y.; Espinosa, N.; Pérez-Bravo, F. DQ2, DQ7 and DQ8 Distribution and Clinical Manifestations in Celiac Cases and Their First-Degree Relatives. *Nutrients* **2015**, *7*, 4955–4965. [CrossRef] [PubMed]
21.   Araya, M.; Mondragón, A.; Pérez-Bravo, F.; Roessler, J.L.; Alarcón, T.; Rios, G.; Bergenfreid, C. Celiac disease in a Chilean population carrying Amerindian traits. *J. Pediatr. Gastroenterol. Nutr.* **2000**, *31*, 381–386. [CrossRef]
22.   Bonamico, M.; Ferri, M.; Mariani, P.; Nenna, R.; Thanasi, E.; Luparia, R.P.; Picarelli, A.; Magliocca, F.M.; Mora, B.; Bardella, M.T.; Verrienti, A.; et al. Serologic and genetic markers of celiac disease: A sequential study in the screening of first degree relatives. *J. Pediatr. Gastroenterol. Nutr.* **2006**, *42*, 150–154. [CrossRef]
23.   Cintado, A.; Sorell, L.; Galván, J.A.; Martínez, L.; Castañeda, C.; Fragoso, T.; Camacho, H.; Ferrer, A.; Companioni, O.; Benitez, J.; et al. HLA DQA1*0501 and DQB1*02 in Cuban celiac patients. *Hum. Immunol.* **2006**, *67*, 639–642. [CrossRef]
24.   El-Akawi, Z.J.; Al-Hattab, D.M.; Migdady, M.A. Frequency of HLA-DQA1*0501 and DQB1*0201 alleles in patients with coeliac disease, their first-degree relatives and controls in Jordan. *Ann. Trop. Paediatr.* **2010**, *30*, 305–309. [CrossRef] [PubMed]
25.   Farré, C.; Humbert, P.; Vilar, P.; Varea, V.; Aldeguer, X.; Carnicer, J.; Carballo, M.; Gassull, M.A. Serological markers and HLA-DQ2 haplotype among first-degree relatives of celiac patients. *Dig. Dis. Sci.* **1999**, *44*, 2344–2349. [CrossRef] [PubMed]
26.   Karinen, H.; Kärkkäinen, P.; Pihlajamäki, J.; Janatuinen, E.; Heikkinen, M.; Julkunen, R.; Kosma, V.M.; Naukkarinen, A.; Laakso, M. HLA genotyping is useful in the evaluation of the risk for coeliac disease in the 1st-degree relatives of patients with coeliac disease. *Scand. J. Gastroenterol.* **2006**, *41*, 1299–1304. [CrossRef]
27.   Martins, R.C.; Gandolfi, L.; Modelli, I.C.; Almeida, R.C.; Castro, L.C.; Pratesi, R. Serologic screening and genetic testing among brazilian patients with celiac disease and their first degree relatives. *Arq. Gastroenterol.* **2010**, *47*, 257–262. [CrossRef]
28.   Megiorni, F.; Mora, B.; Bonamico, M.; Barbato, M.; Nenna, R.; Maiella, G.; Lulli, P.; Mazzilli, MC. HLA-DQ and risk gradient for celiac disease. *Hum. Immunol.* **2009**, *70*, 55–59. [CrossRef]
29.   Mishra, A.; Prakash, S.; Kaur, G.; Sreenivas, V.; Ahuja, V.; Gupta, S.D.; Makharia, G.K. Prevalence of celiac disease among first-degree relatives of Indian celiac disease patients. *Dig. Liver Dis.* **2016**, *48*, 255–259. [CrossRef]
30.   Rubio-Tapia, A.; Van Dyke, C.T.; Lahr, B.D.; Zinsmeister, A.R.; El-Youssef, M.; Moore, S.B.; Bowman, M.; Burgart, L.J.; Melton III, L.J.; Murray, J.A. Predictors of family risk for celiac disease: A population-based study. *Clin. Gastroenterol. Hepatol.* **2008**, *6*, 983–987. [CrossRef]
31.   Singla, S.; Kumar, P.; Singh, P.; Kaur, G.; Rohtagi, A.; Choudhury, M. HLA Profile of Celiac Disease among First-Degree Relatives from a Tertiary Care Center in North India. *Ind. J. Pediatr.* **2016**, *83*, 1248–1252. [CrossRef]
32.   Srivastava, A.; Yachha, S.K.; Mathias, A.; Parveen, F.; Poddar, U.; Agrawal, S. Prevalence, human leukocyte antigen typing and strategy for screening among Asian first-degree relatives of children with celiac disease. *J. Gastroenterol. Hepatol.* **2010**, *25*, 319–324. [CrossRef]
33.   Vaquero, L.; Caminero, A.; Nuñez, A.; Hernando, M.; Iglesias, C.; Casqueiro, J.; Vivas, S. Coeliac disease screening in first-degree relatives on the basis of biopsy and genetic risk. *Eur. J. Gastroenterol. Hepatol.* **2014**, *26*, 263–267. [CrossRef]
34.   Dorn, S.D.; Matchar, D.B. Cost-effectiveness analysis of strategies for diagnosing celiac disease. *Dig. Dis. Sci.* **2008**, *53*, 680–688. [CrossRef] [PubMed]
35.   Megiorni, F.; Pizzuti, A. HLA-DQA1 and HLA-DQB1 in Celiac disease predisposition: Practical implications of the HLA molecular typing. *J. Biomed. Sci.* **2012**, *19*, 88. [CrossRef]
36.   Vader, W.; Stepniak, D.; Kooy, Y.; Mearin, L.; Thompson, A.; van Rood, J.J.; Spaenij, L.; Koning, F. The HLA-DQ2 gene dose effect in celiac disease is directly related to the magnitude and breadth of gluten specific T cell responses. *Proc. Natl. Acad. Sci. USA* **2003**, *100*, 12390–12395. [CrossRef]

37. Sollid, L.M. Coeliac disease: Dissecting a complex inflammatory disorder. *Nat. Rev. Immunol.* **2002**, *2*, 647–655. [CrossRef]
38. Poddighe, D.; Capittini, C.; Gaviglio, I.; Brambilla, I.; Marseglia, G.L. HLA-DQB1*02 allele in children with Celiac Disease: Potential usefulness for screening strategies. *Int. J. Immunogenet.* **2019**, in press. [CrossRef]
39. Fernández-Fernández, S.; Borrell, B.; Cilleruelo, M.L.; Tabares, A.; Jiménez-Jiménez, J.; Rayo, A.I.; Perucho, T.; García-García, M.L. Prevalence of Celiac Disease in a Long-Term Study of a Spanish At-Genetic-Risk Cohort from the General Population. *J. Pediatr. Gastroenterol. Nutr.* **2019**, *68*, 364–370. [CrossRef]
40. Cilleruelo, M.L.; Fernández-Fernández, S.; Jiménez-Jiménez, J.; Rayo, A.I.; de Larramendi, C.H. Prevalence and Natural History of Celiac Disease in a Cohort of At-risk Children. *J. Pediatr. Gastroenterol. Nutr.* **2016**, *62*, 739–745. [CrossRef] [PubMed]
41. Wessels, M.M.S.; de Rooij, N.; Roovers, L.; Verhage, J.; de Vries, W.; Mearin, M.L. Towards an individual screening strategy for first-degree relatives of celiac patients. *Eur. J. Pediatr.* **2018**, *177*, 1585–1592. [CrossRef]
42. Makharia, G.K.; Catassi, C. Celiac Disease in Asia. Gastroenterol. *Clin. N. Am.* **2019**, *48*, 101–113.
43. Poddighe, D.; Rakhimzhanova, M.; Marchenko, Y.; Catassi, C. Pediatric Celiac Disease in Central and East Asia: Current Knowledge and Prevalence. *Medicina* **2019**, *55*, 11. [CrossRef]
44. Singh, P.; Arora, A.; Strand, T.A.; Leffler, DA.; Catassi, C.; Green, P.H.; Kelly, C.P.; Ahuja, V.; Makharia, G.K. Global Prevalence of Celiac Disease: Systematic Review and Meta-analysis. *Clin. Gastroenterol. Hepatol.* **2018**, *16*, 823–836. [CrossRef]

6

Neurological Manifestations of Neuropathy and Ataxia in Celiac Disease

Elizabeth S. Mearns [1,†], Aliki Taylor [2,†], Kelly J. Thomas Craig [1,*,†], Stefanie Puglielli [1], Allie B. Cichewicz [1], Daniel A. Leffler [3], David S. Sanders [4], Benjamin Lebwohl [5] and Marios Hadjivassiliou [4]

[1] IBM Watson Health, Cambridge, MA 02142, USA; elizabethmearns@gmail.com (E.S.M.); stefanie.puglielli@gmail.com (S.P.); allie.cichewicz@gmail.com (A.B.C.)
[2] Takeda Development Centre Europe Ltd., London WC2B 4AE, UK; aliki28@me.com
[3] Takeda Pharmaceuticals International Co, Cambridge, MA 02139, USA; daniel.leffler@takeda.com
[4] Royal Hallamshire Hospital and University of Sheffield, Sheffield S10 2RX, UK; david.sanders@sth.nhs.uk (D.S.S.); m.hadjivassiliou@sheffield.ac.uk (M.H.)
[5] Department of Medicine, Celiac Disease Center, Columbia University Medical Center, New York, NY 10032, USA; bl114@cumc.columbia.edu
* Correspondence: kelly.jean.craig@ibm.com
† These authors contributed equally to this work.

Abstract: Celiac disease (CD) is an immune-mediated gastrointestinal disorder driven by innate and adaptive immune responses to gluten. Patients with CD are at an increased risk of several neurological manifestations, frequently peripheral neuropathy and gluten ataxia. A systematic literature review of the most commonly reported neurological manifestations (neuropathy and ataxia) associated with CD was performed. MEDLINE, Embase, the Cochrane Library, and conference proceedings were systematically searched from January 2007 through September 2018. Included studies evaluated patients with CD with at least one neurological manifestation of interest and reported prevalence, and/or incidence, and/or clinical outcomes. Sixteen studies were included describing the risk of gluten neuropathy and/or gluten ataxia in patients with CD. Gluten neuropathy was a neurological manifestation in CD (up to 39%) in 13 studies. Nine studies reported a lower risk and/or prevalence of gluten ataxia with a range of 0%–6%. Adherence to a gluten-free diet appeared to improve symptoms of both neuropathy and ataxia. The prevalence of gluten neuropathy and gluten ataxia in patients with CD varied in reported studies, but the increased risk supports the need for physicians to consider CD in patients with ataxia and neurological manifestations of unknown etiology.

Keywords: celiac disease; gluten neuropathy; gluten ataxia; prevalence; incidence; gluten-free diet

1. Introduction

Celiac disease (CD) is a chronic, immune-mediated enteropathy in which dietary gluten triggers an inflammatory reaction of the small intestine in genetically predisposed individuals [1–3]. The clinical presentation of the disease varies broadly and may include an array of intestinal symptoms and extra-intestinal manifestations, such as iron-deficiency anemia, osteoporosis, dermatitis herpetiformis, and neurologic disorders [4].

Over the last several decades, the clinical presentation of CD has changed [5] with the proportion of patients presenting with classical CD symptoms decreasing and a corresponding increase in the frequency of extra-intestinal symptoms in children and adults [5–7]. This increasing proportion of extra-intestinal symptoms at presentation can result in lengthened diagnostic delay [8]. Active case-finding to facilitate prompt detection of CD and life-long adherence to a strict gluten-free diet (GFD) among patients with confirmed CD is recommended to reduce symptoms and the likelihood of disease of potentially serious manifestations [1].

Manifestations of CD can include a broad spectrum of musculoskeletal, neurological, cardiovascular, and autoimmune disorders. Most notably, peripheral neuropathies and gluten ataxia are frequent neurological manifestations of CD [9,10]. Many patients who present with neurological manifestations of CD have no gastrointestinal symptoms [11]. Peripheral neuropathy in patients with CD presents with tingling, pain, and numbness from nerve damage, initially in the hands and feet. Otherwise known as gluten neuropathy, it is defined as apparently sporadic idiopathic neuropathy in the absence of an alternative etiology and in the presence of serological evidence of gluten sensitivity. It is a slowly progressive disease with a mean age at onset of 55 years. Only one-third of patients have evidence of enteropathy on biopsy, but the presence or absence of enteropathy does not predetermine the effect of a GFD [12].

CD patients with ataxia often present with difficulty with arm and leg control, gait instability, poor coordination, loss of fine motor skills such as writing, problems with talking, and visual issues. Gluten ataxia usually has an insidious onset with a mean age at onset of 53 years [11]. Patients with gluten ataxia can show signs of cerebellar atrophy which can be irreversible and difficult to treat. Other neurological symptoms include encephalopathy, myopathy, myelopathy, ataxia with myoclonus, and chorea [9,10]. Gluten ataxia was first defined in 1996 as apparently idiopathic sporadic ataxia in patients with positive anti-gliadin antibodies (AGA). CD patients with gluten ataxia also often have oligoclonal bands in their cerebrospinal fluid, evidence of perivascular inflammation in the cerebellum, and anti-Purkinje cell antibodies [13].

Although these neurological manifestations of CD have been described over the last 30 years in the literature, there are still diagnostic delays often resulting in permanent neurological disability. Such delays are attributed to "controversies" arising from some variation in reported prevalence and poor understanding of the use of appropriate serological testing [14–16]. To examine the recent evidence, a systematic literature review was conducted to evaluate the prevalence and outcomes of the two most commonly reported neurological manifestations of CD: gluten neuropathy and gluten ataxia.

2. Materials and Methods

A systematic review of literature indexed in MEDLINE (via PubMed), Embase, and the Cochrane Library from January 2007 to August 2018 was performed in accordance with Preferred Reporting Items for Systematic Reviews and Meta-Analyses (PRISMA) guidelines [17]. The search strategy conducted in MEDLINE (via PubMed) is provided in Table 1. Manual backwards citation tracking of references from included studies and systematic review articles was performed to identify additional relevant studies. Searches were also performed in proceedings of the past three meetings (2015–2018) of the following conferences: Digestive Disease Week, American College of Gastroenterology, and United European Gastroenterology Week.

Table 1. MEDLINE (via PubMed.com) Search Strategy.

Search No.	Search Terms	Search Results (28 August 2018)
1	celiac*[tiab] OR coeliac*[tiab] OR celiac disease[MeSH]	31,137
2	((coeliac OR celiac) AND (trunk* OR axis OR node*)) OR "coeliac artery" OR "celiac artery"	7348
3	#1 NOT #2	25,521
4	(cerebellar ataxia[MeSH] OR "cerebellar ataxia"[tiab] OR ((cerebellum* OR cerebellar) AND ataxi*) OR "gluten ataxia" OR "gluten-sensitive ataxia")	17,238
5	neuropathy[tiab] OR neuropathies[tiab] OR neuropathic[tiab]	88,749
6	#3 AND #4	141
7	#3 AND #5	213
8	#6 OR #7	309
9	case reports[pt]	1,893,340
10	#8 NOT #9	238
11	mice OR mouse OR murine OR rodent*	1,754,334
12	#10 NOT #11	227
13	review[pt] NOT (systematic OR Cochrane OR meta-analy*)	2,162,485
14	#12 NOT #13	160
15	#14; Filter: published 2007 or later	99
16	#15; Filter: abstract	96

Footnotes: *, wildcard search term; #, search number. Abbreviations: tiab, title/abstract; pt, publication type.

To be included, studies (primary studies or systematic reviews with or without meta-analyses) had to be conducted in patients with CD, published from 2007 or later (or last three meetings for conference abstracts) in English, and report the incidence, prevalence, and/or clinical outcomes of ataxia and/or neuropathy. Neuropathy, which is often used synonymously with peripheral neuropathy, is classified according to the type of damage to the nerve. In this systematic review, the terms "neuropathy" and "peripheral neuropathy" are stated as the authors have used them in their studies, recognizing that "neuropathy" may include a wider range of symptoms than peripheral neuropathy, which would represent a large proportion of neuropathy cases overall.

A single investigator screened titles and abstracts to determine if the citation met inclusion criteria, with validation by a second reviewer required for exclusion. Two investigators independently reviewed all potentially relevant full-text citations, with discrepancies resolved by a third reviewer. Screening, data extraction, and validation were performed using DistillerSR (Evidence Partners Inc., Kanata, Ottawa, Canada). One investigator abstracted all data using a standardized tool, and a second reviewer verified entries.

Two independent investigators assessed the quality of included studies using the Oxford Levels of Evidence Instrument [18]. Reviewers used the "Differential diagnosis/symptom prevalence study" section to assess the overall grade of the evidence. Details regarding the categorization of the study designs are available in Table 2.

Table 2. Oxford Levels of Evidence & Grades of Recommendation.

Level	Differential Diagnosis/Symptom Prevalence Study
1a	Systematic review (with homogeneity) of prospective cohort studies
1b	Prospective cohort study with good follow-up
1c	All or none case-series
2a	Systematic review (with homogeneity) of 2b and better studies
2b	Retrospective cohort study, or poor follow-up
2c	Ecological studies
3a	Systematic review (with homogeneity) of 3b and better studies
3b	Non-consecutive cohort study, or very limited population
4	Case-series or superseded reference standards
5	Expert opinion without explicit critical appraisal, or based on physiology, bench research or "first principles"

Grade	Levels of Individual Studies
A	Consistent level 1 studies
B	Consistent level 2 or 3 studies or extrapolations from level 1 studies
C	Level 4 studies or extrapolations from level 2 or 3 studies
D	Level 5 evidence or troublingly inconsistent or inconclusive studies of any level

Table adapted from the Oxford Centre for Evidence-Based Medicine [18].

3. Results

The searches identified 441 citations, 299 conference abstracts, and 1 additional citation identified through backwards citation tracking. After removal of duplicates and screening of titles and abstracts screening, 45 were eligible for full-text review. A total of 16 studies met all eligibility criteria and were included in the systematic review (Figure 1, Table 3) [10,19–33]. Nine studies on gluten ataxia [10,20–23,26,28,31,32] and 13 articles on gluten neuropathy were included [10,19,20,22,24–30,32,33].

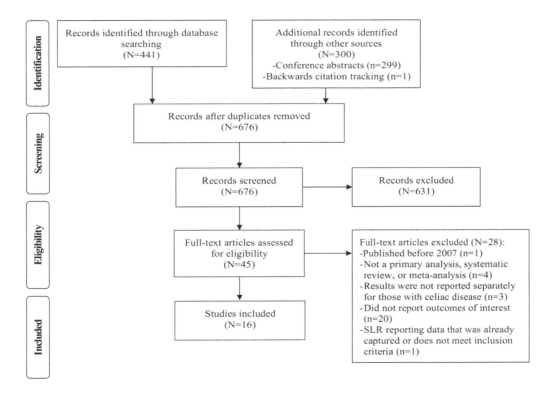

Figure 1. Flow Diagram Showing the Results of the Literature Search.

Table 3. Characteristics of Included Studies.

Author (year)	Study Design	Country	Population	Neurological Complication
Briani and Doria et al. (2008) [19]	Prospective, single-center, cross-sectional	Italy	Patients with CD	Neuropathy
Briani and Zara et al. (2008) [20]	Prospective, single-center, cross-sectional	Italy	Unselected, consecutive patients with CD treated at the University of Padova	Ataxia, neuropathy
Burk et al. (2013) [21]	Prospective, single-center, cross-sectional	Germany	Patients with CD on a GFD recruited from advertisements in the official journal of the German Celiac Society or personal contact	Ataxia
Cakir et al. (2007)[22]	Prospective, multi-center, cross-sectional	Turkey	Children with CD treated at the outpatient follow-up program of celiac patients in the pediatric gastroenterology and nutrition division of Ege University Hospital from 1998–2002	Ataxia, neuropathy
Diaconu et al. (2013) [23]	Prospective, single-center, cross-sectional	Romania	Children (2–18 years) diagnosed with CD from 2000–2010	Ataxia
Hadjivassiliou et al. (2016) [10]	Retrospective, single-center, cohort	UK	Patients with CD and neurological manifestations presenting to the Neuroscience Department at Royal Hallamshire Hospital from 1994–2014	Ataxia, neuropathy
Hadjivassiliou et al. (2017) [31]	Prospective, single-center, observational case series	UK	Patients diagnosed with gluten ataxia at the Sheffield Ataxia Centre	Ataxia
Isikay et al. (2015) [24]	Prospective, single-center, cross-sectional, case-control	Turkey	Asymptomatic children with CD diagnosed at a pediatric gastroenterology outpatient clinic from September 2012–August 2014	Ataxia, neuropathy
Jericho et al. (2017) [25]	Retrospective, single-center, chart review	US	Patients with CD registered at the University of Chicago Celiac Center clinic from January 2002–October 2014	Ataxia, neuropathy
Ludvigsson et al. (2007) [26]	Retrospective, multi-center, database	Sweden	Patients in the Swedish national inpatient register with a hospital-based discharge diagnosis of CD from 1964–2003	Ataxia, neuropathy
Mukherjee et al. (2010) [27]	Retrospective, single-center, database	US	Patients with CD from a prospectively generated database at a university-based referral center	Neuropathy
Ruggieri et al. (2008) [28]	Prospective, single-center, cross-sectional	Italy	Children with CD and neurological dysfunction evaluated at the gluten sensitivity clinic at the Department of Pediatrics at the University of Catania from January 1991–December 2004	Ataxia, neuropathy
Sangal et al. (2017) [32]	Retrospective, single-center, medical record review	Not reported	Children with and without gluten-related disorders between July 2013 and May 2016	Ataxia, neuropathy
Shen et al. (2012) [29]	Questionnaire-based, multi-center, cross-sectional, case-control	US	Patients with CD recruited from the Celiac Disease Center at Columbia University and support groups in New York and California	Neuropathy
Thawani et al. (2015) [30]	Retrospective, multi-center	Sweden	Patients with CD from one of Sweden's pathology departments from June 1969-February 2008	Neuropathy
Thawani et al. (2017) [33]	Retrospective, nationwide registry	Sweden	Patients diagnosed with T1DM between 1964 and 2009, with and without CD (based on biopsies between 1969 and 2008) in the Swedish National Patient Register	Neuropathy

Abbreviations: CD, celiac disease; GFD, gluten-free diet; T1DM, type 1 diabetes mellitus; US, United States; UK, United Kingdom.

The PRISMA flow diagram depicts the flow of information through the different phases of this systematic review. It maps out the number of records identified, included and excluded, and the reasons for exclusions.

Of the studies included, 50% (eight out of 16) were full-text, prospective analyses that reported global prevalence or incidence rates of gluten neuropathy and gluten ataxia [19–24,28,29]. See Box 1 for the definitions of CD, gluten ataxia, and gluten neuropathy. Most studies were performed in Europe (9; Germany, Italy, Romania, Sweden, and United Kingdom (UK)), while four were from the United States (US), two from Turkey, and one multinational study. Findings reported on adults (5), children (5), and both children and adults (6). Clinical outcomes of CD manifestations were reported in 50% (8 out of 16) of the included studies, while the remainder only addressed epidemiology.

Box 1. Definitions of gluten-sensitivity spectrum disorders used in this study.

> *celiac disease* – autoimmune disorder whereby gluten ingestion damages the portion of the small intestine responsible for nutrient absorption; also referred to as gluten-sensitive enteropathy.
> *gluten ataxia* – autoimmune disorder whereby gluten ingestion damages the cerebellum, which controls gait and muscle coordination, and fine control of voluntary movements is compromised.
> *gluten neuropathy* – autoimmune disorder whereby gluten ingestion damages the nerves of the peripheral nervous system, which disrupts communication from the brain and spinal cord to the rest of the body.

3.1. Gluten Neuropathy

Thirteen articles reported gluten neuropathy as a manifestation of CD [10,19,20,22,24–30,32,33]. Estimates of the prevalence of neuropathy in these patients ranged from 0% to 39%, with an increased prevalence/risk in older and female patients. In retrospective and prospective studies of patients with CD in the US and Europe, prevalence of neuropathy ranged from 4% to 23% of adults [20,25,27], 0% to 7% of children [22,24,25,28,32], and 0.7% to 39% of combined/unspecified populations [20,29,30,32]. While these ranges appear to overlap, a few studies directly compared the prevalence and risk of neuropathy by age and indicated that neuropathy occurs more frequently in older populations [27]. In a retrospective US study of adults (n = 171) and children (n = 157) with CD, gluten neuropathy was reported in 23% of adults with a follow-up period of >24 months between 2002 and 2014; however, no cases were reported in children [25]. Another retrospective US study found that significantly more elderly patients aged ≥65 years (11%) had gluten neuropathy compared with younger patients aged 18–30 years (4%; p = 0.023) [27]. Similar to young adults, gluten neuropathy was identified in 3 to 4.5% of children with CD in two studies [28,32]. Another questionnaire-based US study found that the risk of gluten neuropathy rose significantly with every ten-year increase in age (OR, 1.13; 95% CI, 1.04–1.23; p = 0.006). This study also reported a higher risk of gluten neuropathy in females (OR, 1.71; 95% CI, 1.25–2.33; p = 0.001) [29].

Gluten neuropathy may account for approximately one-quarter of neurological manifestations in those with CD. In two studies (one retrospective (n = 228) and one prospective (n = 72)) examining patients with CD and neurological conditions, gluten neuropathy accounted for 19% to 30% of neurological manifestations [10,20]. Patients with CD have a higher risk of gluten neuropathy and experience more severe neuropathic symptoms compared with non-CD controls (p < 0.01) [29]. In three studies (two retrospective and one questionnaire-based) from the US and Sweden, patients with CD had a significantly higher (2.3–5.6 times) risk of peripheral neuropathy compared with control populations [26,29,30]. The risk of polyneuropathy appears highest (4.4–5.6 times) during the first year of follow-up after CD diagnosis [26,30], compared with overall risk, or risk excluding the first year of follow-up (2.3–3.4 times) [26,30]. The risk estimate for neuropathy was only marginally affected after adjustment for education, socioeconomic status, type 1 diabetes mellitus (T1DM), type 2 diabetes mellitus (T2DM), thyroid disease, rheumatologic diseases, pernicious anemia, vitamin deficiencies, and alcoholic disorders (Hazard Ratio (HR), 2.3; 95% Confidence Interval (CI), 1.9–2.7) [30]. Notably, two of these studies adjusted their design to control for the rate of T1DM, as peripheral neuropathy is a long-term manifestation of T1DM [26,30]. However, Thawani et al. (2017) observed there was no significant increased risk of neuropathy for biopsy-confirmed CD patients with T1DM after examining neuropathy incidence in the first five years of CD diagnosis when compared to patients with T1DM only [33].

Symptoms from gluten neuropathy improve when patients with CD follow a GFD, although the diet may not prevent its development, and longer adherence to a GFD may not completely reverse neuropathy. One retrospective US study found that among patients who developed gluten neuropathy ($n = 39$), there was a significant improvement on a GFD ($p < 0.05$) [25]. Two prospective Italian studies also reported that in patients with gluten neuropathy, dietary adherence led to improvement in neuropathy and non-adherence led to worsening [20,28]. However, it should be noted that only one to two patients developed neuropathy in each of these Italian studies. While a GFD may improve symptoms of gluten neuropathy, one questionnaire-based US study found that duration of the diet (<5 vs. 5–9 vs. $\geq$10 years) did not significantly change the proportion of patients who developed the manifestation [29]. Similar proportions of patients developed neuropathy regardless of whether patients were reported to be following a GFD [10,22,25]. In the studies that did document GFD status, the extent of GFD adherence was not reported, limiting assessment of the relationship between neuropathy and degree of gluten exposure.

The severity of gluten neuropathy is variable. With a follow-up period of >20 years, one retrospective British study found that patients with CD on a GFD who developed gluten neuropathy, severity was mild (confined to the legs) in 27%, moderate (involvement of arms but sparing radial nerve) in 40%, and severe (involvement of radial nerve) in 33% [10]. A questionnaire-based US study suggested that the severity of neuropathy is not associated with duration on the GFD [29].

3.2. Gluten Ataxia

Upon physical examination for neurological deficits in patients with CD, estimates of the prevalence of gluten ataxia varied from 0% to 6% [20–23,28,32]. However, in studies among CD patients with neurological manifestations, gluten ataxia was reported in 19% to 41% of patients [10,23]. While studies tended to use similar definitions of ataxia, prevalence estimates varied. Six of the ten included studies used standard neurological exams with combinations of either magnetic resonance imaging (MRI) or magnetic resonance spectroscopy (MRS), or computed tomography (CT) to confirm the diagnosis of ataxia by examination of the vermis, eliminating other potential common causes of ataxia such as thyroid dysfunction, vitamin E deficiency, toxicity, and genetic forms of ataxia (spinocerebellar and Friedrich's) [20–23,28,31].

Of the prospective European studies that used diagnostic CT or MRI/MRS, gluten ataxia was diagnosed in two studies [21,23]. One study of adults ($n = 72$) [21] and one of children ($n = 48$) [23] each reported a prevalence of 6% in patients with CD. The study of 48 children attributed the prevalence of gluten ataxia and the presence of the comorbidities of mental retardation and developmental delays to nutritional deficiencies and toxic effects of severe malnutrition [23]. The other three studies utilizing CT or MRI to define ataxia, one in adults ($n = 71$) [20] and two in children ($n = 27$ and $n = 835$) [22,28], reported that no patients (0%) developed ataxia.

Two included retrospective studies did not report a prevalence of gluten ataxia [10,26]. One study used International Classification of Diseases (ICD, 7–10) codes to identify the symptom of ataxia (excluding trauma or toxicity as main diagnoses) or hereditary ataxia to determine the risk of ataxia in patients with CD [26]. The remaining study had less transparency in the diagnosis of ataxia as the diagnostic criteria were not described, where authors reported that a standard neurological assessment was performed and only reported on the severity of ataxia [10].

One British study suggested that most cases (69%) of gluten ataxia in patients with CD are mild, and patients could walk without assistance [10]. Of the remaining ataxia cases, 17% were moderate (requiring walking aids/support), and 14% were severe (needing a wheelchair). All patients were reported to be following a GFD [10].

In the nine included studies [10,20–23,26,28,31,32], gluten ataxia accounted for up to half of all neurological manifestations observed in people with CD. Definitive conclusions cannot be made regarding age-related differences in CD-associated ataxia from included studies, but available data suggest that gluten ataxia accounts for a smaller proportion of neurological manifestations in children with CD compared with adults.

The risk of gluten ataxia appears to vary over time after CD diagnosis. A retrospective population-based registry study from Sweden evaluated the risk of gluten ataxia in patients with a hospital-based diagnosis of CD (n = 14,371), and found a greater risk of ataxia compared with controls without CD when patients were followed during the first year after discharge (HR, 2.6; 95% CI, 1.0–6.5; p = 0.042) [26]. However, if the first year of follow-up was excluded, the higher risk of ataxia was no longer statistically significant (HR, 1.9; 95% CI, 0.6–6.2; p > 0.05) based upon 14,371 patients with CD and 70,155 reference individuals [26].

The observed effect of GFD on ataxia may be dependent upon the methodological tests to monitor adherence to a GFD and the metrics utilized to assess neurological improvement. A quantitative assessment of the effect of GFD on gluten ataxia was provided by cerebellar MRS in Hadjivassiliou et al. (2017) [31]. In this study, CD patients with gluten ataxia (n = 117) were reviewed for response to GFD: 63 were on strict GFD with the elimination of AGAs, 35 were on GFD but still positive for AGAs, and 19 patients were not on a GFD. GFD adherence was monitored by serological assessments. On MRS, there was a significant improvement in the cerebellum in 62 out of 63 (98%) patients on a strict GFD, in nine of 35 (26%) patients on GFD with positive AGAs, but in only one of 19 (5%) patients not on GFD. Notably, the presence of enteropathy (CD), usually required for the diagnosis of CD, in addition to positive serology, was not found to be a prerequisite for improvement in the cerebellum. The authors concluded that patients with positive serology results and negative duodenal biopsy should still be treated with strict GFD and noted that improved cerebellar function with GFD adherence was associated with clinical improvement [31]. In contrast, a prospective Romanian study in 48 children reported that none of the patients with gluten ataxia had improved symptoms while on a GFD [23]. However, Diaconu et al. (2014) did not state how GFD adherence was monitored and ataxia assessments were self-reported by the parents of the children affected [23].

3.3. Quality Assessment

Based on Oxford Levels of Evidence, the evidence in this review has an overall grade of B. Only one study provided Level 1b evidence [19]. Seven studies [10,25–27,30,32,33] were retrospective cohort studies, which represented Level 2b evidence. One study was a prospective case series, representing level 4 evidence [31]. The remaining seven studies [20–24,28,29] were cross-sectional studies, which we have categorized as Level 2c. The levels of evidence for individual studies are shown in Table 4.

Table 4. Quality Assessment of Included Studies.

Study Identifier	Oxford Level of Evidence
Briani and Doria et al. (2008) [19]	2c. Ecological study *
Briani and Zara et al. (2008) [20]	1b. Prospective cohort study
Burk et al. (2013) [21]	2c. Ecological study *
Cakir et al. (2007) [22]	2c. Ecological study *
Diaconu et al. (2013) [23]	2c. Ecological study *
Hadjivassiliou et al. (2016) [10]	2b. Retrospective cohort study
Hadjivassiliou et al. (2017) [31]	4. Case-series or superseded reference standards
Isikay et al. (2015) [24]	2c. Ecological study *
Jericho et al. (2017) [25]	2b. Retrospective cohort study
Ludvigsson et al. (2007) [26]	2b. Retrospective cohort study
Mukherjee et al. (2010) [27]	2b. Retrospective cohort study
Ruggieri et al. (2008) [28]	2c. Ecological study *
Sangal et al. (2017) [32]	2b. Retrospective cohort study
Shen et al. (2012) [29]	2c. Ecological study *
Thawani et al. (2015) [30]	2b. Retrospective cohort study
Thawani et al. (2017) [33]	2b. Retrospective cohort study

*, Note that this was a cross-sectional study, not an ecological study; there is no Oxford Level of Evidence for cross-sectional studies [18].

4. Discussion

This systematic review demonstrates that gluten neuropathy was reported more often than gluten ataxia (81.25% of included studies reported neuropathy), although the prevalence of gluten neuropathy varied widely (0%–39%). Both ataxia and neuropathy were more prevalent in patients with CD compared with controls. Symptoms of neuropathy were most commonly categorized as moderate, affecting extremities. Prevalence of gluten ataxia in patients with diagnosed CD varied from 0–6%; symptoms were often described as mild, in which patients were still able to walk, although in some cases could be very severe and persistent. The variations in prevalence rates across studies of both gluten ataxia and gluten neuropathy may be related to study design and inclusion criteria, retrospective nature of data collection, quality of assessment of adherence to a GFD, clinical assessment of neurological symptoms, and the age of the populations included.

The prevalence of idiopathic neuropathy in the general population is low but the risk is increased in CD. A literature review of 28 studies reported the prevalence of neuropathy in the general middle-aged and elderly population between 0.1% and 3.3% [34]. Increased neuropathy prevalence was reported in a US study published in 2003 using retrospective data from 400 patients with neuropathy, whereby neuropathy rates for CD were between 2.5% and 8% (compared to 1% in the healthy population) [35]. In a large Swedish population-based study that examined the risk of neurological disease, polyneuropathy was found to be significantly associated with CD (odds ratio 5.4; 95% CI 3.6–8.2) [36]. In further support of this, an age- and sex-matched control study, identified in this review, comparing patients with CD to controls found that CD was associated with a 2.5-fold increased risk of later neuropathy [30]. The highest risk for gluten neuropathy was just after diagnosis of CD, but there was also a consistent excess risk of neuropathy beyond five years after a diagnosis of CD. Two other included studies compared patients with CD of different ages and found that younger patients were less likely to experience neuropathy [25,27]. However, these studies examined established patients with CD and their findings may be an underestimation of risk of neuropathy in young patients. The presentation of atypical symptoms, such as neurological complications, at time of CD diagnosis in children, reported neuropathy prevalence of 10.5% in this small study population [32].

Similar to trends for neuropathy, the prevalence of ataxia in the general population is very low, but this risk is increased in patients with CD. A UK based population-based study estimated the prevalence of late-onset cerebellar ataxia as 0.01% in the general population [37]. Three studies identified in this review reported no cases (0%) of ataxia in both adults and children [20,22,28]; however, estimates of ataxia prevalence ranged from 0-6% across all ages [21,23,32]. In studies that determined ataxia prevalence in children, neurological manifestations were the initial symptoms of CD in 25%–33.33% of patients, and ataxia accounted for 5.26%–18.8% of those cases. [23,32]. The risk of ataxia in those with CD was estimated to be 1.9- to 2.6-fold compared with controls during the first year after diagnosis [26].

Although the prevalence of ataxia in CD is thought to be low, it may be underestimated. A recent UK study of 500 patients diagnosed with progressive ataxia and evaluated over a period of 13 years, found that 101 of 215 (47%) patients with idiopathic sporadic ataxia had serological evidence of gluten reactivity [38]. A study of 1500 patients with cerebellar ataxia referred to the Sheffield Ataxia Centre, UK assessed over 20 years found that 20% had a family history of ataxia, and the remaining 80% had sporadic ataxia. Of sporadic ataxias, gluten ataxia was the most common cause (25%); followed by genetic causes (13%), alcohol excess (12%), and a cerebellar variant of multiple system atrophy (11%) [39]. In a review of gluten sensitivity by Hadjivassiliou et al. (2010) [11], many studies reported that a high proportion of patients with sporadic ataxias (12%–47%) tested positive for AGA compared with 2%–12% of healthy controls [11,38–48]. These studies suggest that even though ataxia is rare, gluten ataxia is a common subtype of sporadic ataxia.

Adherence to a strict GFD can result in clinical improvement in both gluten neuropathy and gluten ataxia. Publications which met criteria for inclusion in this review unanimously support a beneficial effect of the GFD on neuropathy, however, a benefit in ataxia is less clear. Some studies report that ataxia persists in patients on a GFD, while others demonstrated improvement on GFD [10,21,23,31].

This heterogeneity is most likely due to differences in study design, including the assessment of GFD adherence and ataxia symptoms. Severity of ataxia can be assessed with a variety of instruments including self-report and clinician determination using scales for the assessment and rating of ataxia (e.g., Brief Ataxia Rating Scale (BARS), Scale for the Assessment and Rating of Ataxia (SARA), International Cooperative Ataxia Rating Scale (ICARS), modified ICARS (MICARS)), and imaging studies (e.g., MRS, MRI, EEG). Objective quantitation of motor deficits in ataxia is fundamental for measurement of clinical severity but was not commonly reported in studies examining the association between improvements of ataxia and GFD adherence. One study by Hadjivassiliou et al. (2017) utilized a quantitative methodology via MRS to monitor ataxia severity by cerebellar atrophy and assessed GFD adherence with AGA testing [31]. This study demonstrated a beneficial effect of strict GFD adherence on ataxia and benefits were seen in all AGA positive individuals, regardless of baseline enteropathy [31].

It is important to clarify the differences between CD and gluten sensitivity in the context of gluten ataxia and gluten neuropathy. This systematic review primarily concentrated on patients with CD and these two common neurological manifestations. These manifestations, however, may exist in the presence of AGA alone (gluten sensitivity) without evidence of enteropathy (CD), and such patients benefit equally from GFD. Indeed Hadjivassiliou et al. (2016) demonstrated there are no distinguishing features (e.g., type of neurological manifestation, severity, and response to GFD) between those patients with neurological manifestations and CD and those with just positive AGA (no enteropathy) [10]. Despite this, the majority of immunological laboratories have abandoned the use of native AGA assays due to poor specificity in diagnosing CD. Estimation of specificity, however, is based on the presence of a gold standard, in this case, the presence of enteropathy. Given that sensitivity to gluten exists in the absence of enteropathy, then AGA remains probably the only serological marker in diagnosing the whole spectrum of extraintestinal manifestations. Another important consideration when using AGA is the serological cut-off for positive AGA. Such assays are calibrated using serology from patients with CD as the gold standard, and consequently, the serological cut-off tends to be high. It has recently been shown that by recalibrating the serological cut-off of a commercially available AGA assay based on the ability to diagnose GA, the sensitivity of AGA in diagnosing CD became 100% [49].

There were a small number of studies identified that did not meet our inclusion criteria but described the association between gluten neuropathy and enteropathy, and the effects of strict GFD on gluten neuropathy. Of note, a study published by Hadjivassiliou et al. (2006) reported that of 100 patients with clinical immunological characteristics of gluten neuropathy, 29% of patients had evidence of enteropathy [50]. A prospective study published in 2006, followed 35 patients with gluten neuropathy, 25 of which were assigned to strict adherence to a GFD with the remaining ten patients as controls. Strict GFD adherence was defined by the elimination of AGA after one year. When asked, 16/25 patients on the GFD said their neuropathy was better compared to 0/10 in the control group. Eight out of ten patients in the control group stated that their neuropathy was worse [12]. Gluten neuropathy can be associated with significant chronic pain and negatively impact mental health. A recent study assessed neuropathic pain in 60 patients with gluten neuropathy. Neuropathic pain was present in 33 patients and painless neuropathy was more common in patients on a strict GFD (55.6% versus 21.2%, $p = 0.006$). Patients with painful gluten neuropathy presented with significantly worse mental health status [12]. Multivariate analysis showed that, after adjusting for age, gender and mental health index-5, strict GFD was associated with an 89% reduction in risk of peripheral neuropathic pain ($p = 0.006$) [51].

Gluten ataxia and neuropathy were selected for this review because they are the most common neurological manifestations in CD. However, there are other neurological manifestations not assessed (a systematic review of movement disorders related to gluten sensitivity by Vinagre-Aragon et al. (2017) is available [52] for reference). A prospective study reported that up to 22% of patients with CD ($n = 71$) developed some form of neurologic or psychiatric dysfunction (headache, depression, entrapment syndromes, peripheral neuropathy, and epilepsy) [20]. In a British study published in 1998,

57% of patients with neurological dysfunction of unknown cause had serological evidence of gluten sensitivity, compared with 12% of healthy blood donors [53]. Neurological manifestations can have a significant impact on patients' quality of life, and a greater understanding of these complications is needed.

There are several limitations to this systematic review. Both clinical and methodological heterogeneity among reviewed studies limited comparisons of the data. Across all studies included, it is not possible to determine whether factors such as the timing of diagnosis, presentation of CD, or differences diagnostic techniques, affect rates of ataxia and peripheral neuropathy. Lastly, there is potential for publication bias and missed eligible articles in any literature review. However, this risk is assumed to be minimal due to strict adherence to standards for systematic search methodology.

5. Conclusions

In conclusion, this systematic review provides important evidence on the substantially increased risk of gluten ataxia and gluten neuropathy in patients with CD, although estimates across studies vary. These results indicate that adherence to a GFD appears to improve symptoms of both neuropathy and ataxia. The scarcity of data from this global search highlights the need for additional well-designed studies to improve the understanding of neurological manifestations in patients with CD. Given that these results suggest an increased risk of ataxia and neuropathy among patients with CD, clinicians should evaluate for gluten sensitivity in patients with ataxia and neuropathy of unknown origin.

Author Contributions: Conceptualization: E.S.M., A.T., D.A.L., M.H.; Formal analysis: S.P., K.J.T.C., A.B.C.; Funding Acquisition: K.J.T.C.; Methodology: E.S.M., A.B.C., S.P., K.J.T.C.; Project Administration: E.S.M., K.J.T.C.; Supervision: E.S.M., A.T., K.J.T.C.; Validation: K.J.T.C., S.P., A.B.C.; Writing—original draft: E.S.M., A.T., K.J.T.C., S.P.; Writing—review & editing: all authors.

Acknowledgments: The authors would like to thank Lynne Stoecklein for assisting with screening of titles/abstracts and full texts, data collection, and language editing; Talia Boulanger for the conceptualization and design of the systematic review; Jennifer Drahos for critical reading and feedback; and Nicole Fusco for assisting in data collection and proofreading.

References

1.   Rubio-Tapia, A.; Hill, I.D.; Kelly, C.P.; Calderwood, A.H.; Murray, J.A. ACG clinical guidelines: Diagnosis and management of celiac disease. *Am. J. Gastroenterol.* **2013**, *108*, 656–676. [CrossRef] [PubMed]
2.   Tonutti, E.; Bizzaro, N. Diagnosis and classification of celiac disease and gluten sensitivity. *Autoimmun. Rev.* **2014**, *13*, 472–476. [CrossRef]
3.   Ludvigsson, J.F.; Leffler, D.A.; Bai, J.C.; Biagi, F.; Fasano, A.; Green, P.H.; Hadjivassiliou, M.; Kaukinen, K.; Kelly, C.P.; Leonard, J.N.; et al. The Oslo definitions for coeliac disease and related terms. *Gut* **2013**, *62*, 43–52. [CrossRef] [PubMed]
4.   Green, P.H.; Lebwohl, B.; Greywoode, R. Celiac disease. *J. Allergy Clin. Immunol.* **2015**, *135*, 1099–1106. [CrossRef] [PubMed]
5.   Reilly, N.R.; Green, P.H. Epidemiology and clinical presentations of celiac disease. *Semin. Immunopathol.* **2012**, *34*, 473–478. [CrossRef]
6.   Roma, E.; Panayiotou, J.; Karantana, H.; Constantinidou, C.; Siakavellas, S.I.; Krini, M.; Syriopoulou, V.P.; Bamias, G. Changing pattern in the clinical presentation of pediatric celiac disease: A 30-year study. *Digestion* **2009**, *80*, 185–191. [CrossRef]
7.   Ludvigsson, J.F.; Rubio-Tapia, A.; van Dyke, C.T.; Melton, L.J., 3rd; Zinsmeister, A.R.; Lahr, B.D.; Murray, J.A. Increasing incidence of celiac disease in a North American population. *Am. J. Gastroenterol.* **2013**, *108*, 818–824. [CrossRef] [PubMed]
8.   Fuchs, V.; Kurppa, K.; Huhtala, H.; Collin, P.; Maki, M.; Kaukinen, K. Factors associated with long diagnostic delay in celiac disease. *Scand. J. Gastroenterol.* **2014**, *49*, 1304–1310. [CrossRef]
9.   Leffler, D.A.; Green, P.H.; Fasano, A. Extraintestinal manifestations of coeliac disease. *Nat. Rev. Gastroenterol. Hepatol.* **2015**, *12*, 561–571. [CrossRef] [PubMed]
10.   Hadjivassiliou, M.; Rao, D.G.; Grinewald, R.A.; Aeschlimann, D.P.; Sarrigiannis, P.G.; Hoggard, N.; Aeschlimann, P.; Mooney, P.D.; Sanders, D.S. Neurological Dysfunction in Coeliac Disease and Non-Coeliac Gluten Sensitivity. *Am. J. Gastroenterol.* **2016**, *111*, 561–567. [CrossRef] [PubMed]

11. Hadjivassiliou, M.; Sanders, D.S.; Grunewald, R.A.; Woodroofe, N.; Boscolo, S.; Aeschlimann, D. Gluten sensitivity: From gut to brain. *Lancet Neurol.* **2010**, *9*, 318–330. [CrossRef]

12. Hadjivassiliou, M.; Kandler, R.H.; Chattopadhyay, A.K.; Davies-Jones, A.G.; Jarratt, J.A.; Sanders, D.S.; Sharrack, B.; Grunewald, R.A. Dietary treatment of gluten neuropathy. *Muscle Nerve* **2006**, *34*, 762–766. [CrossRef] [PubMed]

13. Hadjivassiliou, M.; Williamson, C.A.; Woodroofe, N. The immunology of gluten sensitivity: Beyond the gut. *Trends Immunol.* **2004**, *25*, 578–582. [CrossRef] [PubMed]

14. Rampertab, S.D.; Pooran, N.; Brar, P.; Singh, P.; Green, P.H. Trends in the presentation of celiac disease. *Am. J. Med.* **2006**, *119*, 355.e9–355.e14. [CrossRef] [PubMed]

15. Green, P.H. The many faces of celiac disease: Clinical presentation of celiac disease in the adult population. *Gastroenterology* **2005**, *128*, S74–S78. [CrossRef] [PubMed]

16. Lionetti, E.; Catassi, C. The role of environmental factors in the development of celiac disease: What is new? *Diseases* **2015**, *3*, 282–293. [CrossRef] [PubMed]

17. Moher, D.; Liberati, A.; Tetzlaff, J.; Altman, D.G. Preferred reporting items for systematic reviews and meta-analyses: The PRISMA statement. *Ann. Intern. Med.* **2009**, *151*, 264–269. [CrossRef] [PubMed]

18. Oxford Centre for Evidence-Based Medicine—Levels of Evidence. March 2009. Available online: http://www.cebm.net/blog/2009/06/11/oxford-centre-evidence-based-medicine-levels-evidence-march-2009/ (accessed on 16 January 2018).

19. Briani, C.; Doria, A.; Ruggero, S.; Toffanin, E.; Luca, M.; Albergoni, M.P.; Odorico, A.D.; Grassivaro, F.; Lucchetta, M.; Lazzari, F.D.; et al. Antibodies to muscle and ganglionic acetylcholine receptors (AchR) in celiac disease. *Autoimmunity* **2008**, *41*, 100–104. [CrossRef] [PubMed]

20. Briani, C.; Zara, G.; Alaedini, A.; Grassivaro, F.; Ruggero, S.; Toffanin, E.; Albergoni, M.P.; Luca, M.; Giometto, B.; Ermani, M.; et al. Neurological complications of celiac disease and autoimmune mechanisms: A prospective study. *J. Neuroimmunol.* **2008**, *195*, 171–175. [CrossRef]

21. Burk, K.; Farecki, M.L.; Lamprecht, G.; Roth, G.; Decker, P.; Weller, M.; Rammensee, H.G.; Oertel, W. Neurological symptoms in patients with biopsy proven celiac disease. *Mov. Disord.* **2009**, *24*, 2358–2362. [CrossRef]

22. Cakir, D.; Tosun, A.; Polat, M.; Celebisoy, N.; Gokben, S.; Aydogdu, S.; Yagci, R.V.; Tekgul, H. Subclinical neurological abnormalities in children with celiac disease receiving a gluten-free diet. *J. Pediatr. Gastroenterol. Nutr.* **2007**, *45*, 366–369. [CrossRef]

23. Diaconu, G.; Burlea, M.; Grigore, I.; Anton, D.T.; Trandafir, L.M. Celiac disease with neurologic manifestations in children. *Revista Medico-Chirurgicala A Societatii de Medici si Naturalisti din Iasi* **2014**, *117*, 88–94.

24. Isikay, S.; Isikay, N.; Kocamaz, H.; Hizli, S. Peripheral neuropathy electrophysiological screening in children with celiac disease. *Arq. Gastroenterol.* **2015**, *52*, 134–138. [CrossRef]

25. Jericho, H.; Sansotta, N.; Guandalini, S. Extraintestinal Manifestations of Celiac Disease: Effectiveness of the Gluten-Free Diet. *J. Pediatr. Gastroenterol. Nutr.* **2017**, *65*, 75–79. [CrossRef]

26. Ludvigsson, J.F.; Olsson, T.; Ekbom, A.; Montgomery, S.M. A population-based study of coeliac disease, neurodegenerative and neuroinflammatory diseases. *Aliment. Pharmacol. Ther.* **2007**, *25*, 1317–1327. [CrossRef]

27. Mukherjee, R.; Egbuna, I.; Brar, P.; Hernandez, L.; McMahon, D.J.; Shane, E.J.; Bhagat, G.; Green, P.H. Celiac disease: Similar presentations in the elderly and young adults. *Dig. Dis. Sci.* **2010**, *55*, 3147–3153. [CrossRef]

28. Ruggieri, M.; Incorpora, G.; Polizzi, A.; Parano, E.; Spina, M.; Pavone, P. Low prevalence of neurologic and psychiatric manifestations in children with gluten sensitivity. *J. Pediatr.* **2008**, *152*, 244–249. [CrossRef]

29. Shen, T.C.; Lebwohl, B.; Verma, H.; Kumta, N.; Tennyson, C.; Lewis, S.; Scherl, E.; Swaminath, A.; Capiak, K.M.; DiGiacomo, D.; et al. Peripheral neuropathic symptoms in celiac disease and inflammatory bowel disease. *J. Clin. Neuromuscul. Dis.* **2012**, *13*, 137–145. [CrossRef]

30. Thawani, S.P.; Brannagan, T.H., 3rd; Lebwohl, B.; Green, P.H.; Ludvigsson, J.F. Risk of Neuropathy Among 28,232 Patients with Biopsy-Verified Celiac Disease. *JAMA Neurol.* **2015**, *72*, 806–811. [CrossRef]

31. Hadjivassiliou, M.; Grunewald, R.A.; Sanders, D.S.; Shanmugarajah, P.; Hoggard, N. Effect of gluten-free diet on cerebellar MR spectroscopy in gluten ataxia. *Neurology* **2017**, *89*, 705–709. [CrossRef]

32. Sangal, K.; Camhi, S.; Lima, R.; Kenyon, V.; Fasano, A.; Leonard, M. Prevalence of neurological symptoms in children with gluten related disorders. *J. Pediatr. Gastroenterol. Nutr.* **2017**, *65*, S328–S329. [CrossRef]

33. Thawani, S.; Brannagan, T.H., 3rd; Lebwohl, B.; Mollazadegan, K.; Green, P.H.R.; Ludvigsson, J.F. Type 1 Diabetes, Celiac Disease, and Neuropathy-A Nationwide Cohort Study. *J. Clin. Neuromuscul. Dis.* **2017**, *19*, 12–18. [CrossRef]

34. Hanewinckel, R.; Drenthen, J.; van Oijen, M.; Hofman, A.; van Doorn, P.A.; Ikram, M.A. Prevalence of polyneuropathy in the general middle-aged and elderly population. *Neurology* **2016**, *87*, 1892–1898. [CrossRef]

35. Chin, R.L.; Sander, H.W.; Brannagan, T.H.; Green, P.H.; Hays, A.P.; Alaedini, A.; Latov, N. Celiac neuropathy. *Neurology* **2003**, *60*, 1581–1585. [CrossRef]

36. Luostarinen, L.; Himanen, S.L.; Luostarinen, M.; Collin, P.; Pirttila, T. Neuromuscular and sensory disturbances in patients with well treated coeliac disease. *J. Neurol. Neurosurg. Psychiatry* **2003**, *74*, 490–494. [CrossRef]

37. Muzaimi, M.B.; Thomas, J.; Palmer-Smith, S.; Rosser, L.; Harper, P.S.; Wiles, C.M.; Ravine, D.; Robertson, N.P. Population based study of late onset cerebellar ataxia in south east Wales. *J. Neurol. Neurosurg. Psychiatry* **2004**, *75*, 1129–1134. [CrossRef]

38. Hadjivassiliou, M. Immune-mediated acquired ataxias. *Handb. Clin. Neurol.* **2012**, *103*, 189–199. [CrossRef]

39. Hadjivassiliou, M.; Boscolo, S.; Tongiorgi, E.; Grunewald, R.A.; Sharrack, B.; Sanders, D.S.; Woodroofe, N.; Davies-Jones, G.A. Cerebellar ataxia as a possible organ-specific autoimmune disease. *Mov. Disord.* **2008**, *23*, 1370–1377. [CrossRef]

40. Abele, M.; Burk, K.; Schols, L.; Schwartz, S.; Besenthal, I.; Dichgans, J.; Zuhlke, C.; Riess, O.; Klockgether, T. The aetiology of sporadic adult-onset ataxia. *Brain* **2002**, *125*, 961–968. [CrossRef]

41. Abele, M.; Schols, L.; Schwartz, S.; Klockgether, T. Prevalence of antigliadin antibodies in ataxia patients. *Neurology* **2003**, *60*, 1674–1675. [CrossRef]

42. Burk, K.; Bosch, S.; Muller, C.A.; Melms, A.; Zuhlke, C.; Stern, M.; Besenthal, I.; Skalej, M.; Ruck, P.; Ferber, S.; et al. Sporadic cerebellar ataxia associated with gluten sensitivity. *Brain* **2001**, *124*, 1013–1019. [CrossRef]

43. Bushara, K.O.; Goebel, S.U.; Shill, H.; Goldfarb, L.G.; Hallett, M. Gluten sensitivity in sporadic and hereditary cerebellar ataxia. *Ann. Neurol.* **2001**, *49*, 540–543. [CrossRef]

44. Hadjivassiliou, M.; Grunewald, R.; Sharrack, B.; Sanders, D.; Lobo, A.; Williamson, C.; Woodroofe, N.; Wood, N.; Davies-Jones, A. Gluten ataxia in perspective: Epidemiology, genetic susceptibility and clinical characteristics. *Brain* **2003**, *126*, 685–691. [CrossRef]

45. Ihara, M.; Makino, F.; Sawada, H.; Mezaki, T.; Mizutani, K.; Nakase, H.; Matsui, M.; Tomimoto, H.; Shimohama, S. Gluten sensitivity in Japanese patients with adult-onset cerebellar ataxia. *Intern. Med.* **2006**, *45*, 135–140. [CrossRef]

46. Luostarinen, L.K.; Collin, P.O.; Peraaho, M.J.; Maki, M.J.; Pirttila, T.A. Coeliac disease in patients with cerebellar ataxia of unknown origin. *Ann. Med.* **2001**, *33*, 445–449. [CrossRef]

47. Pellecchia, M.T.; Scala, R.; Filla, A.; De Michele, G.; Ciacci, C.; Barone, P. Idiopathic cerebellar ataxia associated with celiac disease: Lack of distinctive neurological features. *J. Neurol. Neurosurg. Psychiatry* **1999**, *66*, 32–35. [CrossRef]

48. Anheim, M.; Degos, B.; Echaniz-Laguna, A.; Fleury, M.; Grucker, M.; Tranchant, C. Ataxia associated with gluten sensitivity, myth or reality? *Rev. Neurol.* **2006**, *162*, 214–221. [CrossRef]

49. Hadjivassiliou, M.; Grünewald, R.; Sanders, D.; Zis, P.; Croall, I.; Shanmugarajah, P.; Sarrigiannis, P.; Trott, N.; Wild, G.; Hoggard, N. The Significance of Low Titre Antigliadin Antibodies in the Diagnosis of Gluten Ataxia. *Nutrients* **2018**, *10*, 1444. [CrossRef]

50. Hadjivassiliou, M.; Grunewald, R.A.; Kandler, R.H.; Chattopadhyay, A.K.; Jarratt, J.A.; Sanders, D.S.; Sharrack, B.; Wharton, S.B.; Davies-Jones, G.A. Neuropathy associated with gluten sensitivity. *J. Neurol. Neurosurg. Psychiatry* **2006**, *77*, 1262–1266. [CrossRef]

51. Zis, P.; Sarrigiannis, P.G.; Rao, D.G.; Hadjivassiliou, M. Gluten neuropathy: Prevalence of neuropathic pain and the role of gluten-free diet. *J. Neurol.* **2018**, *265*, 2231–2236. [CrossRef]

52. Vinagre-Aragon, A.; Zis, P.; Grunewald, R.A.; Hadjivassiliou, M. Movement Disorders Related to Gluten Sensitivity: A Systematic Review. *Nutrients* **2018**, *10*, 34. [CrossRef]

53. Hadjivassiliou, M.; Gibson, A.; Davies-Jones, G.A.; Lobo, A.J.; Stephenson, T.J.; Milford-Ward, A. Does cryptic gluten sensitivity play a part in neurological illness? *Lancet* **1996**, *347*, 369–371. [CrossRef]

7

Translation, Cultural Adaptation and Evaluation of a Brazilian Portuguese Questionnaire to Estimate the Self-Reported Prevalence of Gluten-Related Disorders and Adherence to Gluten-Free Diet

Jesús Gilberto Arámburo-Gálvez [1,2], Itallo Carvalho Gomes [3], Tatiane Geralda André [3], Carlos Eduardo Beltrán-Cárdenas [1], María Auxiliadora Macêdo-Callou [4], Élida Mara Braga Rocha [4], Elaine Aparecida Mye-Takamatu-Watanabe [5], Vivian Rahmeier-Fietz [5], Oscar Gerardo Figueroa-Salcido [1,2], Feliznando Isidro Cárdenas-Torres [1], Noé Ontiveros [6,*] and Francisco Cabrera-Chávez [1,*]

[1] Unidad Academica de Ciencias de la Nutrición y Gastronomia, Universidad Autónoma de Sinaloa, Culiacán, Sinaloa 80019, Mexico; gilberto.aramburo.g@gmail.com (J.G.A.-G.); carlos.1.beltran@hotmail.com (C.E.B.-C.); gerardofs95@hotmail.com (O.G.F.-S.): feliznandoc@hotmail.com (F.I.C.-T.)

[2] Posgrado en Ciencias de la Salud, División de Ciencias Biológicas y de la Salud, Universidad de Sonora, Hermosillo, Sonora 83000, Mexico

[3] Programa de Maestría en Ciencias en Enfermeria, Facultad de Enfermería, Los Mochis, Sinaloa 81220, Mexico; carvalhoitallo@gmail.com (I.C.G.); tatianegrandre@gmail.com (T.G.A.)

[4] Faculdade de Juazeiro do Norte, Juazeiro do Norte, Ceará 63010-215, Brazil; auxiliadora.callou@fjn.edu.br (M.A.M.-C.); elidamara@usp.br (É.M.B.R.)

[5] Universidade Estadual de Mato Grosso do Sul, Dourados, Mato Grosso do Sul 79804-970, Brazil; swatanab@terra.com.br (E.A.M.-T.-W.); vivian@uems.br (V.R.-F.)

[6] Division of Sciences and Engineering, Department of Chemical, Biological, and Agricultural Sciences (DC-QB), Clinical and Research Laboratory (LACIUS, URS), University of Sonora, Navojoa 85880, Sonora, Mexico

[*] Correspondence: noe.ontiveros@unison.mx (N.O.); fcabrera@uas.edu.mx (F.C.-C.)

Abstract: *Background*: A Spanish version of a questionnaire intended to estimate, at the population level, the prevalence rates of self-reported gluten-related disorders and adherence to gluten-free diets has been applied in four Latin American countries. However, idiom issues have hampered the questionnaire application in the Brazilian population. Thus, the aim of the present study was to carry out a translation, cultural adaptation, and evaluation of a Brazilian Portuguese questionnaire to estimate the self-reported prevalence of gluten-related disorders and adherence to gluten-free diets in a Brazilian population. *Materials and Methods*: Two bilingual Portuguese–Spanish health professionals carried out the translation of the original Spanish version of the questionnaire to Brazilian-Portuguese. Matching between the two translations was evaluated using the WCopyFind.4.1.5 software. Words in conflict were conciliated, and the conciliated version of the Brazilian Portuguese instrument was evaluated to determine its clarity, comprehension, and consistency. A pilot study was carried out using an online platform. *Results*: The two questionnaires translated into Brazilian Portuguese were highly matched (81.8%–84.1%). The questions of the conciliated questionnaire were clear and comprehensible with a high agreement among the evaluators ($n = 64$) (average Kendall's W score was 0.875). The participants did not suggest re-wording of questions. The answers to the questions were consistent after two applications of the questionnaire (Cohen's k = 0.869). The pilot online survey yielded low response rates (9.0%) highlighting the need for face-to-face interviews. *Conclusions*: The translation and evaluation of a Brazilian Portuguese questionnaire to estimate the self-reported prevalence rates of gluten-related disorders and adherence to gluten-free diets was carried out. The instrument is clear, comprehensible, and generates reproducible results in the target population. Further survey studies involving face-to-face interviews are warranted.

Keywords: celiac disease; gluten-free diet; gluten-related disorders; NCGS; self-report; survey studies

1. Introduction

The spectrum of gluten-related disorders (GRD) involves celiac disease (CD), wheat allergy and non-celiac gluten sensitivity (NCGS). Patients under this spectrum should follow a gluten-free diet (GFD) to avoid the gastrointestinal and/or extraintestinal symptoms triggered by gluten. In fact, survey studies have proven that following a GFD can improve the health-related quality of life in CD patients in spite of the difficulties of following the diet [1]. Different from wheat allergy and NCGS, untreated CD could affect the nutritional status and predispose to other conditions such as osteoporosis [2,3], anemia [4], and intestinal T-cell lymphoma [5]. On its own, following a GFD without medical/dietitian advice can predispose not only to deficiencies in micronutrients, but also to low fiber intake [6,7] increasing the risk of dyslipidemia [8,9]. Notably, recent survey-based studies carried out in Latin American countries have shown that both CD and NCGS are largely underdiagnosed in Mexico, Colombia, and El Salvador, and that most people following a GFD are doing it for reasons other than health related benefits, as well as without medical advice [10–12]. This is not the case in Argentina, a country that has implemented programs for the detection of CD and for ameliorating the economic burden of following a GFD [13]. The questionnaire utilized in these studies is a Spanish version, and this has hampered its application in the Brazilian population. Recently, an Italian instrument [14] designed to estimate the prevalence of NCGS in clinical settings has been translated to Brazilian Portuguese [15], but a validated questionnaire intended to evaluate, at population level, the self-reported prevalence of GRD and adherence to a GFD in Brazilians is not available yet. Thus, as part of an attempt to expose the magnitude and relevance of the underdiagnosis of GRD and the adherence to GFD in the Latin American region, the aim of the present work is to generate and test a Brazilian Portuguese version of a validated Spanish questionnaire designed to estimate the self-reported prevalence of GRD and adherence to a GFD.

2. Materials and Methods

2.1. Questionnaire

The questionnaire is based on a previously designed and tested instrument that is utilized in Spanish-speaking populations [10–13]. The questionnaire includes 2 sections. The first section was designed for those who report adverse reactions after wheat/gluten ingestion, and the second one for those who do not report them. The participants should answer questions related to the symptoms triggered after gluten ingestion, time of appearance of the symptoms, adherence to a GFD or gluten avoidance and the motivations of doing so, among other questions (Supplementary Material Section S1).

2.2. Translation and Back-Translation

The translation process of the questionnaire was carried out as previously described, with minor changes [16,17]. The procedure was as follows: two health professionals, Portuguese–Spanish bilingual, but also Brazilian Portuguese native speakers, realized the translation of the questionnaire from Spanish to Brazilian Portuguese (TBP1 and TBP2). The matches between translations were analyzed using the WCopyFind.4.1.5 software (Charlottesville, VA, USA) to determine literal match by words (ignoring phrases, all punctuations, outer punctuations, numbers, letter case, and skipping non-words, selecting Brazilian-Portuguese as the base language). After conciliation of the words in conflict (words that did not match) by the Spanish-Portuguese translators, a conciliate version of the questionnaire was elaborated and back-translated to Spanish by two Spanish-Portuguese bilingual professionals who were also Spanish native speakers. The match between the back-translated questionnaires (from Brazilian Portuguese to Spanish; two versions) and the match between each back-translated version with the original Spanish version of the questionnaire were evaluated as previously described (selecting Mexican Spanish as the base language). All matches were reported as percentage.

2.3. Questionnaire Clarity, Comprehension and Wording of Questions Evaluation

Clarity and comprehension of the conciliated questionnaire in Brazilian Portuguese was evaluated as previously described [10,16]. A digital version of the Brazilian Portuguese questionnaire was constructed using the SurveyMonkey platform (San Mateo, CA, USA). Brazilian Portuguese native speakers ($n = 64$) received a text message with the link to the questionnaire. Afterwards, participants proceeded to evaluate the clarity and comprehension of all the questions.

The evaluation was initially performed using a numerical scale from 0 to 10 (0 = very easy to understand; 10 = very difficult to understand). Questions rated with values ≤3 were considered as clear and comprehensible, therefore, rewording was not required [10]. Results were reported with 95% confidence intervals. Furthermore, clarity/comprehension was evaluated using a cognitive survey that evaluated each item/question in a three-point ordinal scale; 1: Clear and comprehensible, 2: Difficult to understand, and 3: Incomprehensible [16]. Agreement among participants was evaluated using the Kendall's W coefficient of concordance, ranging from 0 (no agreement) to 1 (complete agreement). A W value ≥ 0.66 was considered as an adequate agreement among the participants. Additionally, to ensure the comprehension of each question, the participants were to answer the following question: In case you do not understand the question, how would you write it? This option was provided if the participants did not correctly understand some questions, or if they thought that there was a more comprehensible way to write the item.

2.4. Questionnaire Test-Retest Consistency

The questionnaire reproducibility was evaluated in a cohort of subjects who reported adverse reactions to wheat/gluten ($n = 12$), as well as in another cohort who reported adverse reactions to foods other than gluten ($n = 8$). Participants answered the questionnaire twice. The time period interval between the first and second application of the questionnaire was at least one week. The reproducibility of the questionnaire was evaluated with Cohen's k coefficient tests.

2.5. Pilot Survey

After the clarity/comprehension and consistency evaluation process, a digital version of the conciliated Brazilian-Portuguese questionnaire (Supplementary Material Section S2) was sent to 966 Brazilian health sciences students from Faculdade do Juazeiro do Norte in Juazeiro do Norte, Ceará, Brazil using the SurveyMonkey platform (San Mateo, CA, USA). The first page of the survey showed a general description of the project and presented the consent form. All data were collected in June 2019. Inclusion criteria were as follows: subjects must be aged ≥ 18 years old, and able to read and answer the questionnaire by themselves. Exclusion criteria were as follows: subjects being < 18 years old or not being able to complete the questionnaire by themselves. Individuals were classified according to previously published definitions on GRD [12] (Supplementary Material Section S3).

2.6. Statistical Analysis and Ethical Issues

Statistical analysis was carried out using PASW statistics version 25.0 (SPSS Inc., Chicago, IL, USA). Total numbers, percentages, and 95% confidence intervals (CI) were analyzed according to a set of descriptive statistics. A p value < 0.05 was considered as statistically significant. OpenEpi software version 3.03a (Atlanta, GA, USA) was used to estimate the prevalence rates (95% CI) per 100 inhabitants. This study was approved by the Research Ethics Committee of the Faculdade do Juazeiro do norte (Número do Parecer: 3.382.689).

3. Results

3.1. Questionnaire Translation and Back-Translation

The complete flow chart and the results of the evaluation of translation, clarity, comprehensibility, and consistency of the questionnaire are shown in Figure 1. Two native Brazilian Portuguese speakers carried out the translations from Spanish to Brazilian Portuguese. Translations to Brazilian-Portuguese (TBP1 and 2) had more than 80% of an overall match between them (TBP1 matched 81.8% with TBP2 and TBP2 matched 84.1% with TBP1). Most of the items in conflict were synonymous in Brazilian Portuguese with the same meaning in Spanish language. After agreement by the translators, the best synonymous were selected to have a conciliated version of the questionnaire translated to Brazilian Portuguese. The back-translations (two versions) of the conciliated Brazilian Portuguese version of the instrument matched 93.7% and 85.4% with the original Spanish version.

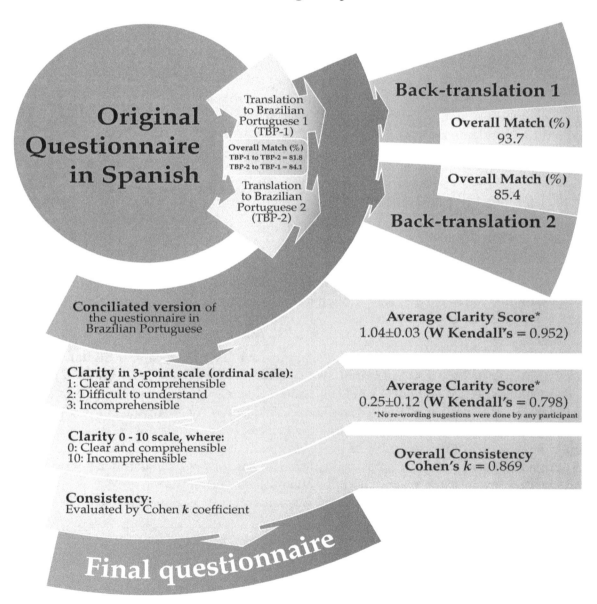

Figure 1. Flow chart of the translation of the questionnaire and the results of the evaluations on matches (between translations 1 and 2 from Spanish to Brazilian Portuguese, and between back-translations to Spanish compared to the original questionnaire), clarity, comprehension, and consistency.

3.2. Questionnaire Clarity/Comprehension

Sixty-four Brazilian Portuguese native speakers (38 females, 26 males; 18–55 years old) evaluated clarity/comprehensibility using a continuous scale (0: clear and comprehensible, 10: incomprehensible). On the bases of this evaluation, the average of the clarity score was 0.25 (CI, 95%: 0.03–0.53; values ranged from 0 to 9) and the Kendall's W score was 0.798. Using the three-point ordinal scale, the average of the clarity score was 1.04. This value is very close to "clear and comprehensible" and, according to the Kendall's W score obtained (0.952), involves a high concordance among the individuals' answers to the questions. Importantly, when the participants were asked for the questions' re-writing to improve the understanding, neither re-wording nor suggestions for changes were reported.

3.3. Questionnaire Consistency

Twenty participants who reported adverse reactions to gluten or to other foods answered the questionnaire twice (12 females and 8 males). The concordance between the first and the second application of the questionnaire was measured individually, and the average of Cohen's k coefficient was 0.869 (Figure 1). This k value can be interpreted as an almost perfect concordance.

3.4. Pilot Study

A total of 966 health sciences students received the link to answer the questionnaire. The response rate was 9.0% (n = 87), but 13 subjects had to be excluded due to their proportioned incomplete demographic data or responses. Thus, a total of 74 valid questionnaires were considered for prevalence estimations. The proportion of male/female was 24.3%: 75.6% (male: 18; female: 56). Average age was 25 ± 6.6 years. The most commonly self-reported, physician-diagnosed conditions were psychiatric diseases (9.45%; IC 95%), irritable bowel syndrome (8.1%; IC 95% 3.88–18.52), diabetes, lactose intolerance, and allergies (6.75%; IC 2.23–15.07, each). However, due to the reduced number of participants, risk analysis between Self-Reported Gluten Sensitivity (SR-GS) and non-Self-Reported Gluten Sensitivity (non-SR-GS) conditions could not be calculated.

Prevalence rates estimations of GRD and other adverse foods reactions are shown in the Table 1. Adverse reactions to wheat/gluten were reported by 16.21% of the participants, though, only two fulfilled criteria for SR-GS (2.70%) (Supplementary Material Section S3). The prevalence rates of wheat allergy and NCGS were 1.35% each. No male fulfilled the criteria for either wheat allergy or NCGS. Physician diagnosis of CD was not reported in this pilot study. The prevalence rate of adherence to a GFD was higher in females than in males, while the prevalence rate of wheat/gluten avoiders was slightly higher in males than in females (p > 0.05).

The characteristics of the individuals following a GFD are shown in Figure 2. It should be noted that almost all participants who were following a GFD (75%) and those that were avoiding wheat/gluten containing foods (75%) fulfilled criteria for non-SR-GS. Regarding the motivations for following a GFD, in the non-SR-GS group the most frequent motivation was weight control (50%), while in the SR-GS group was the symptomatic relapse. Similar results were obtained in the wheat/gluten avoiders group. All participants who were following a GFD reported to be under the supervision of a dietitian to follow the diet. Ten individuals reported recurrent gastrointestinal and/or extra-intestinal symptoms triggered after the ingestion of wheat/gluten containing foods. Bloating (80%), abdominal pain (80%), nausea (60%), stomachache (60%), and reflux (60%) were the most commonly reported gastrointestinal symptoms. On the other hand, lack of wellbeing (60%), tiredness (40%), and muscular pain (40%) were the most commonly reported extra-intestinal symptoms.

Table 1. Self-reported prevalence rates.

Assessment	(+) Cases	Mean Age in Years (Range)	Prevalence by Gender (95% CI)	p-Value	General Prevalence (95% CI)
Adverse reaction to foods	$n = 24$ $M = 6$ $F = 18$	27 (19–47)	$M = 33.33$ (13.34–59.01) $F = 32.14$ (20.28–45.96)	0.999	32.43 (22.0–44.32)
Adverse reaction to wheat/gluten	$n = 12$ $M = 3$ $F = 9$	30 (20–47)	$M = 16.66$ (3.57–41.42) $F = 16.07$ (7.62–28.33)	0.999	16.21 (8.67–26.61)
Self-Reported Gluten sensitivity (SR-GS)	$n = 2$ $M = 0$ $F = 2$	27 (20–34)	$M = 0$ (0.0–18.53) $F = 3.57$ (0.43–12.31)	0.999	2.70 (0.32–9.42)
SR-PD Celiac disease	$n = 0$	—	—	—	—
Wheat allergy	$n = 1$ $M = 0$ $F = 1$	20 (N/D)	$M = 0$ (0.0–18.53) $F = 1.29$ (0.22–6.99)	0.999	1.35 (0.03–7.30)
NCGS	$n = 1$ $M = 0$ $F = 1$	34 (N/D)	$M = 0$ (0.0–18.53) $F = 1.29$ (0.22–6.99)	0.999	1.35 (0.03–7.30)
Adherence to GFD	$n = 8$ $M = 1$ $F = 7$	25 (20–41)	$M = 1.29$ (0.22–6.99) $F = 9.09$ (4.47–17.6)	0.671	10.81 (4.78–20.19)
Avoid wheat/gluten-containing foods	$n = 12$ $M = 3$ $F = 9$	26 (20–41)	$M = 16.66$ (3.57–41.42) $F = 16.07$ (7.62–28.33)	0.999	16.21 (8.67–26.61)

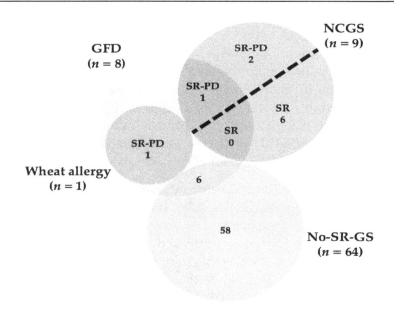

Figure 2. Characteristics of the participants who were following a GFD. SR-PD: Self-reported Physician-Diagnosed; SR: Self-reported; GFD: Gluten-free Diet; NCGS: Non-Celiac Gluten Sensitivity; Non-SR-GS: Non-self-reported Gluten Sensitivity.

4. Discussion

Survey-based studies are useful to estimate the prevalence rates of several conditions and set the ground for further epidemiological studies based on objective diagnostic criteria. The results of survey studies can be interpreted in different ways. Particular attention needed to be given to the most underdiagnosed conditions and those conditions for which there is a lack of sensitive and specific biomarkers, such as CD and NCGS, respectively. In this context, a questionnaire intended to evaluate the self-reported prevalence of GRD and the adherence to a GFD in Spanish-speaking populations was applied in four Latin American countries [10–13]. However, idiom issues hampered the application of this instrument in Brazilian Portuguese speakers, the largest population in South America. To fill this gap, the questionnaire was translated to Brazilian Portuguese and systematically tested. The translations of the questionnaire from Spanish to Brazilian Portuguese matched in high percentage and most of the items in conflict were words with the same meaning. The similarity between Spanish and Portuguese is the highest among romance languages [18], thus allowing for the facilitation of the translation of the questionnaire and, at the same time, it could improve the matching among the translations carried out by different translators. Back-translation is a process necessary to verify the accuracy of the original translation [19] and to reduce any discrepancies between the original version of the instrument and the back-translated version [20]. The overall matching between the back-translated versions with the original Spanish version indicates a high similarity between them. This supports the notion that the conciliated version of the questionnaire in Brazilian-Portuguese mirrors the original Spanish version.

Precision evaluation of the words utilized in a questionnaire is essential to avoid misinterpretation or incomprehension of the formulated questions [21]. In the present study, the outcome of the clarity/comprehension evaluation using a continuous scale was excellent (0.25; where 0 means clear and comprehensible). This indicated that the conciliated version of the questionnaire in Brazilian Portuguese language was clear and comprehensible. Importantly, the participants did not suggest re-writing of questions. These results are similar to those reported in the clarity/comprehension evaluation of the original Spanish version of the questionnaire [10]. To corroborate the clarity/comprehension data obtained in the present study, additional tests based on a three-point ordinal scale were carried out. The results of these tests corroborate that the Brazilian-Portuguese version of the questionnaire was clear and comprehensible. Additionally, the average of the Kendall's W coefficient for the clarity/comprehension evaluation highlighted a very high agreement among the evaluations of the participants [22].

The consistency in the answers to each question of the questionnaire by the same individual was also evaluated. The questionnaire was applied twice at different moments, allowing at least one-week intervals to pass between the two applications. The consistency evaluated as the k coefficient value was 0.869, which can be considered an excellent agreement between the two applications of the questionnaire [23]. This result is similar to that reported for the original Spanish version of the instrument [10].

Online survey studies have gained attention, as the staff requirement to collect data and printing costs can be kept to a minimum. Under these bases, a pilot online survey study was carried out using the instrument generated. However, a very low response rate was reported (9.0%). In line with this, several survey-based studies, conducted using internet platforms, have reported similar and even lower response rates [24]. On the contrary, previous studies have reported high response rates (53.3 to 92.0%) using the Spanish version of the questionnaire utilized in this pilot study, but conducting the survey on the bases of face-to-face interviews in public places instead of using internet platforms [10–13]. The prevalence data generated in the present online pilot survey study should be interpreted with caution, as the response rate was quite low, and the sample was limited to Brazilian health sciences students. The same applies for the data related to the gastrointestinal and extra-intestinal symptoms reported. The main contribution of the online pilot survey study carried out in the present work is that it highlights the need to perform face-to-face interviews to successfully utilize the Brazilian-Portuguese version of the questionnaire intended to evaluate the self-reported prevalence of GRD and adherence to a GFD.

5. Conclusions

In this study, a questionnaire intended to estimate the prevalence of self-reported GRD and adherence to a GFD was translated to Brazilian Portuguese and tested. The questionnaire was clear, comprehensible, and generated reproducible results in the target population. The questionnaire should ideally be applied preferentially on the bases of face-to-face interviews instead of using online platforms. This strategy can help to improve the response rate and minimize bias in order to generate representative results. The present study provides an instrument to estimate the prevalence of self-reported GRD and adherence to a GFD in Brazilian Portuguese native speakers, a community that represents almost half of the South America population.

Author Contributions: Conceptualization, N.O. and F.C.-C.; data curation, J.G.A.-G. and C.E.B.-C.; formal analysis, O.G.F.-S., F.I.C.-T., N.O. and F.C.-C.; investigation, J.G.A.-G., M.A.M.-C., É.M.B.R., E.A.M.-T.-W., V.R.-F., O.G.F.-S., F.I.C.-T., N.O. and F.C.-C.; methodology, J.G.A.-G., I.C.G., T.G.A., C.E.B.-C., M.A.M.-C., É.M.B.R., E.A.M.-T.-W., V.R.-F., O.G.F.-S. and F.I.C.-T.; resources, N.O. and F.C.-C.; visualization, F.I.C.-T., N.O. and F.C.-C.; writing—original draft, J.G.A.-G., N.O. and F.C.-C.; writing—review and editing, I.C.G., T.G.A., C.E.B.-C., M.A.M.-C., É.M.B.R., E.A.M.-T.-W., V.R.-F., O.G.F.-S., F.I.C.-T., N.O. and F.C.-C.

Acknowledgments: We acknowledge the technical support by Yolanda Irene Aguilar Hinojosa and Jose Pedro Mendes Alves Palmela. We acknowledge the postgraduate fellowships given to I.C.G., T.G.A., and F.I.C.-T., by the Mexican Council for Science and Technology (CONACyT).

References

1. Casellas, F.; Rodrigo, L.; Lucendo, A.J.; Fernández-Bañares, F.; Molina-Infante, J.; Vivas, S.; Rosinach, M.; Dueñas, C.; López-Vivancos, J. Benefit on health-related quality of life of adherence to gluten-free diet in adult patients with celiac disease. *Rev. Española Enferm. Dig.* **2015**, *107*, 196–201.
2. Walker, M.D.; Williams, J.; Lewis, S.K.; Bai, J.C.; Lebwohl, B.; Green, P.H.R. Measurement of forearm bone density by dual energy x-ray absorptiometry increases the prevalence of osteoporosis in men with celiac disease. *Clin. Gastroenterol. Hepatol.* **2019**, 1–8. [CrossRef] [PubMed]
3. Ganji, R.; Moghbeli, M.; Sadeghi, R.; Bayat, G.; Ganji, A. Prevalence of osteoporosis and osteopenia in men and premenopausal women with celiac disease: A systematic review. *Nutr. J.* **2019**, *18*, 9. [CrossRef] [PubMed]
4. Freeman, H.J. Iron deficiency anemia in celiac disease. *World J. Gastroenterol.* **2015**, *21*, 9233–9238. [CrossRef] [PubMed]
5. Malamut, G.; Chandesris, O.; Verkarre, V.; Meresse, B.; Callens, C.; Macintyre, E.; Bouhnik, Y.; Gornet, J.M.; Allez, M.; Jian, R.; et al. Enteropathy associated T cell lymphoma in celiac disease: A large retrospective study. *Dig. Liver Dis.* **2013**, *45*, 377–384. [CrossRef] [PubMed]
6. Wild, D.; Robins, G.G.; Burley, V.J.; Howdle, P.D. Evidence of high sugar intake, and low fibre and mineral intake, in the gluten-free diet. *Aliment. Pharmacol. Ther.* **2010**, *32*, 573–581. [CrossRef]
7. Taetzsch, A.; Das, S.K.; Brown, C.; Krauss, A.; Silver, R.E.; Roberts, S.B. Are gluten-free diets more nutritious? An evaluation of self-selected and recommended gluten-free and gluten-containing dietary patterns. *Nutrients* **2018**, *10*, 1881. [CrossRef]
8. Narayan, S.; Lakshmipriya, N.; Vaidya, R.; Bai, M.R.; Sudha, V.; Krishnaswamy, K.; Unnikrishnan, R.; Anjana, R.M.; Mohan, V. Association of dietary fiber intake with serum total cholesterol and low density lipoprotein cholesterol levels in Urban Asian-Indian adults with type 2 diabetes. *Indian J. Endocrinol. Metab.* **2014**, *18*, 624–630.
9. Zhou, Q.; Wu, J.; Tang, J.; Wang, J.-J.; Lu, C.-H.; Wang, P.-X. Beneficial effect of higher dietary fiber intake on plasma HDL-C and TC/HDL-C ratio among chinese rural-to-urban migrant workers. *Int. J. Environ. Res. Public Health* **2015**, *12*, 4726–4738. [CrossRef]
10. Ontiveros, N.; López-Gallardo, J.A.; Vergara-Jiménez, M.J.; Cabrera-Chávez, F. Self-reported prevalence of symptomatic adverse reactions to gluten and adherence to gluten-free diet in an adult mexican population. *Nutrients* **2015**, *7*, 6000–6015. [CrossRef]
11. Cabrera-Chávez, F.; Granda-Restrepo, D.M.; Arámburo-Gálvez, J.G.; Franco-Aguilar, A.; Magaña-Ordorica, D.; de Jesús Vergara-Jiménez, M.; Ontiveros, N. Self-reported prevalence of gluten-related disorders and adherence to gluten-free diet in colombian adult population. *Gastroenterol. Res. Pract.* **2016**, *2016*, 4704309. [CrossRef] [PubMed]
12. Ontiveros, N.; Rodríguez-Bellegarrigue, C.I.; Galicia-Rodríguez, G.; de Jesús Vergara-Jiménez, M.; Zepeda-Gómez, E.M.; Arámburo-Galvez, J.G.; Gracia-Valenzuela, M.H.; Cabrera-Chávez, F. Prevalence of self-reported gluten-related disorders and adherence to a gluten-free diet in salvadoran adult population. *Int. J. Environ. Res. Public Health* **2018**, *15*, 786. [CrossRef] [PubMed]

13. Cabrera-Chávez, F.; Dezar, G.V.A.; Islas-Zamorano, A.P.; Espinoza-Alderete, J.G.; Vergara-Jiménez, M.J.; Magaña-Ordorica, D.; Ontiveros, N. Prevalence of self-reported gluten sensitivity and adherence to a gluten-free diet in argentinian adult population. *Nutrients* **2017**, *9*, 81. [CrossRef] [PubMed]

14. Volta, U.; Bardella, M.T.; Calabrò, A.; Troncone, R.; Corazza, G.R. An Italian prospective multicenter survey on patients suspected of having non-celiac gluten sensitivity. *BMC Med.* **2014**, *12*, 85. [CrossRef] [PubMed]

15. Gadelha De Mattos, Y.A.; Zandonadi, R.P.; Gandolfi, L.; Pratesi, R.; Nakano, E.Y.; Pratesi, C.B. Self-reported non-celiac gluten sensitivity in Brazil: Translation, cultural adaptation, and validation of Italian questionnaire. *Nutrients* **2019**, *11*, 781. [CrossRef]

16. Gusi, N.; Badía, X.; Herdman, M.; Olivares, P.R. Traducción y adaptación cultural de la versión española del cuestionario EQ-5D-Y en niños y adolescentes. *Aten. Primaria* **2009**, *41*, 19–23. [CrossRef] [PubMed]

17. Casellas, F.; Rodrigo, L.; Molina-Infante, J.; Vivas, S.; Lucendo, A.J.; Rosinach, M.; Dueñas, C.; Fernández-Bañares, F.; López-Vivancos, J. Transcultural adaptation and validation of the Celiac Disease Quality of Life (CD-QOL) survey, a specific questionnaire to measure quality of life in patients with celiac disease. *Rev. Española Enferm. Dig.* **2013**, *105*, 585–593. [CrossRef]

18. Henriques, E.R. Text intercomprehension by native speakers of portuguese and spanish. *DELTA* **2000**, *16*, 263–295. [CrossRef]

19. Paegelow, R.S. Back translation revisited: Differences that matter (and those that do not). *ATA Chron.* **2008**, *1*, 22.

20. Chen, H.Y.; Boore, J.R.P. Translation and back-translation in qualitative nursing research: Methodological review. *J. Clin. Nurs.* **2010**, *19*, 234–239. [CrossRef]

21. Kazi, A.M.; Khalid, W. Questionnaire designing and validation. *J. Pak. Med. Assoc.* **2012**, *62*, 514–516. [PubMed]

22. Schmidt, R.C. Managing Delphi surveys using nonparametric statistical techniques. *Decis. Sci.* **1997**, *28*, 763–774. [CrossRef]

23. Landis, J.R.; Koch, G.G. An application of hierarchical kappa-type statistics in the assessment of majority agreement among multiple observers. *Biometrics* **1977**, *33*, 363–374. [CrossRef] [PubMed]

24. Van Mol, C. Improving web survey efficiency: The impact of an extra reminder and reminder content on web survey response. *Int. J. Soc. Res. Methodol.* **2016**, *20*, 317–327. [CrossRef]

Gluten-Induced Extra-Intestinal Manifestations in Potential Celiac Disease—Celiac Trait

Alina Popp [1,2] **and Markku Mäki** [2,*]

[1]   University of Medicine and Pharmacy "Carol Davila" and National Institute for Mother and Child Health "Alessandrescu-Rusescu", Bucharest 020395, Romania; alina.popp@uta.fi

[2]   Faculty of Medicine and Health Technology, Tampere University and Tampere University Hospital, 33520 Tampere, Finland

*   Correspondence: markku.maki@uta.fi

Abstract: Celiac disease patients may suffer from a number of extra-intestinal diseases related to long-term gluten ingestion. The diagnosis of celiac disease is based on the presence of a manifest small intestinal mucosal lesion. Individuals with a normal biopsy but an increased risk of developing celiac disease are referred to as potential celiac disease patients. However, these patients are not treated. This review highlights that patients with normal biopsies may suffer from the same extra-intestinal gluten-induced complications before the disease manifests at the intestinal level. We discuss diagnostic markers revealing true potential celiac disease. The evidence-based medical literature shows that these potential patients, who are "excluded" for celiac disease would in fact benefit from gluten-free diets. The question is why wait for an end-stage disease to occur when it can be prevented? We utilize research on dermatitis herpetiformis, which is a model disease in which a gluten-induced entity erupts in the skin irrespective of the state of the small intestinal mucosal morphology. Furthermore, gluten ataxia can be categorized as its own entity. The other extra-intestinal manifestations occurring in celiac disease are also found at the latent disease stage. Consequently, patients with celiac traits should be identified and treated.

Keywords: gluten; latent celiac disease; potential celiac disease; extra-intestinal manifestations; mild enteropathy; early developing celiac disease; genetic gluten intolerance; natural history; celiac trait

1. Introduction

Celiac disease is an autoimmune systemic disorder in genetically susceptible persons perpetuated by the daily ingestion of gluten cereals (wheat, rye, and barley) with manifestations in the small intestine and organs outside the gut. Patients diagnosed with celiac disease show gluten-induced and gluten-dependent duodenal mucosal lesions (i.e., the typical crypt hyperplastic lesion with villous atrophy). Clinically these newly diagnosed patients may or may not be suffering from gastrointestinal symptoms. A gluten-driven extra-intestinal manifestation is often the only clue for the disease. In the primary care and within different medical disciplines, physicians should suspect celiac disease and perform case finding by serum autoantibody screening. Positive serology is often the only way to identify potential patients for a diagnostic upper intestinal endoscopy [1–3]. In fact, less than half of all adult patients diagnosed with celiac disease complain of gastrointestinal symptoms at an initial diagnosis [4]. This knowledge comes from Finland, where adult celiac disease diagnoses have increased 20 times in recent decades and 0.8% of the total population has a biopsy-confirmed diagnosis [5–7].

Patients diagnosed with celiac disease including a duodenal mucosal lesion may suffer from a number of extra-intestinal diseases [2,3]. Dermatitis herpetiformis manifests outside the gut, is gluten driven and dependent [8,9], has the same genetic background, and occurs within the same families as celiac disease [9,10]. In fact, one identical twin may have celiac disease while the other suffers from dermatitis herpetiformis [11]. Other gluten-driven extra-intestinal manifestations in celiac disease include osteopenia, osteoporosis, fractures [12–14], permanent tooth enamel defects [6,15], arthritis, and arthralgia [16–18] as well as further central and peripheral nervous system [19–22], liver [23–25], and reproductive system involvements [26,27]. Even autoimmune diseases may be gluten driven [28,29], and there is a risk for malignant complications, especially non-Hodgkin lymphoma, in untreated celiac disease [30,31].

By definition, celiac disease is excluded in patients who have normal small intestinal mucosal morphology at their first diagnostic endoscopy if they have been following a normal gluten-containing diet. However, it seems evident that this is not accurate. In a review in 2001, we wrote that gluten-induced extra-intestinal manifestations may develop at the latent disease stage when the mucosa is still morphologically normal [32], citing several observations [19,33–36]. Today such patients are often referred to as having "potential celiac disease" because they are found to be "normal" on biopsy [37]. Meanwhile, dermatitis herpetiformis is our model disease, in which an extra-intestinal manifestation is treated with a gluten-free diet irrespective of the mucosal finding (diseased or not). We reviewed the literature for evidence for extra-intestinal gluten-dependent manifestations in patients "excluded" for celiac disease. In this paper, we also discuss tools for identifying these "potential" treatable patients.

2. Latent or Potential Celiac Disease

The "pre-celiac" state has been described in patients with dermatitis herpetiformis, in whom small intestinal mucosal deterioration was shown to occur after adding extra gluten to the diet [38–40]. An extra gluten load also induced mucosal lesions in healthy individuals [39,41]. The concept of latent celiac disease, without having an extra load of gluten, was shown to be part of the gluten sensitivity spectrum and natural history of celiac disease [42–45]. Specifically, this was shown in Finland in celiac patients who, by chance, had previously undergone a small intestinal biopsy that was reported as normal or who were followed up because of positive serum autoantibody results.

We chose to use the term "latent celiac disease", which is similar to Weinstein [38], when referring to patients with a normal biopsy who later exhibited mucosal deterioration and were diagnosed as celiac disease patients. For us, "latent" means existing but not manifest (i.e., the disease exists but is not manifest at the mucosal level). Based on our early descriptions, Ferguson et al. (1993) defined latent celiac disease as follows: "This term should only be applied to patients who fulfill the following conditions: (i) have a normal jejunal biopsy while taking a normal diet, (ii) at some other time, before or since, have had a flat jejunal biopsy which recovers on a gluten free diet" [46]. Following the first reports on existing celiac disease latency, a numbers of other results have been published, with early papers by Troncone [47] and Corazza et al. [48]. It is now clear that oral tolerance towards gluten can be kept for longer periods, even for decades and into older age [49].

The term "potential celiac disease" has been used interchangeably with latent celiac disease, and this has led to confusion in the celiac disease literature. Thus, the Oslo task force discouraged the use of the term "latent celiac disease", and individuals with a normal outcome from a small intestinal biopsy but who are at increased risk of developing celiac disease based on positive celiac disease serology should be referred to as having potential celiac disease [37]. These "potential patients" are not treated as celiac. The question is, what should a gluten-triggered and gluten-dependent treatable disease outside the gut be called, when the extra-intestinal manifestation occurs at the latent stage of the disease and when conventional diagnostic biopsy criteria have excluded celiac disease? We infer that such patients should not be categorized as having potential celiac disease. Rather, they require proper treatment [50,51].

In Figure 1, we summarize the lifespan natural history of celiac gluten sensitivity, where each line represents a single individual. The term celiac gluten sensitivity encompasses celiac traits, latent celiac disease, genetic gluten intolerance, mild enteropathy celiac disease, early developing celiac disease, and celiac disease itself [1,32,50–53]. The gluten-induced mucosal damage develops rapidly or gradually from normal mucosal morphology to a manifest mucosal lesion. The tolerance towards gluten is individual, and it may be broken after only months or years (childhood celiac disease) but also at adolescence, adulthood, and even after decades of gluten ingestion in old age. The latent celiac disease patients, the "true potential" patients in Figure 1 (i.e., normal on biopsy showing villus height crypt depth ratio >2), are classified as having celiac disease only when the disease has deteriorated to the degree of a manifest mucosal lesion (i.e., villus height crypt depth ratio <2).

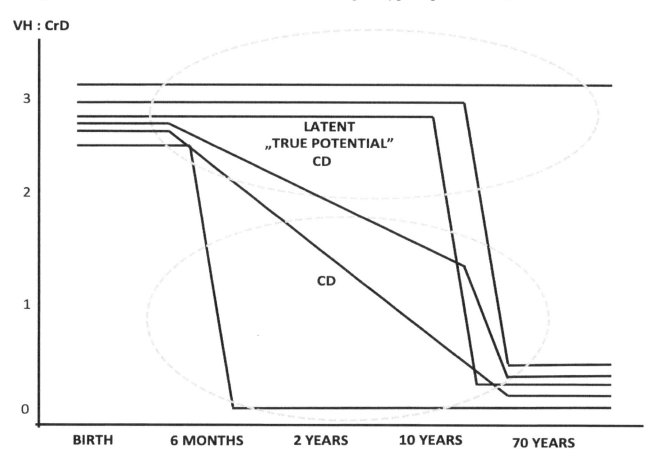

Figure 1. Natural history of developing celiac disease (CD) at the small intestinal mucosal level. Each line represents one individual. We are born with a normal mucosal morphology, a villus height (VH), and a crypt depth (CrD) ratio of approximately three and villi three times taller than crypts are deep. Upon gluten ingestion, mucosal injury proceeds rapidly or gradually at different ages, in childhood or only at an older age. Before developing a manifest mucosal lesion (diseased mucosa on biopsy, VH:CrD <2) every CD patient belongs to the category latent "true potential" CD (normal on biopsy, VH:CrD >2).

3. Markers of Existing Early Disease

An existing gluten-dependent disease without evidence of enteropathy until a later age - latent celiac disease - includes in its definition the susceptibility genes for celiac disease and the genes encoding the *human leukocyte antigen* (HLA) DQ2 or DQ8 molecules [1,32,54]. This is a check that clinicians may perform when there are symptoms and signs suggestive of celiac disease, but the biopsy is normal or does not show clear crypt hyperplasia. It shows only inflammation and descriptive mild villus atrophy. Positivity for DQ2 or DQ8 does not mean very much, since 30% to 40% of the citizens in the country are positive, but double negative means that no celiac disease will develop.

Patients positive for *celiac disease serology* with normal biopsies should be considered to have potential celiac disease [37]. However, gliadin antibody positivity, which is a frequent finding in celiac disease control patients and even in healthy individuals, does not correlate with celiac disease susceptibility genes [55]. Currently, tissue transglutaminase autoantibody (TG2-ab) testing is used to screen for celiac disease. It should be noted, however, that not all serum TG2-abs predict celiac disease [56]. TG2-abs have been described in other autoimmune diseases as well as in infections, tumors, myocardial damage, liver disorders, and psoriasis [54]. These antibodies are not associated with endomysial autoantibodies and may occur in persons negative both for HLA DQ2 and DQ8. The serum endomysial antibody test is the gold standard, and the presence of these autoantibodies predicts impending celiac disease [1,45,50,53,55]. In celiac disease in patients with extra-intestinal manifestations, other autoantibodies play a role in diagnosis and potentially in disease mechanisms [57].

At the mucosal level, inflammation, as measured as the density of intraepithelial T cells (*IELs*), is a very unspecific finding, but is also gluten-dependent in cases of celiac disease [58]. Marsh 1 lesions with increased IELs were shown to have a sensitivity of 59% and specificity of 57% in predicting forthcoming celiac disease [59]. However, when searched for, an autoimmune insult to the morphologically normal intestinal mucosa is, in fact, present. A high density of $\gamma\delta$ *T-cell-receptor-bearing IELs* in patients with morphologically normal mucosa who also carry the susceptibility genes for celiac disease seems to be a prerequisite for developing celiac disease [43,60,61]. Yet, even if an increased density of $\gamma\delta$ T cells is found in latent celiac disease, such a finding is not pathognomonic for the disease [59,61]. In the small intestine, the gluten-dependent autoantibodies target extracellular TG2 and may be detected as *IgA deposits* in biopsy tissues at the latent disease stage [62–64] (Figure 2). In fact, the IgA deposits in the duodenal biopsies accurately predicted forthcoming celiac disease better than IELs, $\gamma\delta^+$ IELs, or serum autoantibodies [59]. The detection of intestinal TG2-abs by phage-antibody libraries is another possibility for diagnosis [52]. However, intestinal TG2-ab production is not only found in celiac disease [65]. Again, when finding an increased density of $\gamma\delta^+$ IELs or IgA deposits in a patient with normal small intestinal mucosal morphology, it is recommended to check whether the patient belongs to the "celiac family" (i.e., are carrying either the HLA DQ2 or DQ8 molecules).

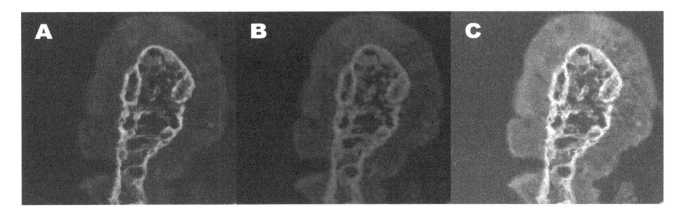

Figure 2. Small intestinal mucosal immunoglobulin (Ig) A deposits are shown in a villus tip from a dermatitis herpetiformis patient with normal mucosal morphology. IgA is stained with green (**A**), transglutaminase 2 (TG2) with red (**B**), and subepithelial colocalisation of IgA and TG2 can be seen in yellow (**C**).

4. Extraintestinal Manifestations

4.1. Dermatitis Herpetiformis

In dermatitis herpetiformis, a gluten-induced and gluten-dependent manifestation occurs outside the gut even in the absence of intestinal mucosal villous atrophy [8,66]. Today, up to 30% of patients with dermatitis herpetiformis have a normal small intestinal mucosal lining [67]. Typically, the disease manifests with itchy papules and vesicles on the elbows, knees and buttocks, and overt gastrointestinal symptoms are rare [67,68]. When patients without enteropathy are challenged with extra gluten, their small intestinal mucosae deteriorate in a way typical of celiac disease [38–40]. When no enteropathy is present, patients only test positively for serum TG2-abs and endomysial antibodies in 40% of cases [67]. However, the patients could be serum endomysial autoantibody positive already while having normal small intestinal mucosa prior to any evidence of skin eruptions [44]. If searched for, the autoimmune effect to the morphologically normal intestinal mucosa caused by an environmental trigger—the daily ingestion of gluten—is, in fact, present. Mucosal inflammatory markers (i.e., the high density of $\gamma\delta^+$ IELs) shows this [35]. Furthermore, in patients who are negative for serum autoantibodies, the antibodies are found at the mucosal level targeting extracellular TG2 [62,69,70], which is a finding typical for an existing disease that is not manifest at the mucosal architectural level (Figure 2).

We infer that patients with gluten-triggered extra-intestinal manifestations, who are now classified as having dermatitis herpetiformis but show a normal small intestinal mucosa, do not belong to the category of potential celiac disease. These patients may even be suffering from osteoporosis and experience bone fractures. Clearly, it is a treatable disease [67,68,71]. In the following, we use parallel reasoning for patients having other gluten-dependent extra-intestinal manifestations occurring at the latent stage of celiac disease.

4.2. Central and Peripheral Nervous System

Gluten-induced neurological manifestations including gluten ataxia are common in adult celiac disease [19–22] and occur in children [2]. Hadjivassiliou et al. noticed that gluten sensitivity was found in patients with neurological disease, and they screened the patients with gliadin antibodies [72]. They also showed that neurological complications occurred during the latent stage of celiac disease. Their use of gliadin antibodies created some skepticism toward the findings, but today gluten ataxia has become a gluten-induced entity in itself, similar to dermatitis herpetiformis [20,73]. In fact, it was shown that gluten ataxia might respond to a strict gluten-free diet even in the absence of an enteropathy [74,75]. Serum transglutaminase 6 antibodies are used for detecting gluten ataxia in patients with and without small intestinal mucosal lesions. Negative seroconversion results from a gluten-free diet [75]. Further evidence that gluten ataxia without enteropathy belongs to the celiac spectrum comes from the finding that TG2-specific autoantibody deposits were detected in the intestinal mucosa [74]. The patients were HLA DQ2-positive or DQ8-positive. All of the control ataxia patients were negative for celiac-type HLA, and they had no IgA deposits in the mucosa [74]. In one gluten ataxia patient, similar TG2-targeted IgA deposits were found in the small vessels of the brain [74]. In a different cohort of idiopathic ataxia patients, the TG2-targeted IgA deposits were again detected, even in the absence of circulating TG2-abs [76].

Gluten-induced peripheral nervous system involvement often expresses as a symmetrical sensorimotor axonal peripheral neuropathy [77]. In patients with or without enteropathy, neuropathies cannot be differentiated based on clinical, genetic, or immunological grounds [78,79].

4.3. Bone Disease

Bone diseases, osteopenia, osteoporosis, and even fractures are highly prevalent in untreated celiac disease [14,80,81]. Strict gluten-free diets improve bone health in celiac disease and are an effective therapy for long-term bone mineral recovery [13,82].

Latent celiac disease patients, before manifesting an overt disease, might suffer from gluten-dependent symptoms as well as osteopenia and osteoporosis [62,83–86]. Kaukinen et al. showed that eight of 10 patients without villous atrophy had a bone disease, and they all were DQ2 positive [83]. On biopsy, it was shown that they belonged to the celiac spectrum since they had increased densities of $\gamma\delta^+$ IELs. Furthermore, their initial TG2 and endomysial antibodies normalized with a gluten-free diet. Dickey et al. again measured bone mineral density in 31 endomysial antibody-positive patients who were excluded for celiac disease (i.e., classified as having Marsh 0 or Marsh 1 lesions). They found osteopenia to be present in 30% and osteoporosis in 10% of these patients, and the degree of bone disease did not differ from that found in patients diagnosed with overt celiac disease. Negative seroconversion followed upon implementation of a gluten-free diet in the 26 of the 27 patients with normal biopsies. On the contrary, eight patients continued their gluten-containing diet, and seven of them evolved toward villous atrophy compatible with celiac disease within one to two years [84]. Kurppa et al. proved that the gluten-free diet had a positive effect on the bone mineral density in endomysial antibody-positive patients with normal villous morphology, which is similar to those with celiac-type enteropathy [85]. Zanini et al. concluded that celiac disease patients with mild enteropathy have various markers of existing malabsorption including bone disease, and, thus, require treatment with a gluten-free diet [86].

Patients with true potential celiac disease are also a risk of fractures. Pasternack et al. showed that dermatitis herpetiformis patients reported earlier fractures in 45 out of 222 cases at diagnosis. Altogether, 16% of the fractures had occurred in patients with normal small intestinal histology, 35% occurred in patients with partial villous atrophy, and 49% occurred in patients with subtotal villous atrophy in Reference [71].

4.4. Liver Diseases

Celiac disease may initially present as a monosymptomatic liver disease, such as cryptogenic hypertransaminasaemia or autoimmunue-type of liver damage [23–25,87]. There are few reports of liver injury in potential or latent celiac disease. Zanini et al. observed that celiac disease with mild enteropathy and positive celiac disease-related serology is not a mild disease. Moreover, they showed alanine aminotransferase serum values to be elevated in 9/121 (8%), γ-glutamyltransferase in 5/102 (5%), and alkaline phosphatase in 6/101 (6%) of patients. The authors concluded that these patients should also be treated [86].

4.5. Other Extraintestinal Manifestations

4.5.1. Permanent Tooth Dental Enamel Defects

Adult patients with celiac disease and dermatitis herpetiformis, as well as children with dermatitis herpetiformis, show celiac-type dental enamel defects in their permanent dentition [15,88–90]. Typical enamel defects were found in all healthy family members of celiac disease patients found to have manifest mucosal lesions. Furthermore, these celiac-type enamel defects occurred without small intestinal changes and were strongly associated with the HLA DR3 [34]. Importantly, these permanent tooth enamel defects are induced by gluten ingestion in early childhood, when the enamel is developing (i.e., at the latent stage of celiac disease and dermatitis herpetiformis).

4.5.2. Malignancies

In 1986, Freeman and Chiu reported that intestinal lymphoma might appear at the latent stage of celiac disease when the mucosa is morphologically normal [33]. However, it is not known whether untreated patients without a manifest mucosal lesion carry an increased risk of malignancy. However, there are many complications, including malignancies, that may occur in adulthood when the patient is undiagnosed by ingesting gluten. Celiac disease patients diagnosed at an adult and elderly age have not had manifest mucosal lesions from early childhood (Figure 1) [42–45,48,49].

Figure 3 indicates that all the extra-intestinal manifestations induced by gluten in untreated celiac disease can be detected in the latent stage of the disease.

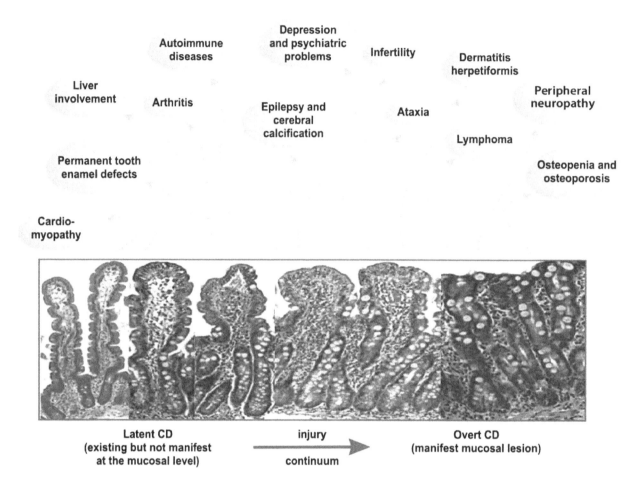

Figure 3. Celiac trait. Gluten-induced extra-intestinal manifestations exist in both patients with normal (latent celiac disease, CD) and diseased small intestinal mucosa (overt CD). Drawing adapted from the "cooking pot" of splashing extra-intestinal manifestations, which is first presented at the International Celiac Disease Symposium in Dublin 1992, and from drawings in references No. 34, 53, and 54.

5. Celiac Trait

Celiac disease diagnosis requires a gluten-induced small intestinal mucosal lesion. As indicated in Figure 3, the so-called "flat" lesion is the end stage of the mucosal injury. Figure 3 also summarizes our review and shows that, when there is a gluten-induced and gluten-dependent extra-intestinal manifestation in celiac disease, the manifestation can be found in patients before the mucosa is diseased or when it shows only minor non-specific changes. For susceptible persons, upon gluten ingestion, celiac disease develops gradually from normal mucosal morphology through mucosal inflammation, crypt hyperplasia, and villous atrophy to the "flat" mucosal lesions [91]. When the mucosa is morphologically normal and, for example, bones are already fracturing due to gluten ingestion, we should not call this condition potential celiac disease [38]. Moreover, we should not wait for the manifest mucosal lesion to develop (i.e., celiac disease). The patient deserves accurate treatment early. The benefit of treating these patients may be due to correction of micronutrient deficiencies having an impact on extra-intestinal manifestations [58]. We suggest that the term celiac trait be used in these cases [1,32,51].

Author Contributions: Both authors searched the literature and contributed equally in writing the review.

References

1.   Mäki, M.; Collin, P. Celiac disease. *Lancet* **1997**, *349*, 1755–1759. [CrossRef]

2. Laurikka, P.; Nurminen, S.; Kivelä, L.; Kurppa, K. Extraintestinal manifestations of celiac disease: Early detection for better long-term outcomes. *Nutrients* **2018**, *10*, 1015. [CrossRef] [PubMed]

3. Pinto-Sanchez, M.I.; Bercik, P.; Verdu, E.F.; Bai, J.C. Extraintestinal manifestations of celiac disease. *Dig. Dis.* **2015**, *33*, 147–154. [CrossRef] [PubMed]

4. Kaukinen, K.; Collin, P.; Mäki, M. Celiac disease-a diagnostic and therapeutic challenge. *Duodecim* **2010**, *126*, 245–254. [PubMed]

5. Collin, P.; Reunala, T.; Rasmussen, M.; Kyrönpalo, S.; Pehkonen, E.; Laippala, P.; Mäki, M. High incidence and prevalence of adult celiac disease: Augmented diagnostic approach. *Scand. J. Gastroenterol.* **1997**, *32*, 1129–1133. [CrossRef] [PubMed]

6. Lohi, S.; Mustalahti, K.; Kaukinen, K.; Laurila, K.; Collin, P.; Rissanen, H.; Lohi, O.; Bravi, E.; Gasparin, M.; Reunanen, A.; et al. Increasing prevalence of celiac disease over time. *Aliment. Pharmacol. Ther.* **2007**, *26*, 1217–1225. [CrossRef] [PubMed]

7. Virta, L.J.; Kaukinen, K.; Collin, P. Incidence and prevalence of diagnosed celiac disease in Finland: Results of effective case finding in adults. *Scand. J. Gastroenterol.* **2009**, *44*, 933–938. [CrossRef] [PubMed]

8. Fry, L.; Riches, D.J.; Seah, P.P.; Hoffbrand, A.V. Clearance of skin lesions in dermatitis herpetiformis after gluten withdrawal. *Lancet* **1973**, *301*, 288–291. [CrossRef]

9. Reunala, T.; Kosnai, I.; Karpati, S.; Kuitunen, P.; Török, E.; Savilahti, E. Dermatitis herpetiformis: Jejunal findings and skin response to gluten-free diet. *Arch. Dis. Child.* **1984**, *59*, 517–522. [CrossRef]

10. Reunala, T.; Mäki, M. Dermatitis herpetiformis: A genetic disease. *Eur. J. Dermatol.* **1993**, *3*, 519–526.

11. Hervonen, K.; Karell, K.; Holopainen, P.; Collin, P.; Partanen, J.; Reunala, T. Concordance of dermatitis herpetiformis and celiac disease in monozygous twins. *J. Investig. Dermatol.* **2000**, *115*, 990–993. [CrossRef] [PubMed]

12. Molteni, N.; Caraceni, M.P.; Bardella, M.T.; Ortolani, S.; Gandolini, G.G.; Bianchi, P. Bone mineral density in adult celiac patients and the effect of gluten-free diet from childhood. *Am. J. Gastroenterol.* **1990**, *85*, 51–53. [PubMed]

13. Mustalahti, K.; Collin, P.; Sievänen, H.; Salmi, J.; Mäki, M. Osteopenia in patients with clinically silent celiac disease warrants screening. *Lancet* **1999**, *354*, 744–745. [CrossRef]

14. Heikkilä, K.; Pearce, J.; Mäki, M.; Kaukinen, K. Celiac disease and bone fractures: A systematic review and meta-analysis. *J. Clin. Endocrinol. Metab.* **2015**, *100*, 25–34. [CrossRef] [PubMed]

15. Trotta, L.; Biagi, F.; Bianchi, P.I.; Marchese, A.; Vattiato, C.; Balduzzi, D.; Collesano, V.; Corazza, G.R. Dental enamel defects in adult celiac disease: Prevalence and correlation with symptoms and age at diagnosis. *Eur. J. Intern. Med.* **2013**, *24*, 832–834. [CrossRef] [PubMed]

16. Mäki, M.; Hällström, O.; Verronen, P.; Reunala, T.; Lahdeaho, M.L.; Holm, K.; Visakorpi, J.K. Reticulin antibody, arthritis, and celiac disease in children. *Lancet* **1988**, *1*, 479–480. [CrossRef]

17. Collin, P.; Korpela, M.; Hällström, O.; Viander, M.; Keyriläinen, O.; Mäki, M. Rheumatic complaints as a presenting symptom in patients with celiac disease. *Scand. J. Rheumatol.* **1992**, *21*, 20–23. [CrossRef] [PubMed]

18. Daron, C.; Soubrier, M.; Mathieu, S. Occurrence of rheumatic symptoms in celiac disease: A meta-analysis: Comment on the article "Osteoarticular manifestations of celiac disease and non-celiac gluten hypersensitivity" by Dos Santos and Lioté. *Jt. Bone Spine* **2017**, *84*, 645–646. [CrossRef]

19. Gobbi, G.; Bouquet, F.; Greco, L.; Lambertini, A.; Tassinari, C.A.; Ventura, A.; Zaniboni, M.G. Celiac disease, epilepsy and cerebral calcifications. The Italian Working Group on Celiac Disease and Epilepsy. *Lancet* **1992**, *340*, 439–443.

20. Hadjivassiliou, M.; Grunewald, R.A.; Chattopadhyay, A.K.; Davies-Jones, G.A.; Gibson, A.; Jarrat, J.A.; Kandler, R.H.; Lobo, A.; Powell, T.; Smith, C.M. Clinical, radiological, neurophysiological, and neuropathological characteristics of gluten ataxia. *Lancet* **1998**, *352*, 1582–1585. [CrossRef]

21. Luostarinen, L.; Pirttilä, T.; Collin, P. Celiac disease presenting with neurological disorders. *Eur. Neurol.* **1999**, *42*, 132–135. [CrossRef] [PubMed]

22. Zis, P.; Sarrigiannis, P.G.; Rao, D.G.; Hadjivassiliou, M. Gluten neuropathy: Prevalence of neuropathic pain and the role of gluten-free diet. *J. Neurol.* **2018**, *265*, 2231–2236. [CrossRef] [PubMed]

23. Volta, U.; De Franceschi, L.; Lari, F.; Molinaro, N.; Zoli, M.; Bianchi, F.B. Celiac disease hidden by cryptogenic hypertransaminasaemia. *Lancet* **1998**, *352*, 26–29. [CrossRef]

24. Kaukinen, K.; Halme, L.; Collin, P.; Färkkilä, M.; Mäki, M.; Vehmanen, P.; Partanen, J.; Höckerstedt, K. Celiac disease in patients with severe liver disease: Gluten-free diet may reverse hepatic failure. *Gastroenterology* **2002**, *122*, 881–888. [CrossRef] [PubMed]

25. Korpimäki, S.; Kaukinen, K.; Collin, P.; Haapala, A.-M.; Holm, P.; Laurila, K.; Kurppa, K.; Saavalainen, P.; Haimila, K.; Partanen, J.; et al. Gluten-sensitive hypertransaminasemia in celiac disease: An infrequent and often subclinical finding. *Am. J. Gastroenterol.* **2011**, *106*, 1689–1696. [CrossRef] [PubMed]

26. Sher, K.S.; Jayanthi, V.; Probert, C.S.; Stewart, C.R.; Mayberry, J.F. Infertility, obstetric and gynaecological problems in celiac sprue. *Dig. Dis.* **1994**, *12*, 186–190. [CrossRef]

27. Tersigni, C.; Castellani, R.; de Waure, C.; Fattorossi, A.; De Spirito, M.; Gasbarrini, A.; Scambia, G.; Di Simone, N. Celiac disease and reproductive gdisorders: Meta-analysis of epidemiologic associations and potential pathogenic mechanisms. *Hum. Reprod. Update* **2014**, *20*, 582–593. [CrossRef]

28. Ventura, A.; Magazzu, G.; Greco, L. Duration of exposure to gluten and risk for autoimmune disorders in patients with celiac disease. *Gastroenterology* **1999**, *117*, 297–303. [CrossRef]

29. Cosnes, J.; Cellier, C.; Viola, S.; Colombel, J.F.; Michaud, L.; Sarles, J.; Hugot, J.P.; Ginies, J.L.; Dabadie, A.; Mouterde, O. Groupe D'Etude et de Recherche Sur la Maladie Coeliaque. Incidence of autoimmune diseases in celiac disease: Protective effect of the gluten-free diet. *Clin. Gastroenterol. Hepatol.* **2008**, *6*, 753–758. [CrossRef]

30. Holmes, G.K.T.; Prior, P.; Lane, M.R.; Pope, D.; Allan, R.N. Malignancy in celiac disease—Effect of a gluten free diet. *Gut* **1989**, *30*, 333–338. [CrossRef]

31. Tio, M.; Cox, M.R.; Eslick, G.D. Meta-analysis: Celiac disease and the risk of all-cause mortality, any malignancy and lymphoid malignancy. *Aliment. Pharmacol. Ther.* **2012**, *35*, 540–551. [CrossRef] [PubMed]

32. Mäki, M. Celiac disease. In *Gastrointestinal Functions*; Delvin, E.E., Lentze, M.J., Eds.; Nestlé Nutrition Workshop Series, Pediatric Program; Lippincott Williams & Wilkins: Vevey, Switzerland, 2001; Volume 46, pp. 257–274. ISBN 0-7817-3208-5.

33. Freeman, H.J.; Chiu, B.K. Multifocal small bowel lymphoma and latent celiac sprue. *Gastroenterology* **1986**, *90*, 1992–1997. [CrossRef]

34. Mäki, M.; Aine, L.; Lipsanen, V.; Koskimies, S. Dental enamel defects in first-degree relatives of celiac disease patients. *Lancet* **1991**, *337*, 763–764. [CrossRef]

35. Savilahti, E.; Reunala, T.; Mäki, M. Increase of lymphocytes bearing the gamma/delta T-cell receptor in the jejunum of patients with dermatitis herpetiformis. *Gut* **1992**, *33*, 206–211. [CrossRef] [PubMed]

36. Mäki, M.; Huupponen, T.; Holm, K.; Hällström, O. Seroconversion of reticulin autoantibodies predicts celiac disease in insulin-dependent diabetes mellitus. *Gut* **1995**, *36*, 239–242. [CrossRef] [PubMed]

37. Ludvigsson, J.F.; Leffler, D.A.; Bai, J.C.; Biagi, F.; Fasano, A.; Green, P.H.; Hadjivassiliou, M.; Kaukinen, K.; Kelly, C.P.; Leonard, J.N.; et al. The Oslo definitions for celiac disease and related terms. *Gut* **2013**, *62*, 43–52. [CrossRef] [PubMed]

38. Weinstein, W.M. Latent celiac sprue. *Gastroenterology* **1974**, *66*, 489–493.

39. Ferguson, A.; Blackwell, J.N.; Barnetson, R.S. Effects of additional dietary gluten on the small-intestinal mucosa of volunteers and of patients with dermatitis herpetiformis. *Scand. J. Gastroenterol.* **1987**, *22*, 543–549. [CrossRef]

40. Chorzelski, T.P.; Rosinska, D.; Beutner, E.H.; Sulej, J.; Kumar, V. Aggressive gluten challenge of dermatitis herpetiformis cases converts them from seronegative to seropositive for IgA-class endomysial antibodies. *J. Am. Acad. Dermatol.* **1988**, *18*, 672–678. [CrossRef]

41. Doherty, M.; Barry, R.E. Gluten-induced mucosal changes in subjects without overt small-bowel disease. *Lancet* **1981**, *1*, 517–520. [CrossRef]

42. Mäki, M.; Holm, K.; Koskimies, S.; Hallstrom, O.; Visakorpi, J.K. Normal small bowel biopsy followed by celiac disease. *Arch. Dis. Child.* **1990**, *65*, 1137–1141. [CrossRef] [PubMed]

43. Mäki, M.; Holm, K.; Collin, P.; Savilahti, E. Increase in γ/δ T cell receptor bearing lymphocytes in normal small bowel mucosa in latent celiac disease. *Gut* **1991**, *32*, 1412–1414. [CrossRef] [PubMed]

44. Mäki, M.; Holm, K.; Lipsanen, V.; Hällström, O.; Viander, M.; Collin, P.; Savilahti, E.; Koskimies, S. Serological markers and HLA genes among healthy first-degree relatives of patients with celiac disease. *Lancet* **1991**, *338*, 1350–1353. [CrossRef]

45. Collin, P.; Helin, H.; Mäki, M.; Hällström, O.; Karvonen, A.L. Follow-up of patients positive in reticulin and gliadin antibody tests with normal small-bowel biopsy findings. *Scand. J. Gastroenterol.* **1993**, *28*, 595–598. [CrossRef] [PubMed]

46. Ferguson, A.; Arranz, E.; O'Mahony, S. Clinical and pathological spectrum of celiac disease—Active, silent, latent, potential. *Gut* **1993**, *34*, 150–151. [CrossRef] [PubMed]

47. Troncone, R. Latent celiac disease in Italy. *Acta Paediatr.* **1995**, *84*, 1252–1257. [CrossRef] [PubMed]

48. Corazza, G.R.; Andreani, M.L.; Biagi, F.; Bonvicini, F.; Bernardi, M.; Gasbarrini, G. Clinical, pathological, and antibody pattern of latent celiac disease: Report of three adult cases. *Am. J. Gastroenterol.* **1996**, *91*, 2203–2207.

49. Vilppula, A.; Kaukinen, K.; Luostarinen, L.; Kerkelä, I.; Patrikainen, H.; Valve, T.; Mäki, M.; Collin, P. Increasing prevalence and high incidence of celiac disease in elderly people: A population-based study. *BMC Gastroenterol.* **2009**, *9*, 49. [CrossRef]

50. Kaukinen, K.; Collin, P.; Mäki, M. Latent celiac disease or celiac disease beyond villous atrophy? *Gut* **2007**, *56*, 1339–1340. [CrossRef]

51. Mäki, M. Lack of consensus regarding definitions of celiac disease. *Nat. Rev. Gastroenterol. Hepatol.* **2012**, *9*, 305–306. [CrossRef]

52. Not, T.; Ziberna, F.; Vatta, S.; Quaglia, S.; Martelossi, S.; Villanacci, V.; Marzari, R.; Florian, F.; Vecchiet, M.; Sulic, A.M.; et al. Cryptic genetic gluten intolerance revealed by intestinal antitransglutaminase antibodies and response to gluten-free diet. *Gut* **2011**, *60*, 1487–1493. [CrossRef] [PubMed]

53. Kurppa, K.; Collin, P.; Viljamaa, M.; Haimila, K.; Saavalainen, P.; Partanen, J.; Laurila, K.; Huhtala, H.; Paasikivi, K.; et al. Diagnosing mild enteropathy celiac disease: A randomized, controlled clinical study. *Gastroenterology* **2009**, *136*, 816–823. [CrossRef] [PubMed]

54. Husby, S.; Koletzko, S.; Korponay-Szabó, I.R.; Mearin, M.L.; Phillips, A.; Shamir, R.; Troncone, R.; Giersiepen, K.; Branski, D.; Catassi, C.; et al. European Society for Pediatric Gastroenterology, Hepatology, and Nutrition Guidelines for the Diagnosis of Celiac Disease. *J. Pediatr. Gastroenterol. Nutr.* **2012**, *54*, 136–160. [CrossRef] [PubMed]

55. Mäki, M. The humoral immune system in celiac disease. *Baillière's Clin. Gastroenterol.* **1995**, *9*, 231–249. [CrossRef]

56. Simon-Vecsei, Z.; Király, R.; Bagossi, P.; Tóth, B.; Dahlbom, I.; Caja, S.; Csősz, É.; Lindfors, K.; Sblattero, D.; Nemes, E.; et al. A single conformational transglutaminase 2 epitope contributed by three domains is critical for celiac antibody binding and effects. *Proc. Natl. Acad. Sci. USA* **2012**, *109*, 431–436. [CrossRef] [PubMed]

57. Yu, X.B.; Uhde, M.; Green, P.H.; Alaedini, A. Autoantibodies in the extraintestinal manifestations of celiac disease. *Nutrients* **2018**, *10*, 1123. [CrossRef] [PubMed]

58. Rostami, K.; Aldulaimi, D.; Holmes, G.; Johnson, M.W.; Robert, M.; Srivastava, A.; Fléjou, J.-F.; Sanders, D.S.; Volta, U.; Derakhshan, M.H.; et al. Microscopic enteritis: Bucharest consensus. *World J. Gastroenterol.* **2015**, *21*, 2593–2604. [CrossRef] [PubMed]

59. Salmi, T.T.; Collin, P.; Järvinen, O.; Haimila, K.; Partanen, J.; Laurila, K.; Korponay-Szabo, I.R.; Huhtala, H.; Reunala, T.; Mäki, M.; et al. Immunoglobulin A autoantibodies against transglutaminase 2 in the small intestinal mucosa predict forthcoming celiac disease. *Aliment. Pharmacol. Ther.* **2006**, *24*, 541–552. [CrossRef] [PubMed]

60. Holm, K.; Mäki, M.; Savilahti, E.; Lipsanen, V.; Laippala, P.; Koskimies, S. Intraepithelial gamma/delta T-cell-receptor lymphocytes and genetic susceptibility to celiac disease. *Lancet* **1992**, *339*, 1500–1503. [CrossRef]

61. Iltanen, S.; Holm, K.; Partanen, J.; Laippala, P.; Mäki, M. Increased density of jejunal γδ+ T cells in patients having normal mucosa—Marker of operative autoimmune mechanisms? *Autoimmunity* **1999**, *29*, 1787–1791. [CrossRef]

62. Korponay-Szabo, I.R.; Halttunen, T.; Szalai, Z.; Laurila, K.; Király, R.; Kovács, J.B.; Fésüs, L.; Mäki, M. In vivo targeting of intestinal and extraintestinal transglutaminase 2 by celiac autoantibodies. *Gut* **2004**, *53*, 641–648. [CrossRef] [PubMed]

63. Kaukinen, K.; Peräaho, M.; Collin, P.; Partanen, J.; Woolley, N.; Kaartinen, T.; Nuutinen, T.; Halttunen, T.; Mäki, M.; Korponay-Szabo, I. Small-bowel mucosal transglutaminase 2-specific IgA deposits in celiac disease without villous atrophy: A prospective and randomized clinical study. *Scand. J. Gastroenterol.* **2005**, *40*, 564–572. [CrossRef] [PubMed]

64. Koskinen, O.; Collin, P.; Korponay-Szabo, I.; Salmi, T.; Iltanen, S.; Haimila, K.; Partanen, J.; Mäki, M.; Kaukinen, K. Gluten-dependent small bowel mucosal transglutaminase 2-specific IgA deposits in overt and mild enteropathy celiac disease. *J. Pediatr. Gastroenterol. Nutr.* **2008**, *47*, 436–442. [CrossRef] [PubMed]

65. Maglio, M.; Ziberna, F.; Aitoro, R.; Discepolo, V.; Lania, G.; Bassi, V.; Miele, E.; Not, T.; Troncone, R.; Auricchio, R. Intestinal production of anti-tissue transglutaminase 2 antibodies in patients with diagnosis other than celiac disease. *Nutrients* **2017**, *9*, 1050. [CrossRef] [PubMed]

66. Reunala, T.; Blomqvist, K.; Tarpila, S.; Halme, H.; Kangas, K. Gluten-free diet in dermatitis herpetiformis. I. Clinical response of skin lesions in 81 patients. *Br. J. Dermatol.* **1977**, *97*, 473–480. [CrossRef] [PubMed]

67. Mansikka, E.; Hervonen, K.; Kaukinen, K.; Collin, P.; Huhtala, H.; Reunala, T.; Salmi, T. Prognosis of dermatitis herpetiformis patients with and without villous atrophy at diagnosis. *Nutrients* **2018**, *10*, 641. [CrossRef] [PubMed]

68. Reunala, T.; Salmi, T.T.; Hervonen, K.; Kaukinen, K.; Collin, P. Dermatitis herpetiformis: A common extraintestinal manifestation of celiac disease. *Nutrients* **2018**, *10*, 602. [CrossRef]

69. Salmi, T.T.; Hervonen, K.; Laurila, K.; Collin, P.; Mäki, M.; Koskinen, O.; Huhtala, H.; Kaukinen, K.; Reunala, T. Small bowel transglutaminase 2-specific IgA deposits in dermatitis herpetiformis. *Acta Derm. Venereol.* **2014**, *94*, 393–397. [CrossRef]

70. Salmi, T.; Collin, P.; Korponay-Szabo, I.R.; Laurila, K.; Partanen, J.; Huhtala, H.; Kiraly, R.; Lorand, L.; Reunala, T.; Mäki, M.; et al. Endomysial antibody-negative celiac disease: Clinical characteristics and intestinal autoantibody deposits. *Gut* **2006**, *55*, 1746–1753. [CrossRef]

71. Pasternack, C.; Mansikka, E.; Kaukinen, K.; Hervonen, K.; Reunala, T.; Collin, P.; Huhtala, H.; Mattila, V.M.; Salmi, T. Self-reported fractures in dermatitis herpetiformis compared to celiac disease. *Nutrients* **2018**, *10*, 351. [CrossRef]

72. Hadjivassiliou, M.; Gibson, A.; Davies-Jones, G.A.; Lobo, A.J.; Stephenson, T.J.; Milford-Ward, A. Does cryptic gluten sensitivity play a part in neurological illness? *Lancet* **1996**, *347*, 369–371. [CrossRef]

73. Hadjivassiliou, M.; Grünewald, R.A.; Sanders, D.S.; Zis, P.; Croall, I.; Shanmugarajah, P.D.; Sarrigiannis, P.G.; Trott, N.; Wild, G.; Hoggard, N. The significance of low titre antigliadin antibodies in the diagnosis of gluten ataxia. *Nutrients* **2018**, *10*, 1444. [CrossRef] [PubMed]

74. Hadjivassiliou, M.; Davies-Jones, G.A.B.; Sanders, D.S.; Grunewald, R.A. Dietary treatment of gluten ataxia. *J. Neurol. Neurosurg. Psychiatry* **2003**, *74*, 1221–1224. [CrossRef] [PubMed]

75. Hadjivassiliou, M.; Mäki, M.; Sanders, D.S.; Williamson, C.A.; Grunewald, R.A.; Woodroofe, N.M.; Korponay-Szabo, I.R. Antibody targeting of brain and intestinal trasnglutaminase in gluten ataxia. *Neurology* **2006**, *66*, 373–377. [CrossRef] [PubMed]

76. Hadjivassiliou, M.; Aeschlimann, P.; Sanders, D.S.; Mäki, M.; Kaukinen, K.; Grünewald, R.A.; Bandmann, O.; Woodroofe, N.; Haddock, G.; Aeschlimann, D.P. Transglutaminase 6 antibodies in the diagnosis of gluten ataxia. *Neurology* **2013**, *80*, 1740–1745. [CrossRef] [PubMed]

77. Zis, P.; Sarrigiannis, P.G.; Rao, D.G.; Hadjivassiliou, M. Quality of life in patients with gluten neuropathy: A case-controlled study. *Nutrients* **2018**, *10*, 662. [CrossRef] [PubMed]

78. Hadjivassiliou, M.; Grünewald, R.A.; Kandler, R.H.; Chattopadhyay, A.K.; Jarratt, J.A.; Sanders, D.S.; Sharrack, B.; Wharton, S.B.; Davies-Jones, G.A. Neuropathy associated with gluten sensitivity. *J. Neurol. Neurosurg. Psychiatry* **2006**, *77*, 1262–1266. [CrossRef]

79. Hadjivassiliou, M.; Kandler, R.H.; Chattopadhyay, A.K.; Davies-Jones, A.G.; Jarratt, J.A.; Sanders, D.S.; Sharrack, B.; Grünewald, R.A. Dietary treatment of gluten neuropathy. *Muscle Nerve* **2006**, *34*, 762–766. [CrossRef]

80. Larussa, T.; Suraci, E.; Nazionale, I.; Abenavoli, L.; Imeneo, M.; Luzza, F. Bone mineralization in celiac disease. *Gastroenterol. Res. Pract.* **2012**, 198025. [CrossRef]

81. Zanchetta, M.B.; Longobardi, V.; Bai, J.C. Bone and celiac disease. *Curr. Osteoporos. Rep.* **2016**, *14*, 43–48. [CrossRef]

82. Grace-Farfaglia, P. Bones of contention: Bone mineral density recovery in celiac disease—A systematic review. *Nutrients* **2015**, *7*, 3347–3369. [CrossRef] [PubMed]

83. Kaukinen, K.; Mäki, M.; Partanen, J.; Sievänen, H.; Collin, P. Celiac disease without villous atrophy: Revision of criteria called for. *Dig. Dis. Sci.* **2001**, *46*, 879–887. [CrossRef] [PubMed]

84. Dickey, W.; Hughes, D.F.; McMillan, S.A. Patients with serum IgA endomysial antibodies and intact duodenal villi: Clinical characteristics and management options. *Scand. J. Gastroenterol.* **2005**, *40*, 1240–1243. [CrossRef] [PubMed]

85. Kurppa, K.; Collin, P.; Sievänen, H.; Huhtala, H.; Mäki, M.; Kaukinen, K. Gastrointestinal symptoms, quality of life and bone mineral density in mild enteropathic celiac disease: A prospective clinical trial. *Scand. J. Gastroenterol.* **2010**, *45*, 305–314. [CrossRef] [PubMed]

86. Zanini, B.; Caselani, F.; Magni, A.; Turini, D.; Ferraresi, A.; Lanzarotto, F.; Villanacci, V.; Carabellese, N.; Ricci, C.; Lanzini, A. Celiac disease with mild enteropathy is not mild disease. *Clin. Gastroenterol. Hepatol.* **2013**, *11*, 253–258. [CrossRef] [PubMed]

87. Volta, U. Pathogenesis and clinical significance of liver injury in celiac disease. *Clin. Rev. Allergy Immunol.* **2009**, *36*, 62–70. [CrossRef] [PubMed]

88. Aine, L.; Mäki, M.; Collin, P.; Keyriläinen, O. Dental enamel defects in celiac disease. *J. Oral Pathol. Med.* **1990**, *19*, 241–245. [CrossRef]

89. Aine, L.; Reunala, T.; Mäki, M. Dental enamel defects in children with dermatitis herpetiformis. *J. Pediatr.* **1991**, *118*, 572–574. [CrossRef]

90. Aine, L.; Mäki, M.; Reunala, T. Celiac-type dental enamel defects in patients with dermatitis herpetiformis. *Acta Derm. Venereol.* **1992**, *72*, 25–27.

91. Marsh, M.N. Gluten, major histocompatibility complex, and the small intestine. A molecular and immunologic approach to the spectrum of gluten sensitivity ('celiac sprue'). *Gastroenterology* **1992**, *102*, 330–354. [CrossRef]

9

Celiac-Related Autoantibodies and IL-17A in Bulgarian Patients with Dermatitis Herpetiformis

Tsvetelina Velikova [1], Martin Shahid [2], Ekaterina Ivanova-Todorova [3], Kossara Drenovska [2], Kalina Tumangelova-Yuzeir [3], Iskra Altankova [1] and Snejina Vassileva [2,*]

[1] Clinical Immunology, University Hospital Lozenetz, 1407 Sofia, Bulgaria; tsvelikova@medfac.mu-sofia.bg (T.V.); altankova@abv.bg (I.A.)
[2] Department of Dermatology, Faculty of Medicine, Medical University—Sofia, 1431 Sofia, Bulgaria; martin.shahidmd@gmail.com (M.S.); kosara@lycos.com (K.D.)
[3] Laboratory of Clinical Immunology—University Hospital St. Ivan Rilski, 1431 Sofia, Bulgaria; katty_iv@yahoo.com (E.I.-T.); kullhem000@gmail.com (K.T.-Y.)
* Correspondence: snejina.vassileva@gmail.com

Abstract: *Background and objectives*: Dermatitis herpetiformis (DH) is a blistering dermatosis, which shares common immunologic features with celiac disease (CD). The aim of the present study was to explore the performance of a panel of CD-related antibodies and IL-17A in Bulgarian patients with DH. *Materials and Methods:* Serum samples from 26 DH patients at mean age 53 ± 15 years and 20 healthy controls were assessed for anti-tissue transglutaminase (anti-tTG), anti-deamidated gliadin peptides (anti-DGP), anti-actin antibodies (AAA), and IL-17A by enzyme linked immuno-sorbent assay (ELISA), as well as anti-tTG, anti-gliadin (AGA), and anti-Saccharomyces cerevisiae antibodies (ASCA) using immunoblot. *Results:* The average serum levels of anti-tTG, anti-DGP, AGA, AAA, and the cytokine IL-17A were at significantly higher levels in patients with DH compared to the average levels in healthy persons which stayed below the cut-off value ($p < 0.05$). Anti-DGP and anti-tTG antibodies showed the highest diagnostic sensitivity and specificity, as well as acceptable positive and negative predictive value. None of the healthy individuals was found positive for the tested antibodies, as well as for ASCA within the DH group. All tests showed good to excellent correlations (r = 0.5 ÷ 0.9, $p < 0.01$). *Conclusions:* Although the diagnosis of DH relies on skin biopsy for histology and DIF, serologic testing of a panel of celiac-related antibodies could be employed with advantages in the diagnosing process of DH patients. Furthermore, DH patients who are positive for the investigated serologic parameters could have routine monitoring for gastrointestinal complications typical for the gluten-sensitive enteropathy.

Keywords: dermatitis herpetiformis; anti-tTG; anti-DGP; AAA; AGA; IL-17A

1. Introduction

Dermatitis herpetiformis (DH), also known as Duhring-Brocq disease, is a rare subepidermal blistering dermatosis, currently regarded as the specific extraintestinal manifestation of celiac disease (CD) [1,2]. It most commonly affects the skin, while associated gluten sensitive enteropathy (GSE) can be clinically variable to absent. Histologically, DH is characterized by subepidermal blisters with predominant neutrophilic infiltration in the papillary dermis. A pathognomonic finding in DH, detected by direct immunofluorescence (DIF) microscopy on perilesional uninvolved skin, is the presence of granular deposits of immunoglobulin A (IgA) along the dermo-epidermal junction (DEJ) and at the tips of the dermal papillae. Recently, it has been documented that the autoantigen for deposited cutaneous IgA is epidermal transglutaminase (eTG, TG3)—an enzyme closely related, but not identical to the tissue transglutaminase (tTG, TG2) autoantigen-specific for CD [3]. IgA deposits in skin represent antibodies against gut tTG that cross-react with the highly homologous eTG by forming insoluble aggregates in the papillary dermis [4].

The pathophysiology of DH is closely related to that of CD and involves a complex interplay among genetic, environmental, and immune factors. Both diseases occur in gluten-sensitive individuals, heal with a gluten-free diet (GFD), and relapse on gluten challenge [5]. DH and CD share the same genetic background with a high frequency of human leukocyte antigen (HLA)-DQ2 and HLA-DQ8 haplotypes [6,7]. The majority of patients with DH exhibit morphologic small-bowel changes characteristics of CD, ranging from slight villous atrophy to increased density of intraepithelial lymphocytes [1,8]. However, overt enteropathy is reported in less than 10% of patients, and the gastrointestinal symptoms are usually absent or so mild that the DH patients are unaware of them [9]. Last but not least, patients with DH and CD often have the same associated autoimmune diseases, such as juvenile diabetes, hypothyroidism, pernicious anemia, and connective tissue disorders [5].

A hallmark of CD is the loss of tolerance to wheat gluten with enhanced production of various gluten-dependent autoantibodies, as a result from the gluten-induced small-bowel mucosal T-cell activation, which is the cornerstone in the pathogenesis of the celiac pathology [10]. These circulating CD-specific antibodies are widely used to diagnose GSE serologically before proceeding to small-bowel mucosal biopsies. Historically, among the first serum-based antibody tests introduced in CD diagnostics are the antigliadin antibody (AGA) [11,12], the gluten-dependent IgA-class R1-type reticulin (ARA) [13], and endomysial autoantibody (EMA) assays [14]. In 1997, Dieterich and co-workers identified TG2 as the autoantigen of CD [15]. As various TG2-based enzyme-linked immunosorbent assays (ELISA) became available, a new era in celiac disease case finding by serology began [16]. Later research has shown that TG2 was also the specific protein antigen in the ARA and EMA tests [17]. As a result of the constant development of serologic tests for CD, a new generation of assays detecting the presence of antibodies against deamidated gliadin peptides (DGPs) as antigens appeared [18,19]. The accurate diagnosis of DH is essential, similar to CD, as the disease requires a lifelong commitment to a GFD. It relies on few but essential specific criteria, including clinical, histologic, immunopathologic, and serologic celiac-related markers, the latter being detected in DH patients as well [2,20]. Perilesional biopsy with a specific DIF microscopy finding has remained the gold standard along with the presence of suggestive clinical picture and supportive serological results [21].

Furthermore, the predictive accuracy of serological tests depends on the disease prevalence in the population [22]. In this regard, it is of interest to analyze the performance of celiac-related tests in patients from different countries and origin. In a previous report of a series of 78 DH patients from Bulgaria, the prevalence of DH among other autoimmune blistering diseases was 7.45% with a minimum estimated incidence of 0.88 cases per million annually [23].

An early event in blister formation in DH is the accumulation of neutrophils in the papillary dermis, the upregulation of the adhesion molecules, and release of enzymes and inflammatory mediators causing basement membrane damage and subsequent clefting, which could also explain the typical distribution of skin lesions at sites of trauma [24]. Interleukin (IL)-17A is involved in the production of other pro-inflammatory cytokines and matrix metalloproteinases, as well as in the attraction of neutrophils implicated in the pathogenesis of DH [25]. However, the suggested hypothesis for the role of IL-17A in DH pathogenesis needs further investigation.

Our study aimed to explore comparatively the performance of a panel of celiac-related antibodies, such as anti-tTG, AGA, anti-DGP, anti-actin (AAA) antibodies, as well as cytokine IL-17A, in a cross-sectional study of a Bulgarian cohort of DH patients.

2. Material and Methods

2.1. Serum Samples

Sera from 26 newly diagnosed and untreated DH patients (mean age 53 ± 15 years; range 18–72 years) were collected before initiation of a gluten-free diet. All patients attended the Department of Dermatology, Aleksandrovska University Hospital, Sofia and provided written informed consent to participate in the study. The diagnosis of DH was based on (i) clinical presentation and (ii) presence of granular deposits of IgA in the papillary dermis by direct IF microscopy. Sera from 20 healthy individuals at mean age 31 ± 8 (range 21–42 years) served as controls. All sera were stored at −80 °C until assayed. Female-to-male ratio for DH patients was 1:1, and for the control group 1:1.2. Age and sex differences between the studied groups were considered as non-significant ($p > 0.05$). All patients and control subjects were found negative for other autoimmune disease markers (i.e., anti-nuclear antibodies, rheumatoid factor, and anti-neutrophil cytoplasmic antibodies).

This study was performed in accordance with the declaration of Helsinki Principles and approved by the Ethical Committee of the Medical University of Sofia, Bulgaria.

2.2. Immune Serology Testing

Sera taken from all DH patients and control subjects were analyzed by ELISA and immunoblotting (Line Blot) at the Laboratory of Clinical Immunology, University Hospital "St. Ivan Rilski," Sofia.

2.2.1. Immunoenzyme Testing

ELISA commercial kits were used to determine the following celiac-related antibodies and the pro-inflammatory cytokine IL-17A:

- anti-tTG antibodies (Anti-Tissue Transglutaminase Screen IgA + IgG, Orgentec Diagnostika GmbH, cut-off value > 10 U/mL);
- anti-DGP antibodies (Quanta Lite Celiac DGP Screen IgA + IgG, Inova Diagnostics, Inc., San Diego, USA, cut-off > 15 U/mL);
- AAA (Quanta Lite F-Actin IgA ELISA, Inova Diagnostics, Inc., San Diego, USA, cut-off > 20 U/mL);
- IL-17A (Human IL-17A ELISA kit, Diaclone, GenProbe, France, sensitivity < 2.3 pg/mL).

Analyses were performed following the manufacturers' instructions.

2.2.2. Immunoblot Testing

Anti-tTG, AGA, and ASCA were assessed in serum samples by performing line blot testing (Seraline®Zöliakie-3 IgG, Seramun Diagnostica GmbH, Germany). The assay strips were scanned with IvD-registered Seraline Scan software with hardware key (Seramun Diagnostica GmbH, Germany). The results were given as the relative value of intensity.

2.3. Statistical Analysis

Row data were evaluated statistically by the software package for statistical analysis (SPSS) v.19 (SPSS®, IBM 2009). We used descriptive, correlation, and receiver operating characteristics (ROC) curve analysis to evaluate the performance characteristics of the applied tests in diagnosing DH. Results are presented as mean ± SE (standard error) or number (%). Differences between the groups were assessed using unpaired Student's T-test preceded by an evaluation of normality (Kolmogorov–Smirnoff test). The Mann–Whitney U-test was used where appropriate. A P-value of <0.05 was considered statistically significant.

3. Results

3.1. Serum Levels of the Celiac Disease-Related Autoantibodies and the Pro-Inflammatory Cytokine IL-17A

The mean ELISA values of the measured parameters in DH patients and the control group are presented on Figure 1 and Supplementary Table S1. The mean levels of anti-tTG and anti-DGP antibodies were significantly higher in DH patients compared to healthy controls (36.9 ± 20.3 IU/mL versus 2.1 ± 0.4 IU/mL, $p = 0.02$, and 40.7 ± 10.2 IU/mL versus 1.87 ± 0.68, $p < 0.001$, respectively). Similarly, the AAA titers significantly differed between both groups, being moderately higher in DH sera than in the healthy subjects (22.6 ± 3.9 IU/mL versus 9.1 ± 0.9 IU/mL, $p = 0.05$). There was a 60-fold increase in the concentrations of IL-17A in DH patients compared to control sera (5.3 ± 2.2 pg/mL versus 0.08 ± 0.07 pg/mL, $p = 0.031$) (Figure 1A).

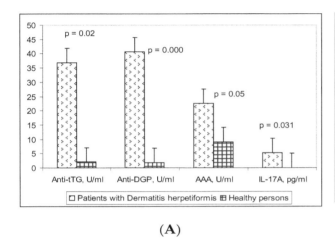

(A)

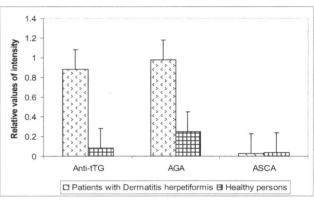

(B)

Figure 1. Mean serum levels of anti-tTG antibodies, anti-DGP, anti-actin antibodies, and IL-17A in the study groups, assessed by (**A**) ELISA and (**B**) line blot.

The mean serum levels of the autoantibodies investigated by Line blot are also demonstrated (Figure 1 and Table S1). There were significantly higher levels of anti-tTG and AGA antibodies in DH patients compared to healthy controls (0.88 ± 0.24 versus 0.08 ± 0.02, $p = 0.003$, and 0.98 ± 0.31 versus 0.25 ± 0.08, $p = 0.030$, respectively). In contrast, no differences were found in the mean levels of ASCA within the studied groups (Figure 1B).

3.2. Performance Characteristics of the Celiac-Related Antibodies Tested in DH Patients

The results of the performance of anti-tTG, anti-DGP antibodies, AAA, and AGA, assessed by ELISA and line blot are shown in Table 1. Antibodies against tTG were found in 11 (42.3%) (IgA + IgG, ELISA) and 12 (46%) (IgG, line blot) patients with DH. Half of the DH patients had AGA IgG (Line blot) in their sera, and 12 (46.4%) were positive for anti-DGP antibodies. The smallest number of patients—9 (34.7%) were found positive for AAA (ELISA).

None of the control sera were tested positive for anti-tTG (ELISA and blot), AAA or AGA, whereas one subject showed positive results for anti-DGP. This defined a specificity of 100% in distinguishing DH from healthy individuals for the test systems applied in our study, excluding anti-DGP antibodies, which exerted a specificity of 95%.

Positive predictive values (PPV) for all tests were 100%, except for anti-DGP—90.9%. The negative predictive values (NPV) of the test remained slightly above 50%, and the highest NPV was observed for AGA (60%) and anti-tTG (Line blot) (59%).

Table 1. Performance characteristics of anti-tTG antibodies, anti-DGP antibodies, AAA, and AGA, assessed by ELISA and line blot in Dermatitis Herpetiformis patients.

	Anti-tTG IgA + IgG (ELISA)	Anti-DGP IgA + IgG (ELISA)	AAA IgG (ELISA)	Anti-tTG IgG (Line Blot)	AGA IgG (Line Blot)
Sensitivity	42.3%	46.4%	34.7%	46%	50%
Specificity	100%	95%	100%	100%	100%
PPV *	100%	90.9%	100%	100%	100%
NPV **	57%	57.1%	54.1%	59%	60%

* PPV, positive predictive value; ** NPV, negative predictive value.

3.3. ROC Curve Analysis of the Celiac Disease-Related Antibodies and IL-17A in DH Patients

The ROC curve analyses of the ELISA tests revealed the best performance of anti-DGP antibodies (AUC 0.939, $p < 0.001$), followed by anti-tTG antibodies testing (AUC 0.864, $p = 0.002$) (Supplementary Table S2). We did not find significant AUC for AAA. According to IL-17 serum levels, our results demonstrated excellent performance of the test (AUC 0.811, $p < 0.05$) (Figure 2A). From the celiac-related antibodies assessed by line blot, anti-tTG testing alone had significant AUC of 0.734, while the other tests showed unsatisfactory performance (Figure 2B).

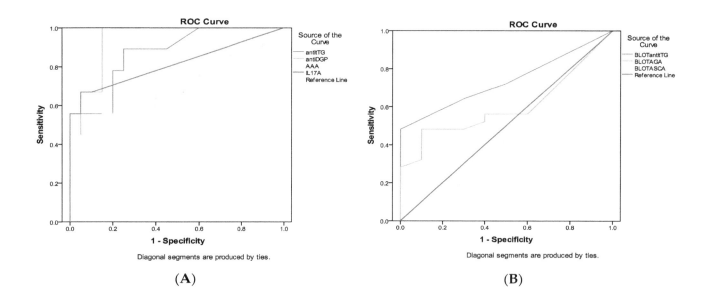

Figure 2. Receiver operating characteristics (ROC) curve analysis of the tested parameters, assessed by (**A**) ELISA and (**B**) line blot.

3.4. Correlation between Tests

The results of all tests showed good to excellent correlation to each other ($r = 0.5 \div 0.9$, $p < 0.01$) (Table 2). The strongest correlations were established for the following pairs of antibodies, all of them assessed by ELISA: anti-tTG—IL-17A ($r = 0.938$, $p < 0.001$), anti-tTG – anti-DGP ($r = 0.894$, $p < 0.001$), and anti-tTG—AAA ($r = 0.863$, $p = 0.001$). In comparison, the correlation between anti-DGP antibodies and IL-17A was evaluated as a weak one ($r = 0.452$, $p = 0.031$). Anti-tTG ELISA levels moderately correlated with anti-tTG assessed by line blot ($r = 0.520$, $p = 0.003$) (Table 2).

Table 2. Correlation between tests. Results are presented as Pearson's coefficient (r) and significance (p).

	Anti-tTG (ELISA)	Anti-DGP (ELISA)	AAA (ELISA)	IL-17A (ELISA)	Anti-tTG (Line Blot)	AGA (Line Blot)
Anti-tTG (ELISA)		r = 0.894 $p < 0.001$	r = 0.863 $p = 0.001$	r = 0.938 $p < 0.001$	r = 0.520 $p = 0.003$	r = 0.507 $p = 0.076$
	anti-DGP (ELISA)		r = 0.502 $p = 0.009$	r = 0.452 $p = 0.031$	r = 0.532 $p = 0.001$	r = 0.346 $p = 0.038$
		AAA (ELISA)		r = 0.692 $p < 0.001$	r = 0.112 $p = 0.500$	r = 0.221 $p = 0.186$
			IL-17A(ELISA)		r = 0.079 $p = 0.676$	r = −0.222 $p = 0.238$
				Anti-tTG (Line blot)		r = 0.678 $p < 0.001$
					AGA (Line blot)	

All Pearson's coefficients were calculated by bivariate correlation, except for the line blot results where the Spearman coefficient was calculated via Chi-square test.

4. Discussion

Growing evidence shows that patients with DH may possess most of the specific autoantibodies that can be found in patients with CD, including circulating autoantibodies against gliadin, tTG, and DGP [1]. On the other hand, conflicting results were obtained by the use of the anti-DGP ELISA for detecting gluten enteropathy in DH patients. Previously reported sensitivities for IgA anti-DGP antibodies vary from 46% to 78% [20,26]. In this study, the relative sensitivities and specificities of a panel of CD-related autoantibodies in Bulgarian patients with DH were compared with the reactivities of control healthy subjects. We included conventional celiac-related antibodies—anti-tTG, anti-DGP, and AGA, as well as AAA, the latter being used for non-invasive evaluation of villous atrophy. ASCA were tested along with other antibodies due to the presence of coated Mannan on the Line blot. Moreover, we were interested in assessing the serum levels of IL-17A in DH patients. We chose not to compare EMA with the other autoantibodies in our celiac-related panel due to the subjective semiquantitative nature of EMA testing that is not easy to standardize.

All investigated celiac-related antibodies—anti-tTG, anti-DGP, and AGA, independent of the used method (ELISA or Line blot), were significantly higher in the DH group compared to the healthy controls. Nevertheless, the sensitivity and specificity of the applied tests were acceptable. We found that 42.3% of our DH patients were positive for anti-tTG (IgA + IgG) assessed by ELISA. When we tested the serum samples for IgG anti-tTG by line blot, we found a higher sensitivity of 46%. Half of the DH patients had IgG AGA (Line blot) in their serum samples, and 46.4% had anti-DGP (ELISA) antibodies. We also defined the specificity of 100% for anti-tTG (ELISA and line blot), AAA, and AGA in discriminating DH from healthy persons, as well as a specificity of 95% for anti-DGP antibodies. These results are in accordance with other studies, demonstrating sensitivity ranges between 47% and 100% and specificity ranging 90% to 100% for celiac-related antibodies in patients with DH [9,27–32]. PPVs for all tests were 100%, except for anti-DGP, which was 90.9% due to one positive healthy individual. Unfortunately, the NPVs of the tests remained slightly above 50%, and the highest NPV was observed for AGA (60%) and anti-tTG (59%) assessed by line blot. However, during the last decade, only a few studies updated this information. Thus, our results contribute to previously published literature data.

Comparing tests by the ROC curve analyses, the best performance was revealed for anti-DGP antibodies, followed by anti-tTG (ELISA) testing and anti-tTG (Line blot) antibodies. Although the specificity of AGA was 50%, the AUC of 0.600 was non-significant and therefore, unreliable.

Among all celiac-related serological tests, IgA anti-tTG antibodies have been considered the most sensitive and specific ones that should be tested in patients with DH symptoms [1]. Since some patients with DH or CD may have selective IgA deficiency, we chose the dual IgG/IgA test system to exclude false-negative results. [27,33]. In our study, the performance of anti-DGP in diagnosing DH was shown to be superior to the anti-tTG antibodies. In previous comparative studies among DH patients, the sensitivity and specificity of anti-DGP were either lower than those of anti-tTG and EMA, similar, or superior to them [34], as it is in the present study. The possible explanations for such discrepancies lie in the fact that anti-DGP and AGA, which are directed against deamidated gliadin peptides and whole gliadin peptide, respectively, are related to the presence of intestinal damage, whereas antibodies against the converting enzyme tTG are linked not only to mucosal but also to skin lesions as well [34]. However, current knowledge has shown that the available serologic armamentarium lacks sensitivity when used in patients with mild or minor enteropathy [35,36]. The similarity of DH and CD related to the enteropathy makes DH a fascinating model of skin CD, where papulovesicular and pruritic rash can be concomitant with a broad spectrum of intestinal damage varying from normal structure to villous atrophy [37]. However, DH is the second gluten-sensitive disorder exhibiting varied histological damage where one can assess the performance of the celiac serology [34]. In the present study, we chose to assess by ELISA anti-tTG and anti-DGP antibodies of both IgA and IgG subclasses. The results obtained allowed us to conclude that the combination of both isotypes of anti-DGP assays has higher specificity than IgA anti-tTG.

There is an insufficient number of investigations regarding anti-actin testing in DH patients. Of the 26 patients with DH in our study, nine were positive for AAA. However, no significant differences were found in the serum levels of AAA in DH patients and healthy controls. Serum levels of IgG AAA were assessed by ELISA in a single study on a series of 10 adult Romanian DH patients. The authors documented sensitivity and specificity of 33.3% and 100%, respectively, for AAA in DH patients [38]. Our results also showed that the AUC for AAA was unacceptable and therefore not reliable for the DH diagnosis.

We did not find differences in the mean levels of ASCA within the studied groups. Although ASCA have been reported to be positive in about 30% of CD patients [39], which was also confirmed by us in a cohort of Bulgarian CD patients [40], there were no data regarding ASCA in DH patients available so far.

Concerning the IL-17A, in a single study Zebrowska et al. documented significantly higher expression of this cytokine in the epidermis (perilesional skin) and the serum of DH and bullous pemphigoid patients, compared to the control group [41]. We also detected 60-fold higher concentrations of IL-17A in DH patients compared to healthy controls ($p = 0.031$). Two studies provided data for the involvement of IL-17A in DH pathogenesis. Juczynska et al. demonstrated increased expression of JAK/STAT proteins in skin lesions in patients with DH and bullous pemphigoid in comparison to perilesional skin and control group [42]. They suggested that pro-inflammatory cytokine network and induction of inflammatory infiltrate in tissues can contribute to the pathogenesis of skin lesions in both diseases. Surprisingly, serum IL-17 demonstrated excellent performance in our study (AUC 0.811, $p = 0.008$), which could be of benefit for the clinical practice.

We found good to excellent correlation ($r = 0.5 \div 0.9$, $p < 0.01$) between the tests. The strongest correlations were established for the following pairs: anti-tTG (ELISA)—IL-17A, anti-tTG (ELISA)—anti-DGP antibodies, and anti-tTG (ELISA)—AAA. These results suggested a good coincidence between the different tests in diagnosing DH. There was a moderate correlation between anti-tTG antibodies estimated by ELISA and by line blot, which is not encouraging regarding the interchangeability between the two methods for anti-tTG detection. Previous studies showed similar correlations between celiac-related antibodies in patients with GSE [40].

This study has some limitations. The relatively small size of the study population might have affected the significance of the results. The lack of data on anti-TG3 is another weak point of the present work. We assume that further research involving a larger number of DH patients and newly emerging test systems for detection of other transglutaminase antibodies (TG3 and/or TG6) would clarify the findings presented in the current study and may have a significant impact on the clinical practice.

5. Conclusions

Serologic tests are important noninvasive screening tool among symptomatic patients with clinical suspicion of DH that can help select patients for diagnostic DIF analysis. Furthermore, such tests are helpful in the resolution of ambiguous and false-negative DIF results. The usability of serologic DH tests is defined by their sensitivity and specificity, which are quite variable based on current data. This is due to scarcity of data from limited populations.

In this respect, serologic testing with a panel of celiac-related antibodies, rather than individual ones, may be successfully employed to support the diagnosis of DH. In our study, the performance of anti-DGP in diagnosing DH was shown to be superior to that of anti-tTG antibodies. In addition, the best performance (ROC curve analysis) was revealed for anti-DGP antibodies followed by anti-tTG ELISA. This is the first such study among Bulgarian patients and hopefully more will follow. Further studies among different populations are needed in order to improve evidence-based results and to decrease interpolation of data.

Author Contributions: Conceptualization: T.V., I.A., and S.V.; data curation: T.V. and K.D.; Formal analysis: T.V., M.S., K.T.-Y., I.A. and S.V.; funding acquisition, T.V. and I.A.; investigation: T.V., K.T.-Y. and I.A.; methodology, T.V., E.I.-T., K.T.-Y., I.A. and S.V.; project administration: T.V. and I.A.; resources: M.S., K.D. and S.V.; supervision: T.V., I.A. and S.V.; validation: T.V. and I.A.; visualization: T.V.; writing—original draft: T.V.; writing—review and editing: M.S., E.I.-T., K.D., I.A. and S.V.

Acknowledgments: This study was supported by grant number 12-D/2013-2014, project № 3-D, from the Medical University, Sofia.

References

1. Antiga, E.; Caproni, M. The diagnosis and treatment of dermatitis herpetiformis. *Clin. Cosmet. Investig. Dermatol.* **2015**, *8*, 257–265. [CrossRef] [PubMed]
2. Caproni, M.; Antiga, E.; Melani, L.; Fabbri, P. The Italian Group for Cutaneous Immunopathology. Guidelines for the diagnosis and treatment of dermatitis herpetiformis. *J. Eur. Acad. Dermatol. Venereol.* **2009**, *23*, 633–638. [CrossRef] [PubMed]
3. Reunala, T.; Salmi, T.T.; Hervonen, K.; Kaukinen, K.; Collin, P. Dermatitis Herpetiformis: A Common Extraintestinal Manifestation of Coeliac Disease. *Nutrients* **2018**, *10*, 602. [CrossRef] [PubMed]
4. Sárdy, M.; Kárpáti, S.; Merkl, B.; Paulsson, M.; Smyth, N. Epidermal transglutaminase (TGase 3) is the autoantigen of dermatitis herpetiformis. *J. Exp. Med.* **2002**, *195*, 747–757. [CrossRef] [PubMed]
5. Collin, P.; Salmi, T.T.; Hervonen, K.; Kaukinen, K.; Reunala, T. Dermatitis herpetiformis: A cutaneous manifestation of coeliac disease. *Ann. Med.* **2017**, *49*, 23–31. [CrossRef] [PubMed]
6. Bonciani, D.; Verdelli, A.; Bonciolini, V.; D'Errico, A.; Antiga, E.; Fabbri, P.; Caproni, M. Dermatitis herpetiformis: From the genetics to the development of skin lesions. *Clin. Dev. Immunol.* **2012**, *2012*, 239691. [CrossRef]
7. Reunala, T. Dermatitis herpetiformis: Coeliac disease of the skin. *Ann. Med.* **1998**, *30*, 416–418. [CrossRef]
8. Savilahti, E.; Reunala, T.; Mäki, M. Increase of lymphocytes bearing the gamma/delta T cell receptor in the jejunum of patients with dermatitis herpetiformis. *Gut* **1992**, *33*, 206–211. [CrossRef]
9. Alonso-Llamazares, J.; Gibson, L.E.; Rogers, R.S. Clinical, pathologic, and immunopathologic features of dermatitis herpetiformis: Review of the Mayo Clinic experience. *Int. J. Dermatol.* **2007**, *46*, 910–919. [CrossRef]
10. Mazzarella, G. Effector and suppressor T cells in celiac disease. *World J. Gastroenterol.* **2015**, *21*, 7349–7356. [CrossRef]
11. Berger, E. *Zur Allergischen Pathogenese der Cöliakie*; Bibliotheca Paediatrica; S Karger Ag: Basel, Switzerland, 1958; pp. 1–55.
12. Rossi, T.M.; Tjota, A. Serologic indicators of celiac disease. *J. Pediatr. Gastroenterol. Nutr.* **1998**, *26*, 205–210. [CrossRef] [PubMed]

13. Seah, P.P.; Fry, L.; Hoffbrand, A.V.; Holborow, E.J. Tissue antibodies in dermatitis herpetiformis and adult coeliac disease. *Lancet* **1971**, *1*, 834–836. [CrossRef]

14. Chorzelski, T.P.; Beutner, E.H.; Sulej, J.; Tchorzewska, H.; Jablonska, S.; Kumar, V.; Kapuscinska, A. IgA anti-endomysium antibody. A new immunological marker of dermatitis herpetiformis and coeliac disease. *Br. J. Dermatol.* **1984**, *111*, 395–402. [CrossRef] [PubMed]

15. Dieterich, W.; Ehnis, T.; Bauer, M.; Donner, P.; Volta, U.; Riecken, E.O.; Schuppan, D. Identification of tissue transglutaminase as the autoantigen of celiac disease. *Nat. Med.* **1997**, *3*, 797–801. [CrossRef] [PubMed]

16. Caja, S.; Mäki, M.; Kaukinen, K.; Lindfors, K. Antibodies in celiac disease: Implications beyond diagnostics. *Cell. Mol. Immunol.* **2011**, *8*, 103–109. [CrossRef]

17. Korponay-Szabó, I.R.; Laurila, K.; Szondy, Z.; Halttunen, T.; Szalai, Z.; Dahlbom, I.; Rantala, I.; Kovács, J.B.; Fésüs, L.; Mäki, M. Missing endomysial and reticulin binding of coeliac antibodies in transglutaminase 2 knockout tissues. *Gut* **2003**, *52*, 199–204. [CrossRef] [PubMed]

18. Molberg, O.; Mcadam, S.N.; Körner, R.; Quarsten, H.; Kristiansen, C.; Madsen, L.; Fugger, L.; Scott, H.; Norén, O.; Roepstorff, P.; et al. Tissue transglutaminase selectively modifies gliadin peptides that are recognized by gut-derived T cells in celiac disease. *Nat. Med.* **1998**, *4*, 713–717. [CrossRef]

19. Kasperkiewicz, M.; Dähnrich, C.; Probst, C.; Komorowski, L.; Stöcker, W.; Schlumberger, W.; Zillikens, D.; Rose, C. Novel assay for detecting celiac disease-associated autoantibodies in dermatitis herpetiformis using deamidated gliadin-analogous fusion peptides. *J. Am. Acad. Dermatol.* **2012**, *66*, 583–588. [CrossRef] [PubMed]

20. Sugai, E.; Smecuol, E.; Niveloni, S.; Vázquez, H.; Label, M.; Mazure, R.; Czech, A.; Kogan, Z.; Mauriño, E.; Bai, J.C. Celiac disease serology in dermatitis herpetiformis. Which is the best option for detecting gluten sensitivity? *Acta Gastroenterol. Latinoam.* **2006**, *36*, 197–201.

21. Fuertes, I.; Mascaró, J.M.; Bombí, J.A.; Iranzo, P. A Retrospective Study of Clinical, Histological, and Immunological Characteristics in Patients with Dermatitis Herpetiformis. The Experience of Hospital Clinic de Barcelona, Spain between 1995 and 2010 and a Review of the Literature. *Actas Dermo-Sifiliográficas Engl. Ed.* **2011**, *102*, 699–705. [CrossRef]

22. Dahele, A.; Gosh, S. The role of serological tests in redefining coeliac disease. *Proc. R. Coll. Phys. Edinb.* **2000**, *30*, 100–113.

23. Shahid, M.; Drenovska, K.; Velikova, T.; Vassileva, S. Dermatitis herpetiformis in Bulgaria: Report of 78 patients. *J. Investig. Dermatol.* **2017**, *137*, S280. [CrossRef]

24. Clarindo, M.V.; Possebon, A.T.; Soligo, E.M.; Uyeda, H.; Ruaro, R.T.; Empinotti, J.C. Dermatitis herpetiformis: Pathophysiology, clinical presentation, diagnosis and treatment. *An. Bras. Dermatol.* **2014**, *89*, 865–877. [CrossRef]

25. Harrington, L.E.; Hatton, R.D.; Mangan, P.R.; Turner, H.; Murphy, T.L.; Murphy, K.M.; Weaver, C.T. Interleukin 17-producing CD4+ effector T cells develop via a lineage distinct from the T helper type 1 and 2 lineages. *Nat. Immunol.* **2005**, *6*, 1123–1132. [CrossRef]

26. Jaskowski, T.D.; Donaldson, M.R.; Hull, C.M.; Wilson, A.R.; Hill, H.R.; Zone, J.J.; Book, L.S. Novel Screening Assay Performance in Pediatric Celiac Disease and Adult Dermatitis Herpetiformis. *J. Pediatr. Gastroenterol. Nutr.* **2010**, *51*, 19–23. [CrossRef]

27. Desai, A.M.; Krishnan, R.S.; Hsu, S. Medical pearl: Using tissue transglutaminase antibodies to diagnose dermatitis herpetiformis. *J. Am. Acad. Dermatol.* **2005**, *53*, 867–868. [CrossRef]

28. Porter, W.M.; Unsworth, D.J.; Lock, R.J.; Hardman, C.M.; Baker, B.S.; Fry, L. Tissue transglutaminase antibodies in dermatitis herpetiformis. *Gastroenterology* **1999**, *117*, 749–750. [CrossRef]

29. Dieterich, W.; Schuppan, D.; Laag, E.; Bruckner-Tuderman, L.; Reunala, T.; Kárpáti, S.; Zágoni, T.; Riecken, E.O. Antibodies to Tissue Transglutaminase as Serologic Markers in Patients with Dermatitis Herpetiformis. *J. Investig. Dermatol.* **1999**, *113*, 133–136. [CrossRef]

30. Kumar, V.; Jarzabek-Chorzelska, M.; Sulej, J.; Rajadhyaksha, M.; Jablonska, S. Tissue Transglutaminase and Endomysial Antibodies—Diagnostic Markers of Gluten-Sensitive Enteropathy in Dermatitis Herpetiformis. *Clin. Immunol.* **2001**, *98*, 378–382. [CrossRef]

31. Koop, I.; Ilchmann, R.; Izzi, L.; Adragna, A.; Koop, H.; Barthelmes, H. Detection of autoantibodies against tissue transglutaminase in patients with celiac disease and dermatitis herpetiformis. *Am. J. Gastroenterol.* **2000**, *95*, 2009–2014. [CrossRef]

32. Caproni, M.; Cardinali, C.; Renzi, D.; Calabrò, A.; Fabbri, P. Tissue transglutaminase antibody assessment in dermatitis herpetiformis. *Br. J. Dermatol.* **2001**, *144*, 196–197. [CrossRef]

33. Sárdy, M.; Csikós, M.; Geisen, C.; Preisz, K.; Kornseé, Z.; Tomsits, E.; Töx, U.; Hunzelmann, N.; Wieslander, J.; Kárpáti, S.; et al. Tissue transglutaminase ELISA positivity in autoimmune disease independent of gluten-sensitive disease. *Clin. Chim. Acta Int. J. Clin. Chem.* **2007**, *376*, 126–135. [CrossRef]

34. Sugai, E.; Hwang, H.J.; Vazquez, H.; Smecuol, E.; Niveloni, S.; Mazure, R.; Maurino, E.; Aeschlimann, P.; Binder, W.; Aeschlimann, D.; et al. New Serology Assays Can Detect Gluten Sensitivity among Enteropathy Patients Seronegative for Anti-Tissue Transglutaminase. *Clin. Chem.* **2010**, *56*, 661–665. [CrossRef] [PubMed]

35. Green, P.H.R.; Rostami, K.; Marsh, M.N. Diagnosis of coeliac disease. *Best Pract. Res. Clin. Gastroenterol.* **2005**, *19*, 389–400. [CrossRef]

36. Rostami, K.; Kerckhaert, J.; Tiemessen, R.; von Blomberg, B.M.; Meijer, J.W.; Mulder, C.J. Sensitivity of antiendomysium and antigliadin antibodies in untreated celiac disease: Disappointing in clinical practice. *Am. J. Gastroenterol.* **1999**, *94*, 888–894. [CrossRef]

37. Marsh, M.N. Gluten, major histocompatibility complex, and the small intestine. A molecular and immunobiologic approach to the spectrum of gluten sensitivity ('celiac sprue'). *Gastroenterology* **1992**, *102*, 330–354. [CrossRef]

38. Samaşca, G.; Băican, A.; Pop, T.; Pîrvan, A.; Miu, N.; Andreica, M.; Cristea, V.; Dejica, D. IgG-F-actin antibodies in celiac disease and dermatitis herpetiformis. *Rom. Arch.* **2010**, *69*, 177–182.

39. Granito, A.; Muratori, L.; Muratori, P.; Guidi, M.; Lenzi, M.; Bianchi, F.B.; Volta, U. Anti-saccharomyces cerevisiae antibodies (ASCA) in coeliac disease. *Gut* **2006**, *55*, 296.

40. Velikova, T.; Spassova, Z.; Tumangelova-Yuzeir, K.; Krasimirova, E.; Ivanova-Todorova, E.; Kyurkchiev, D.; Altankova, I. Serological Update on Celiac Disease Diagnostics in Adults. *Int. J. Celiac Dis.* **2018**, *6*, 20–25. [CrossRef]

41. Zebrowska, A.; Wagrowska-Danilewicz, M.; Danilewicz, M.; Stasikowska-Kanicka, O.; Cynkier, A.; Sysa-Jedrzejowska, A.; Waszczykowska, E. IL-17 Expression in Dermatitis Herpetiformis and Bullous Pemphigoid. *Mediat. Inflamm.* **2013**, *2013*, 967987. [CrossRef]

42. Juczynska, K.; Wozniacka, A.; Waszczykowska, E.; Danilewicz, M.; Wagrowska-Danilewicz, M.; Wieczfinska, J.; Pawliczak, R.; Zebrowska, A. Expression of the JAK/STAT Signaling Pathway in Bullous Pemphigoid and Dermatitis Herpetiformis. *Mediat. Inflamm.* **2017**, *2017*, 6716419. [CrossRef] [PubMed]

10

Fatigue as an Extra-Intestinal Manifestation of Celiac Disease

Lars-Petter Jelsness-Jørgensen [1,2], **Tomm Bernklev** [3,4] and **Knut E. A. Lundin** [5,6,*]

1   Department of Health Science, Østfold University College, N-1757 Halden, Norway; lars.p.jelsness-jorgensen@hiof.no
2   Department of Gastroenterology, Østfold Hospital Trust Kalnes, N-1714 Grålum, Norway
3   Department of Research and Innovation, Vestfold Hospital Trust, N-3103 Tønsberg, Norway; tomm.bernklev@medisin.uio.no
4   Faculty of Medicine, Institute of Clinical Medicine, University of Oslo, N-0318 Oslo, Norway
5   K.G. Jebsen Coeliac Disease Research Centre, University of Oslo, N-0318 Oslo, Norway
6   Department of gastroenterology, Oslo University Hospital Rikshospitalet, N-0372 Oslo, Norway
*   Correspondence: knut.lundin@medisin.uio.no

Abstract: Celiac disease may present with a range of different symptoms, including abdominal problems in a broader sense, iron deficiency and "constant tiredness". All of these symptoms should consequently lead the clinicians to consider celiac disease as a potential etiopathogenetic cause. Although the pathophysiology of celiac disease is well documented, the actual mechanisms for disease presentation(s) are less well understood. We here address the topic of fatigue in celiac disease. A systematic literature search identified 298 papers of which five met the criteria for full evaluation. None of the reviewed papers were of high quality and had several methodological weaknesses. We conclude that there is an unmet need to study the contributing factors and management of fatigue in celiac disease.

Keywords: fatigue; energy; celiac disease; extra-intestinal manifestations

1. Introduction

Celiac disease is by definition an inflammatory disorder in the small intestine that is driven by dietary gluten from wheat, rye and barley [1]. The disease is often also termed an autoimmune disease due to a hallmark of the disease; autoantibodies to the endogenous enzyme tissue transglutaminase TG2. The crucial importance of intestinal inflammation and the most frequent presentation of the disease as a severe malabsorption syndrome led most clinicians to think of the disease as mainly an intestinal disorder. However, we now know that a very large proportion of the patients do not primarily display intestinal complaints, but that their disease presentation is more coloured by extra-intestinal manifestations [2,3]. In a recent review by Leffler et al. [3] this is well described, including anaemia, musculoskeletal, skin, neurological and organ-specific manifestations. Some of these manifestations are caused by the intestinal disorder, others may be caused by systemic inflammation and/or genetic overlap to other immune disorders [4]. Today we consider that symptoms like abdominal problems in the wider sense, unexplained iron deficiency and "constant tiredness" should all prompt the clinicians to consider celiac disease [5,6].

From our own clinical practice, we experience many patients with untreated celiac disease that suffer from fatigue. In most cases fatigue improves with diet, but far from always. In addition, these patients also present with a significant reduction in their health-related quality of life [2]. Fatigue is described as a "persistent, overwhelming sense of tiredness, weakness or exhaustion resulting in a decreased capacity for physical and/or mental work". While fatigue may be a natural and transient part of life, a typical feature in chronic disease is that these symptoms are unrelieved by adequate sleep or rest [7]. The aetiopathogenesis of fatigue in chronic disease appears to result from a complex inter-relationship of biological, psychosocial and behavioural processes [8].

The aim of this review was consequently to address the aspect of fatigue in celiac disease and to systematically summarise the existing literature on this topic.

2. Materials and Methods

Multiple searches were undertaken using MEDLINE, CINAHL, EMBASE, Psychinfo, Academic Search Premiere, and Cochrane. Both medical subject heading (MeSH) searching and free-text searching were used to maximize citation retrieval (Table 1). The searches were performed independently by a university librarian, and one of the co-authors (L.-P.J.-J.).

Table 1. Search terms used for literature search.

Fatigue	Coeliac Disease
Fatigue (MeSH)	Coeliac disease
Mental fatigue	
Chronic fatigue	
Tiredness	
Exhaustion	
Weariness	
Vitality	
Asthenia	
Low energy	

Due to the limited number of publications on fatigue in coeliac disease, no time limit was set for the papers. The searches were performed between April and June 2018, and the most recent search was performed on August 5th, 2018. The searches were limited to "humans", "adult" and English language since there was no scope for translation.

Studies with all types of designs were included if they had measured and reported data on fatigue in patients with celiac disease. Reviews, commentaries, abstracts/posters, case reports, protocols and letters to editors were excluded. The review was conducted in line with the PRISMA guidelines [9].

3. Results

The search yielded 298 references in total, of which 248 were excluded on title (Figure 1). After removing duplicates and screening the remaining 42 papers, a total of 16 papers were examined in full. Of these 16 papers, 11 did not report any specific methodology for fatigue measurement and were consequently excluded. Hence, a total of five papers were included in full review. Figure 1 describes the citation retrieval and the handling process in detail.

3.1. Quality Assessment

The quality of the included papers was assessed using the Joanna Briggs Institute Critical Appraisal Checklist, specific to the methodological design of each paper. The studies were classified as being of high, medium or low quality. A quality score was reduced if the paper did not define fatigue, report the sample size, if the sample size was judged inadequate according to study design, if the response rate was low or not reported, if the questionnaires used were not validated, if the methods and statistical analysis was insufficiently described or if there were indications of selective reporting. Two researchers (T.B./L.-P.J.-J.) performed quality assessment independently to ensure optimal assessment of the included papers. Based on these criteria, all of the reviewed papers had several methodological weaknesses, and none were judged to be of high quality. However, due to the low number of publications on fatigue and celiac disease, none of the papers were excluded from full-review based on quality.

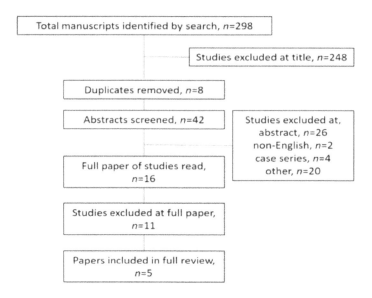

Figure 1. Citation retrieval and handling process.

3.2. Outline of the Included Papers

In total, three papers assessed fatigue as the primary endpoint, one study investigated extra-intestinal symptoms and health-related quality of life (HRQoL), while one study assessed quality of sleep. An overview of the included papers is presented in Table 2.

Table 2. Summary of the included articles.

Study (Ref. No.)	Study Population and Setting	Study Design and Participants	Questionnaires Measuring Fatigue	Strengths and Limitations
Häuser et al., 2006 [10]	A subgroup of members (1000/18,355) from the German Coeliac Society (GZG) ≥18 years was invited to participate. Every 18th person on the membership list was invited in order to ensure a geographically representative sample. Normative data were collected from the handbooks of the SF-36, GBB-24 and HADS-D. Exclusion criteria: <18 years of age	Cross-sectional design Available for analyses: n = 446	SF-36 (Vitality subscale) GBB-24 (Fatigue subscale)	L: Fatigue not specified as aim, merely reported as parts of the questionnaire results L: No definition of fatigue L: Sample consisting of members of a patient society only L: Low response rate S: Normative data for comparison L: Self-reported information on comorbidity L: Single centre study S: Validated instruments used L: Coeliac disease diagnosis self-reported only
Siniscalchi et al., 2005 [11]	Caucasion adults ≥18 years of age from Campania, Italy, were consecutively recruited from an outpatient clinic. Participants divided into two groups (Group 1: Patients on gluten containing diet, Group 2: Patients on gluten-free diet). Control group consisted of volunteers recruited from medical an non-medical hospital staff. Exclusion criteria: <18 years of age, lack of informed consent, major psychiatric disease, active thyroid gland disease	Cross-sectional design Coeliac disease: n = 130 Control group: n = 80	CFS FSS VAS	S: Definition of fatigue. L: Inadequate language L: Groups not comparable due to differences in BMI, Ferritin, Haemoglobin L: No evidence of appropriate matching of groups L: Inadequate statistical control for differences between groups L: Methods used to collect socio-demographic and clinical data is lacking L: Unclear presentation of results L: Procedure for questionnaire handling insufficiently described L: Lack of information about validity and reliability on the study questionnaires, both in Italian and in the target group L: No clear identification and control of potential confounding factors L: Data not presented in line with study aims

Table 2. *Cont.*

Study (Ref. No.)	Study Population and Setting	Study Design and Participants	Questionnaires Measuring Fatigue	Strengths and Limitations
Jordá et al., 2010 [12]	Patients with celiac disease seen between March 2008 and April 2009 were prospectively invited to participate in the study Included patients stratified in two groups (Group 1: Following gluten-free diet, Group 2: Untreated)	Cross-sectional study $n = 51$ Group 1: $n = 38$ Group 2: $n = 13$	D-FIS	L: No definition of fatigue. S: Validated fatigue questionnaire used L: Small sample and small subgroups L: Lack of information on recruitment procedure L: Lack of information concerning the collection of socio-demographic and clinical data L: No information on ethical approval L: No information about response rate or number of patients approached for inclusion L: Characteristics differ between groups
Ciacci et al., 2007 [13]	Patients with CD screened for inclusion at the Department of Clinical and Experimental Medicine, Federico II University—Naples, Italy6 0 patients randomized following a 30-day gluten-free diet	Randomized, double blind, parallel study $n = 60$ (L-Carnitine group $n = 30$, placebo $n = 30$)	Scott-Huskisson VAS VSA SF-36 (Vitality subscale)	S: Definition of fatigue S: Randomized groups S: Allocation concealment S: Clear definition of coeliac disease L: Large number of participants did not complete study ($n = 13$ (22%)) L: Single centre L: Lack of calculation of effect size L: No information on validity/reliability of fatigue questionnaires
Zingone et al., 2010 [14]	Adult coeliac disease patients consecutively recruited from September 2009 to March 2010 from Frederico II University (Naples, Italy) Participants divided into two groups (Group 1: Coeliac patients at diagnosis on gluten containing diet. Group 2: Coeliac patients at follow up on gluten-free diet) Gender- and age-matched control group Inclusion criteria: Informed consent, 19–60 years Exclusion criteria: Major psychiatric disease, cancer, pregnancy or children blow 3 years of age	Case Control study Group 1: $n = 30$ Group 2: $n = 30$ Control group: $n = 30$	Fatigue-VAS	L: Fatigue not specified as aim, merely reported as parts of the questionnaire results. L: No definition of fatigue L: No information about response rate or number of patients approached for inclusion L: Large numeric differences in characteristics between coeliac groups L: No control for confounding variables S: Gender- and age-matched controls

Table legends and abbreviations: L; Limitation., S; Strength., SF-36; Short Form-36 Health Survey., D-FIS; Daily Fatigue Impact Scale., FSS; Fatigue Severity Scale., CFS; Chronic Fatigue Syndrome Questionnaire., GBB-24., Geißener Symptom Check List., VSA; Verbal Scale for Asthenia, VSA. CD; Coeliac disease, HADS-D; Hospital anxiety and depression scale – depression.

3.3. Definition and Measurement of Fatigue

In two out of five papers, a definition or a more detailed description of fatigue was provided. Both Siniscalchi et al. [11] and Ciacci et al. [13] defined fatigue as "difficulty in initiating or sustaining regular activities". However, in none of these studies a reference to the definition were provided.

In total, six different ways of measuring fatigue have been used in the five studies reviewed. Five of these instruments have only been used once. In addition, one study has used the sub-scale vitality from the health-related quality of life questionnaire SF-36.

In a majority of the papers, there is lack of information about the validity and reliability of the instruments used to measure fatigue. While Häuser et al. [10] and Jordá et al. [12] provide references to adequate psychometrical testing of the SF-36, Giessener Symptom Checklist (GBB-24) and Daily Fatigue Impact Scale (D-FIS), none of the Italian studies provide clear reference to adequate testing. In fact, in two of the latter studies one of the instruments seem to have been labeled differently while referring to the same reference by Wessely et al. [15]. While Siniscalchi et al. [11] use the label Chronic Fatigue Syndrome (CFS) questionnaire, Ciacci et al. [13] use the label Verbal Scale for Asthenia. Moreover, when investigating the original study by Wessely et al. [15] in depth, it seems like this instrument was developed for this particular study and that the necessary tests for validity and reliability were not performed, and at least not published.

3.4. Prevalence of Fatigue and Its Associations

None of the reviewed studies present prevalence data, even though one of the aims in the study by Siniscalchi et al. [11] were to evaluate the prevalence of fatigue in celiac disease. When looking at fatigue in patients on normal versus gluten-free diet, results also differ. While Zingone et al. [14] and Siniscalchi et al. [11] found no significant differences, Jordá et al. [12] found that untreated patients reported significantly worse fatigue. In addition, when comparing celiac disease patients and healthy controls, both Häuser et al. [10] and Zingone et al. [14] found impaired scores in celiac disease.

While Zingone et al. [14] found impaired sleep to be associated with increased fatigue, Jordá et al. [12] found that increased fatigue was associated with impaired HRQoL. Merely two studies [11,12] investigated potential socio-demographic and clinical factors associated with fatigue, finding that there is no association between fatigue and factors such as gender, age, or GI symptoms in celiac disease. While Jordá et al. [12] reported that lower haemoglobin levels were correlated with worse scores of the D-FIS fatigue scale, Siniscalchi et al. [11] were not able to identify any association.

3.5. Interventions to Alleviate Fatigue

Only one of the studies were designed as an intervention. The study by Ciacci et al. [13] aimed to investigate the effect on fatigue of a long L-Carnitine treatment in adult celiac disease patients. While there were no reports of serious adverse events, abdominal and skin problems were registered in a total of six patients (10%). Moreover, a large number of patients did not complete the study ($n = 13$), of which three were dropouts. The main finding is that fatigue scores were significantly more improved in the intervention versus placebo group. However, even though fatigue scores in the intervention group displayed a larger decrease than in the placebo group, patients in the intervention group had a higher fatigue scores than the placebo group at baseline (T0). Moreover, the mean fatigue VAS at the end of study (T2) was 2.40 (SD 1.80) versus 2.93 (SD 1.85) in the intervention versus placebo group, respectively. While Ciacci et al. does not report any measures of effect size, calculation of Cohens d [16] on the differences between the intervention and placebo group at T2 reveal a small effect size (0.29).

4. Discussion

In this review we were only able to identify 16 papers that, to some extent, had investigated fatigue in celiac disease. Of these, 11 papers [6,17–26] did not report any specific methodology concerning fatigue assessment. Of the remaining five papers [10–14], in which fatigue assessment had been described methodologically, merely three investigated fatigue as the primary endpoint [11–13]. In addition, critical assessment revealed that none of the included studies held high scientific quality.

A basic problem in fatigue research is the lack of a common accepted definition [27]. Indeed, lack of definition and conceptual clarification was also observed in this review, where only two studies provided a definition of fatigue [11,13]. On the other hand, the fatigue definitions presented in those two papers both lacked a clear reference to existing literature.

Fatigue is frequently reported by patients as well as observed by clinicians in celiac disease [23,25,26]. However, a vast majority of the published literature base their reports merely on clinical consultation rather than rigorous methodological research (i.e., using validated measurement tools). Thus, the actual prevalence of fatigue in celiac disease remains unclear. However, there are indications that the level of fatigue is higher in these patients than in control groups and the background population [10,14]

We were only able to identify one single study that reported on potential socio-demographic and clinical factors associated with fatigue symptoms in celiac disease [11]. Of the factors studied, none were significantly associated with fatigue. However, since data is not shown, it is unclear whether this finding was true for all of the different fatigue measures used in the study. Furthermore, two of the included studies found that fatigue was associated with reduced HRQoL and increased sleep problems, respectively [12,14]. Although there is currently very limited documentation on these associations, this appears to coincide with findings in other patient populations [28–32]. In addition, our review only found one study that was designed as an intervention with fatigue as the primary endpoint. Even though Ciacci et al. [13] conclude that L-Carnitine therapy is safe and effective in ameliorating fatigue in celiac disease, these results should be interpreted with extreme caution. Firstly, the study is hampered by the fact that it does not reach its own power estimates due to a large number of patients not completing the study (21.6%). Secondly, the study does not use fatigue measurement tools that has been adequately tested for validity and reliability. In addition, the absolute difference in mean fatigue VAS between the groups at end of study revealed a small effect size according to Cohen's d [16,33].

Several studies in other populations have shown that anaemia is associated with increased fatigue symptoms [7,34]. The pathogenesis of anaemia-related fatigue remains unclear, but some suggest that abnormalities in energy metabolism play a role in inducing fatigue [35]. Moreover, while some studies have shown that haemoglobin response is associated with meaningful improvements in fatigue, others have not been able to reveal any significant association between the use of erythropoiesis-stimulating agents and fatigue symptom [36,37]. In the current review we were unable to identify studies that specifically looked at anaemia as predictor of fatigue in celiac disease. However, Siniscalchi et al. [11] noted that the included celiac patients in their study had significantly lower haemoglobin levels. A similar observation was reported in Jordá et al. [12]. In the latter study, a significant correlation between worse fatigue scores and lower haemoglobin levels was reported. However, even though Jordá et al. [12] report that their regression analysis show that haemoglobin levels may be involved in the perception of fatigue, the data presented in the paper does not justify such a conclusion. In fact, the dependent variable used in their study was not fatigue, but HRQoL (EQ-5D-VAS). Consequently, the current observation on the potential association between fatigue and anaemia was based on a univariate analysis only.

This review is not without limitations. The fact that we chose to limit our focus to adults and English publications only may have influenced our identification of relevant publications. On the other hand, a strength is the rigorous literature search in several databases, as well as the blinded quality assessment of each of the papers by two of the authors.

5. Conclusions

Although frequently reported in clinical practice, fatigue has been scarcely studied in celiac disease. In addition, existing literature is characterized by significant methodological weaknesses. Consequently, there is an unmet need to understand contributing factors for fatigue as well as the impact of fatigue in celiac disease.

Author Contributions: K.E.A.L. identified the topic of this review and prepared a first draft. L.-P. J.-J. and T.B. performed the literature review and prepared the manuscript. All authors finalized the manuscript.

Acknowledgments: Trine Tingelholm Karlsen (Østfold University College) is acknowledged for her contribution to the literature search.

References

1. Ludvigsson, J.F.; Leffler, D.A.; Bai, J.C.; Biagi, F.; Fasano, A.; Green, P.H.; Hadjivassiliou, M.; Kaukinen, K.; Kelly, C.P.; Leonard, J.N.; et al. The Oslo definitions for coeliac disease and related terms. *Gut* **2013**, *62*, 43–52. [CrossRef] [PubMed]

2. Ludvigsson, J.F.; Bai, J.C.; Biagi, F.; Card, T.R.; Ciacci, C.; Ciclitira, P.J.; Green, P.H.R.; Hadjivassiliou, M.; Holdoway, A.; van Heel, D.A.; et al. Diagnosis and management of adult coeliac disease: Guidelines from the British Society of Gastroenterology. *Gut* **2014**, *63*, 1210–1228. [CrossRef] [PubMed]

3. Leffler, D.A.; Green, P.H.; Fasano, A. Extraintestinal manifestations of coeliac disease. *Nat. Rev. Gastroenterol. Hepatol.* **2015**, *12*, 561–571. [CrossRef] [PubMed]

4. Lundin, K.E.; Wijmenga, C. Coeliac disease and autoimmune disease-genetic overlap and screening. *Nat. Rev. Gastroenterol. Hepatol.* **2015**, *12*, 507–515. [CrossRef] [PubMed]

5. Hin, H.; Bird, G.; Fisher, P.; Mahy, N.; Jewell, D. Coeliac disease in primary care: Case finding study. *BMJ* **1999**, *318*, 164–167. [CrossRef] [PubMed]

6. Sanders, D.S.; Patel, D.; Stephenson, T.J.; Ward, A.M.; McCloskey, E.V.; Hadjivassiliou, M.; Lobo, A.J. A primary care cross-sectional study of undiagnosed adult coeliac disease. *Eur. J. Gastroenterol. Hepatol.* **2003**, *15*, 407–413. [CrossRef] [PubMed]

7. Jelsness-Jorgensen, L.P.; Bernklev, T.; Henriksen, M.; Torp, R.; Moum, B.A. Chronic fatigue is more prevalent in patients with inflammatory bowel disease than in healthy controls. *Inflamm. Bowel Dis.* **2011**, *17*, 1564–1572. [CrossRef] [PubMed]

8. Van Langenberg, D.R.; Gibson, P.R. Systematic review: Fatigue in inflammatory bowel disease. *Aliment. Pharmacol. Ther.* **2010**, *32*, 131–143. [CrossRef] [PubMed]

9. Moher, D.; Liberati, A.; Tetzlaff, J.; Altman, D.G. Preferred reporting items for systematic reviews and meta-analyses: The PRISMA statement. *Ann. Intern. Med.* **2009**, *151*, 264–269. [CrossRef] [PubMed]

10. Hauser, W.; Gold, J.; Stein, J.; Caspary, W.F.; Stallmach, A. Health-related quality of life in adult coeliac disease in Germany: Results of a national survey. *Eur. J. Gastroenterol. Hepatol.* **2006**, *18*, 747–754. [CrossRef] [PubMed]

11. Siniscalchi, M.; Iovino, P.; Tortora, R.; Forestiero, S.; Somma, A.; Capuano, L.; Franzese, M.D.; Sabbatini, F.; Ciacci, C. Fatigue in adult coeliac disease. *Aliment. Pharmacol. Ther.* **2005**, *22*, 489–494. [CrossRef] [PubMed]

12. Jorda, F.C.; Lopez Vivancos, J. Fatigue as a determinant of health in patients with celiac disease. *J. Clin. Gastroenterol.* **2010**, *44*, 423–427. [CrossRef] [PubMed]

13. Ciacci, C.; Peluso, G.; Iannoni, E.; Siniscalchi, M.; Iovino, P.; Rispo, A.; Tortora, R.; Bucci, C.; Zingone, F.; Margarucci, S.; et al. L-Carnitine in the treatment of fatigue in adult celiac disease patients: A pilot study. *Dig. Liver. Dis.* **2007**, *39*, 922–928. [CrossRef] [PubMed]

14. Zingone, F.; Siniscalchi, M.; Capone, P.; Tortora, R.; Andreozzi, P.; Capone, E.; Ciacci, C. The quality of sleep in patients with coeliac disease. *Aliment. Pharmacol. Ther.* **2010**, *32*, 1031–1036. [CrossRef] [PubMed]

15. Wessely, S.; Powell, R. Fatigue syndromes: A comparison of chronic "postviral" fatigue with neuromuscular and affective disorders. *J. Neurol. Neurosurg. Psychiatr.* **1989**, *52*, 940–948. [CrossRef]

16. Cohen, J. *Statistical Power Analysis for The Behavioral Sciences*, 2nd ed.; Lawrence Erlbaum Associates: Mahwah, NJ, USA, 1988.

17. Zarkadas, M.; Cranney, A.; Case, S.; Molloy, M.; Switzer, C.; Graham, I.D.; Butzner, J.D.; Rashid, M.; Warren, R.E.; Burrows, V. The impact of a gluten-free diet on adults with coeliac disease: Results of a national survey. *J. Hum. Nutr. Diet.* **2006**, *19*, 41–49. [CrossRef] [PubMed]

18. Spijkerman, M.; Tan, I.L.; Kolkman, J.J.; Withoff, S.; Wijmenga, C.; Visschedijk, M.C.; Weersma, R.K. A large variety of clinical features and concomitant disorders in celiac disease—A cohort study in the Netherlands. *Dig. Liver Dis.* **2016**, *48*, 499–505. [CrossRef] [PubMed]

19. Silvester, J.A.; Graff, L.A.; Rigaux, L.; Walker, J.R.; Duerksen, D.R. Symptomatic suspected gluten exposure is common among patients with coeliac disease on a gluten-free diet. *Aliment. Pharmacol. Ther.* **2016**, *44*, 612–619. [CrossRef] [PubMed]

20. Jericho, H.; Sansotta, N.; Guandalini, S. Extraintestinal manifestations of celiac disease: Effectiveness of the gluten-free diet. *J. Pediatr. Gastroenterol. Nutr.* **2017**, *65*, 75–79. [CrossRef] [PubMed]

21. Sansotta, N.; Amirikian, K.; Guandalini, S.; Jericho, H. Celiac disease symptom resolution: Effectiveness of the gluten-free diet. *J. Pediatr. Gastroenterol. Nutr.* **2018**, *66*, 48–52. [CrossRef] [PubMed]

22. Catassi, C.; Kryszak, D.; Louis-Jacques, O.; Duerksen, D.R.; Hill, I.; Crowe, S.E.; Brown, A.R.; Procaccini, N.J.; Wonderly, B.A.; Hartley, P.; et al. Detection of Celiac disease in primary care: A multicenter case-finding study in North America. *Am. J. Gastroenterol.* **2007**, *102*, 1454–1460. [CrossRef] [PubMed]

23. Nurminen, S.; Kivela, L.; Huhtala, H.; Kaukinen, K.; Kurppa, K. Extraintestinal manifestations were common in children with coeliac disease and were more prevalent in patients with more severe clinical and histological presentation. *Acta Paediatr.* **2018**. [CrossRef] [PubMed]

24. Barratt, S.M.; Leeds, J.S.; Sanders, D.S. Factors influencing the type, timing and severity of symptomatic responses to dietary gluten in patients with biopsy-proven coeliac disease. *JGLD* **2013**, *22*, 391–396. [PubMed]

25. Ford, S.; Howard, R.; Oyebode, J. Psychosocial aspects of coeliac disease: A cross-sectional survey of a UK population. *Br. J. Health Psychol.* **2012**, *17*, 743–757. [CrossRef] [PubMed]

26. Francavilla, R.; Cristofori, F.; Castellaneta, S.; Polloni, C.; Albano, V.; Dellatte, S.; Indrio, F.; Cavallo, L.; Catassi, C. Clinical, serologic, and histologic features of gluten sensitivity in children. *J. Pediatr.* **2014**, *164*, 463–467. [CrossRef] [PubMed]
27. DeLuca, J. *Fatigue: As a Window to the Brain*, 1st ed.; MIT Press: Cambridge, MA, USA, 2005.
28. Jelsness-Jorgensen, L.P.; Bernklev, T.; Henriksen, M.; Torp, R.; Moum, B.A. Chronic fatigue is associated with impaired health-related quality of life in inflammatory bowel disease. *Aliment. Pharmacol. Ther.* **2011**, *33*, 106–114. [CrossRef] [PubMed]
29. Frigstad, S.O.; Hoivik, M.L.; Jahnsen, J.; Cvancarova, M.; Grimstad, T.; Berset, I.P.; Huppertz-Hauss, G.; Hovde, Ø.; Bernklev, T.; Moum, B.; et al. Fatigue is not associated with vitamin D deficiency in inflammatory bowel disease patients. *WJG* **2018**, *24*, 3293–3301. [CrossRef] [PubMed]
30. Kotterba, S.; Neusser, T.; Norenberg, C.; Bussfeld, P.; Glaser, T.; Dorner, M.; Schürks, M. Sleep quality, daytime sleepiness, fatigue, and quality of life in patients with multiple sclerosis treated with interferon beta-1b: Results from a prospective observational cohort study. *BMC Nephrol.* **2018**, *18*. [CrossRef] [PubMed]
31. Rupp, I.; Boshuizen, H.C.; Jacobi, C.E.; Dinant, H.J.; van den Bos, G.A.M. Impact of fatigue on health-related quality of life in rheumatoid arthritis. *Arthritis Rheum.* **2004**, *51*, 578–585. [CrossRef] [PubMed]
32. Opheim, R.; Fagermoen, M.S.; Bernklev, T.; Jelsness-Jorgensen, L.P.; Moum, B. Fatigue interference with daily living among patients with inflammatory bowel disease. *Qual. Life Res.* **2014**, *23*, 707–717. [CrossRef] [PubMed]
33. Cohen, J. A power primer. *Psychol. Bull.* **1992**, *112*, 155–159. [CrossRef] [PubMed]
34. Romberg-Camps, M.J.; Bol, Y.; Dagnelie, P.C.; Hesselink-van de Kruijs, M.A.; Kester, A.D.; Engels, L.G.; van Deursen, C.; Hameeteman, W.H.A.; Pierik, M.; Pierik, F.; et al. Fatigue and health-related quality of life in inflammatory bowel disease: Results from a population-based study in the Netherlands: The IBD-South Limburg cohort. *Inflamm. Bowel Dis.* **2010**, *16*, 2137–2147. [CrossRef] [PubMed]
35. Sobrero, A.; Puglisi, F.; Guglielmi, A.; Belvedere, O.; Aprile, G.; Ramello, M.; Grossi, F.A.O.U. San Martino—IST, Istituto Nazionale Ricerca sul Cancro (GENOVA) Fatigue: A main component of anemia symptomatology. *Semin. Oncol.* **2001**, *28*, 15–18. [CrossRef]
36. Bohlius, J.; Tonia, T.; Nuesch, E.; Juni, P.; Fey, M.F.; Egger, M.; Bernhard, J. Effects of erythropoiesis-stimulating agents on fatigue- and anaemia-related symptoms in cancer patients: Systematic review and meta-analyses of published and unpublished data. *Br. J. Cancer* **2014**, *111*, 33–45. [CrossRef] [PubMed]
37. Cella, D.; Kallich, J.; McDermott, A.; Xu, X. The longitudinal relationship of hemoglobin, fatigue and quality of life in anemic cancer patients: Results from five randomized clinical trials. *Ann. Oncol.* **2004**, *15*, 979–986. [CrossRef] [PubMed]

11

The Skin in Celiac Disease Patients: The Other Side of the Coin

Ludovico Abenavoli [1,*], Stefano Dastoli [2], Luigi Bennardo [2], Luigi Boccuto [3,4], Maria Passante [2], Martina Silvestri [2], Ilaria Proietti [5], Concetta Potenza [5], Francesco Luzza [1] and Steven Paul Nisticò [2]

[1]   Digestive Physiopathology Unit, Department of Health Sciences, Magna Graecia University of Catanzaro, 88100 Catanzaro, Italy
[2]   Dermatology Unit, Department of Health Sciences, Magna Graecia University of Catanzaro, 88100 Catanzaro, Italy
[3]   JC Self Research Institute, Greenwood Genetic Center, Greenwood, SC 29646, USA
[4]   Clemson University School of Health Research, Clemson University, Clemson, SC 29634, USA
[5]   Dermatology Unit "Daniele Innocenzi", Department of Medical-Surgical Sciences and Biotechnologies, Sapienza University of Rome, Polo Pontino, 04110 Terracina, Italy
*   Correspondence: l.abenavoli@unicz.it

Abstract: Celiac disease (CD) is an autoimmune enteropathy that primarily affects the small intestine and is characterized by atrophy of intestinal villi. The manifestations of the disease improve following a gluten-free diet (GFD). CD is associated with various extra-intestinal diseases. Several skin manifestations are described in CD patients. The present paper reviews all CD-associated skin diseases reported in the literature and tries to analyze the pathogenic mechanisms possibly involved in these associations. Different hypotheses have been proposed to explain the possible mechanisms involved in every association between CD and cutaneous manifestations. An abnormal small intestinal permeability seems to be implicated in various dermatological manifestations. However, most of the associations between CD and cutaneous diseases is based on case reports and case series and a few controlled studies. To better assess the real involvement of the cutaneous district in CD patients, large multicentric controlled clinical trials are required.

Keywords: gluten; gut; enteropathy; gluten-free diet; level of evidences

1. Introduction

Celiac disease (CD) is an autoimmune disorder that occurs in genetically predisposed subjects who develop an immune reaction to gluten [1]. CD primarily involves the small intestine. However, the clinical presentation can be characterized by both intestinal and extra-intestinal manifestations. The incidence of CD is up to 1% in the majority of populations. Genetic factors play an important role in the pathogenesis of CD. The almost totality of the patients with CD possess class II human leukocyte antigen (HLA) -DQ2 and -DQ8, or their variants. However, up to 40% of people with European and Asian origins carries these genes, indicating that the expression of these molecules is necessary, but not sufficient, to develop the disease [2].

The intestinal immune response to gluten is present in two sites: The lamina propria and the epithelium [3]. Both the lamina propria (adaptive) and intraepithelial (innate) immune responses are necessary for the generation of the pathological celiac lesion, but how these two processes interact is not clear [1]. The presentation of CD has shifted from the historically classic malabsorption pediatric symptoms in childhood to non-specific symptoms, which may be present also in adulthood. The symptoms classically include weight loss, chronic diarrhea, and failure to thrive. Non-specific symptoms are more common and include gastrointestinal manifestations, such as bloating, abdominal pain, constipation, as well as extra-intestinal manifestations, as osteoporosis, headache, iron deficiency, and chronic fatigue [4,5].

In the last years, skin diseases are acquiring more and more importance among the extra-intestinal manifestations of CD [4]. The aim of this review is to summarize the association between cutaneous diseases and CD. For this reason, searches were undertaken in the PubMed/Medline database in March 2019 using the following terms: A combined research of "celiac disease" and "skin", "blistering diseases", "cutaneous manifestations", "pemphigus", and other skin disorders. In this way, 7923 articles were found and 100 were selected as reported in Figure 1. In addition, the studies were rated using the Oxford Centre for Evidence Based Medicine 2011 and levels of evidence assigned to each association [6]. The assigned levels of evidence were discussed among members until consensus was reached (Table 1).

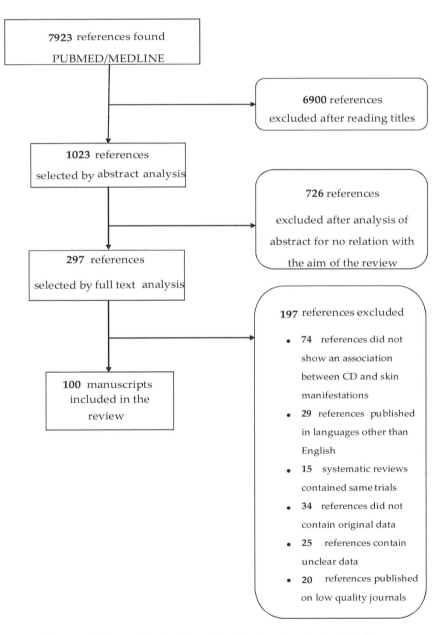

Figure 1. Flow chart of the identified and selected studies.

Table 1. Level of evidences of the association between celiac disease and skin disorders.

Disorders Associated	Level of Evidence
Pemphigus	4
Dermatitis herpetiformis	1A
Linear IgA bullous dermatosis	4
Urticaria	2B
Hereditary angioneurotic edema	4
Atopic dermatitis	4
Cutaneous vasculitis	4
Erythema nodosum	4
Erythema elevatum diutinum	4
Necrolytic migratory erythema	4
Psoriasis	1A
Vitiligo disease	3B
Stomatous Aphtitis	2A
Behçet's disease	4
Oral lichen planus	3B
Dermatomyositis	4
Porphyria	4
Rosacea	2B
Alopecia areata	3B
Acquired hypertrichosis lanuginosa	5
Pyoderma gangrenosum	4
Ichthyosiform dermatoses	4
Pellagra	5
Generalized acquired cutis laxa	5
Skin malignancies	2B

Levels of evidence: 1A Systematic Reviews of Randomized Control Trials; 1B Individual RCT; 2A Systematic Reviews of cohort studies; 2B Individual cohort study; 3A Systematic Reviews of case-control studies; 3B Individual Case-Control Study; 4 Case-series (and poor quality cohort and case-control studies); 5 Expert opinion without explicit critical appraisal.

2. Blistering Diseases

Blistering diseases are characterized by the formation of bullae, blisters, and erosions on the cutaneous surface. Among them pemphigus, dermatitis herpetiformis and linear IgA bullous dermatosis may be related to CD.

2.1. Pemphigus

Pemphigus is a group of autoimmune diseases characterized by the formation of flaccid bullae and erosions of the mucosae and skin [7]. In 2014, an association among pemphigus, epilepsy, and CD was reported [8]. Various case reports associate pemphigus with the positive blood markers of CD, and in particular IgA anti-gliadin (AGA) and anti-endomysium (EMA) antibodies [8,9]. In this case, instauration of a gluten-free diet (GFD) may induce pemphigus disappearance [9].

2.2. Dermatitis Herpetiformis

Dermatitis herpetiformis (DH) or Duhring-Brocq disease is an inflammatory skin disease characterized by a chronic relapsing course and typical histopathological and immunopathological findings. It presents as symmetrical, grouped polymorphic lesions consisting of erythema, urticarial plaques, and papules involving the extensor surfaces of the elbows, knees, shoulders, buttocks, sacral region, neck, face, and scalp. Herpetiform vesicles may occur later and are often immediately excoriated, resulting in erosions, crusted papules, or areas of post-inflammatory dyschromia. Petechial or ecchymotic lesions may occur in the palmoplantar regions and are observed more frequently in children. DH is the most common extra-intestinal manifestation of CD in >85% of cases and it improves significantly with a GFD. In fact, DH and CD share the same HLA haplotypes, DQ2 and DQ8 [10]. Various authors showed the decreasing incidence rate of DH, along with a simultaneous rapid increase in CD. This fits the hypothesis that subclinical, undiagnosed CD is a prerequisite for the development of DH [11].

Moreover, patients with DH have elevated levels of IgA anti-transglutaminase antibodies both TG2 and TG3, which are the most sensitive and specific antibodies to be tested in patients with a suspected DH [12]. At present, a valid hypothesis is that the immune pathogenesis of DH starts from hidden CD in the gut with a TG2, and possibly also a TG3, autoantibody response and evolves into an immune complex deposition of high avidity IgA TG3 antibodies together with the TG3 enzyme in the papillary dermis. This seems to be due to the active TG3 enzyme in the aggregates resulting in covalent cross-linking of the complex to the dermal structures [13].

A small bowel biopsy shows typical CD alterations in almost all these patients, including: Partial-to-total villous atrophy, elongated crypts, decreased villus/crypt ratio, increased mitotic index in the crypts, increased intraepithelial lymphocyte (IEL) density, increased IEL mitotic index, infiltration of plasma cells, lymphocytes, mast cells, and eosinophils and basophils into the lamina propria [14]. The histology of DH is characterized by subepidermal vesicles and blisters associated with the accumulation of neutrophils at the top of dermal papillae. Sometimes, eosinophils can be found within the inflammatory infiltrate, making difficult the differential diagnosis with bullous pemphigoid. The histopathology of DH is not diagnostic as other bullous diseases, including linear IgA dermatosis and epidermolysis bullosa acquisita, which may show similar histologic findings [10]. It is important to obtain a skin fragment near the vesicle for histopathological analysis to identify neutrophilic micro-abscesses. Neutrophils and eosinophils on the top of dermal papillae may form the Piérard micro-abscess, which are typical of this dermatosis, but not pathognomonic. The direct immunofluorescence histology of perilesional skin affected is the gold standard to confirm the diagnosis. It shows the deposition of IgA1 in granular pattern in the lamina lucida of the basement membrane zone. The deposits of IgA in a linear pattern can be found in less than 5% of cases. Indirect immunofluorescence can be used to evaluate the presence of autoantibodies and circulating anti-gliadin, anti-endomysial, anti-reticulin IgA, and anti-epidermal transglutaminase antibodies (anti-tTG) [15]. The first-choice treatment of DH is a strict, life-long GFD which can lead to the resolution of cutaneous and gastrointestinal manifestations with relief in the itching and burning sensation of the vesicle-erythematous-papule.

However, in the first month after the diagnosis or in the inflammatory phases of the disease, in which a GFD alone would not be enough to resolve the cutaneous manifestations, several drugs can be used, including dapsone, steroids or sulfones [10,15].

2.3. Linear IgA Bullous Dermatosis

Linear IgA bullous dermatosis (LABD) is a rare dermatosis characterized by small vesicles and erythematous papules. Pruritus is almost always present with an acute or gradual onset. Up to 24% of the patients affected by LABD also present gluten sensitivity enteropathy and they are responsive to a GFD [16]. LABD and CD often share the same HLA haplotype (i.e., A1, B8, DR3). Although very few case reports have been found in the literature, some authors suggested an association between LABD and gluten sensitivity [16].

3. Urticaria

Urticaria is characterized by intensely pruritic, raised wheals, with or without edema of the deeper cutis. It is usually self-limited, but can be chronic. Chronic urticaria (CU) is defined by recurrent episodes occurring at least twice a week for 6 weeks [17]. The association between CD and CU is widely debated. Ludvigsson and collaborators examined the association between CD and urticaria in 28,900 patients with biopsy-verified CD: 453 patients with CD and no previous diagnosis of urticaria developed urticaria and 79 of these 453 had CU. This confirms that CD is associated with urticaria, especially in its chronic form [17]. CU has been shown to have a genetic association with the human leukocyte antigen HLA-DQ8 alleles. Interestingly, HLAD-Q8 has an association with CD [18]. It has been shown that in CU, there are IgG autoantibodies that inappropriately activate mast cells. The inflammatory response generated in CD probably activates the cells that produce the IgG autoantibodies in CU. It has also been shown that, in patients affected by CD and urticaria, a GFD leads to complete remission of urticaria [19].

4. Hereditary Angioneurotic Edema

Hereditary angioneurotic edema (HANE) is an autosomal dominant genetic disease due to a C1-esterase inhibitor deficiency that leads to an overproduction of bradykinin, causing an increase in vascular permeability. It is characterized by recurrent, marked and diffuse swellings of the subcutaneous and submucosal tissues, painful abdominal attacks, and laryngeal edema with airway obstruction. The symptoms in HANE might be mediated by the activation of the complement system and recent clinical data indicate that the major mediator of angioedema is bradykinin [20]. The therapy consists mainly in the C1-esterase inhibitor concentrate and fresh frozen plasma [20]. The association between CD and hereditary angioneurotic edema, was first reported by Farkas and co-workers [21]. The activation of the pathways of the complement system plays an important role in the pathogenesis of CD and HANE. Gluten ingestion can stimulate complement activity as well as HANE is characterized by an activation of the classic complement pathway [22]. Screening hereditary angioedema patients for CD is warranted if abdominal attacks or neurological symptoms persist despite adequate management. Complement testing is recommended whenever abdominal symptoms persist despite the histological and serological remission of gluten-sensitive enteropathy after the introduction of a GFD [22].

5. Atopic Dermatitis

Atopic dermatitis (AD) is a chronic inflammatory skin disease associated with a heterogeneous group of symptoms and signs. Cutaneous signs and symptoms include erythema, lichenification, prurigo nodules and itch. AD affects 40 million individuals worldwide, and its prevalence is still increasing. Notably, AD appears to be more prevalent among children under five years of age with a decrease in adulthood. The onset of AD occurs primarily in childhood and is thought to precede allergic disorders mediated by IgE sensitization to environmental antigens in the patient affected by atopic triad, as well as AD, asthma, and allergic rhino-conjunctivitis. The complex interaction between genetics, environmental factors, microbiota changes, skin barrier deficiency, immunological derangement, and possibly autoimmunity, contributes to the development of this skin disease [23]. AD has also been linked to CD. Ress and coworkers analyzed the prevalence of CD in children with AD compared with a general pediatric population and showed a four-fold greater risk of developing CD in patients with AD (OR, 4.18; 95% CI, 1.12–15.64). This association may be explained, considering the common cytokine pathways between the two diseases and the screening for CD in patients with AD must be considered in order to prevent the long-term complications of CD [24].

6. Cutaneous Vasculitis

Vasculitis is an inflammatory process affecting the vessel wall and leading to its compromise or destruction with subsequent ischemic and hemorrhagic events. Cutaneous vasculitis is generally characterized by petechiae, palpable purpura and infiltrated erythema indicating dermal superficial, small-vessel vasculitis, or less commonly by nodular erythema, deep ulcers, livedo racemosa, and digital gangrene implicating deep dermal or subcutaneous, muscular-vessel vasculitis [25]. A skin biopsy, extending to subcutis and taken from the earliest, most symptomatic, reddish or purpuric lesion, represents the gold standard for the diagnosis of cutaneous vasculitis. The association between CD and cutaneous vasculitis has been described in several reports [19]. Leukocytoclastic vasculitis (LV), also known as hypersensitivity vasculitis, is a small vessel vasculitis, and it is thought to result from the deposition of circulating immune complexes into the vessel walls, specifically in dermal post-capillary venules, activating the complement pathway. LV is usually limited to the skin and may manifest as palpable purpura, maculopapular rash, bullae, papules, nodules, or ulcers [26]. Meyers et al. reported a case of a young woman, affected by uncontrolled CD, who presented cutaneous LV with the remission of skin lesions after the treatment with a GFD. The coexistence of these two entities might be related to increased intestinal permeability. Exogenous antigens may permeate the damaged CD mucous in larger quantities than normal. This may explain the elevated gluten fraction antibody titer. Moreover, circulating immune complexes are well documented in CD. They probably originate because of the impaired phagocytic function of the reticular endothelium system and subsequently they are deposited in the skin [27,28]. The treatment with a GFD may improve CV lesions in cases associated with CD [28].

7. Erythema Nodosum

Erythema nodosum (EN) is the most common form of panniculitis. It classically presents as tender, warm, erythematous subcutaneous nodules on the bilateral pretibial areas. Although it can occur in both sexes and at any age, it affects predominantly young women [29]. EN associated with CD was reported three times since 1991. It was proposed that the augmented intestinal permeability to various antigens may provoke the skin hypersensitivity reaction [30]. Generally, EN resolves within 8 weeks but as an active disease, it may last up to 18 weeks, and even for a longer period when the antigenic stimulus persists. Furthermore, it has been reported in the literature that CD may coexist with sarcoidosis which is a common cause of EN [31]. EN associated to CD may be far more common than expected. All patients with recurrent or persistent EN of unknown origin should be screened for an underlying CD.

8. Erythema Elevatum Diutinum

Erythema elevatum diutinum (EED) is a rare, chronic and treatable skin condition. The etiology of the disease is unknown, but it has been suggested to be related to high circulating levels of antibodies formed in response to repeated infection. It has many histological mimics and is often associated with several systemic diseases [32]. EED is considered to be a variant of leukocytoclastic vasculitis clinically manifesting as asymptomatic to painful erythematous papules, plaques or nodules, which are usually distributed symmetrically on the extensor surfaces of extremities. It is rarely accompanied by systemic features other than arthritis [32]. Rodriguez-Serna et al. described for the first time, the association between CD and EED in an 11-year-old girl, considering it not a coincidence. With the beginning of the GFD, the cutaneous lesions disappeared and anti-gliadin antibody levels returned to normal. Both conditions have an immune basis in which the increase in IgA appears to play an important role [33]. The pathogenesis of EED is characterized by immune complex deposition, resulting in complement activation, neutrophilic infiltration, and the release of destructive enzymes [32]. Tasanen and others described the presence of granular deposits of IgA and C3 at the derma-epidermal junctions in the affected skin of a patient who presented with EED and CD [34]. Therefore, it is important to evaluate the presence of CD in patients with EED.

9. Necrolytic Migratory Erythema

Necrolytic migratory erythema (NME) is the acronym used for the first time by Wilkinson, to describe the characteristic cutaneous pathology related to glucagonoma. It presents with red-blotch rashes, irregular edges and with vesicles that can be intact or followed by crusting erosions. Frequently, it affects the skin surrounding the lips and upper limbs, more rarely the lower limbs, the abdomen, the groin, the perineum and the buttocks. The affected areas may appear dry or fissured. Initially, the lesion may be exacerbated by pressure or trauma. The phases of lesion development are observed synchronously. Most of the patients have angular cheilitis, stomatitis, glossitis, alopecia, and gastrointestinal symptoms, such as weight loss and diarrhea [35]. NME develops in approximately 70% of patients with glucagonoma syndrome. The etiology is still unclear although a very strong relationship has been noted between hypoaminoacidemia, zinc and a fatty acids deficit due to malabsorption with the severity of NME. A further relationship with NME has been shown in inflammatory autoimmune diseases, such as CD. In fact, the patients affected by CD, who developed the NME, substantially improved the severity of the latter by following a GFD [36].

10. Psoriasis

Psoriasis is a very common chronic inflammatory disease characterized by scaly, well-demarcated, erythematous plaques affecting up to 2% of the general population. The lesions are distributed on different parts of the body, in particular the elbows, knees, trunk, hands and feet [37]. The disease-related quality of life is significantly reduced in patients affected by psoriasis [38]. Psoriatic patients are more likely to have other concomitant autoimmune diseases, such as ulcerative colitis and Crohn disease. CD may be considered as part of these groups. A recent study showed that psoriatic patients have a 2.2-fold risk of being diagnosed with CD compared to healthy controls [39]. A metanalysis showed that IgA AGA, were positive in approximately 14% of psoriatic patients versus 5% of matched controls. Moreover, there was a correlation between the CD antibody positivity and the severity of psoriatic manifestations. Interestingly, the elevated CD antibodies did not always lead to a biopsy-confirmed diagnosis of CD, suggesting that an association between psoriasis and gluten sensitivity, marked by antibody positivity, may be present even in the absence of CD [40]. Psoriasis and CD share different biological mechanisms. Various susceptibility loci are common to both diseases, in particular genes regulating innate and adaptive immune response, such as *RUNX3, TNFAIP3, SOCS1, ELMO1, ETS1, ZMIZ1, UBE2L3.34-36*, and *SH2B3* [41]. Psoriasis and CD have also both been linked to dysregulation in the pathways of Th1, Th17 cells, gamma-delta t-cells and an increased intestinal permeability [42]. Although there are no big clinical trials regarding this argument, a GFD seems to be beneficial for psoriatic patients. Two small clinical trials showed a decrease in serological markers of CD after a GFD and one showed a significant reduction in the psoriasis area severity index. Three case reports also documented the resolution of psoriasis after a GFD [40]. There is also an Italian multicenter study showing that 7 out of 8 patients affected by CD and psoriasis who underwent a GFD showed a significant improvement in the psoriasis area severity index, suggesting a role of gluten in the pathogenesis of both diseases [43].

11. Vitiligo Disease

Vitiligo is an acquired disease characterized by skin depigmentation with the formation of circumscribed white macules, without melanocytes. It predominantly affects the photoexposed areas of the body and the darker phototypes. The disease affects approximately 1% of people in the world and it is often a pathology with inherited characteristics [44]. The etiology is complex and not entirely known. The present dogma suggests that several genetic factors render the melanocyte fragile and susceptible to apoptosis, thus predisposing individuals to developing vitiligo [45]. The association between vitiligo and autoimmune diseases has not yet been fully explained, but genetic data have provided important insights. The susceptibility genes that were identified encode components of the immune system, supporting the hypothesis of a deregulated immune response in vitiligo (HLA class I and II, PTPN22, IL2Rα, GZMB, FOXP3, BACH2, CD80, and CCR6) [46]. The relationship between vitiligo and CD is controversial. The study of Shahmoradi et al. analyzed the frequency of celiac autoantibodies in a group of vitiligo patients compared with the control, involving 128 individuals, 64 vitiligo patients and 64 individuals as the control group [47]. Both IgA EMA and anti-transglutaminase antibodies were measured by the ELISA method in the serum of all participants. The serum of the two vitiligo patients was positive for antibodies. All control groups were seronegative for these antibodies ($p < 0.05$). This study may indicate that both of these autoimmune diseases may be stimulated by a common signal in the immune system that is triggered by a gluten rich diet [47].

12. Behçet's Disease

Behçet's disease (BD) is a chronic-relapsing inflammatory pathology of unknown etiology, characterized by frequent episodes of oral and/or genital ulcers, iritis, associated with various systemic manifestations such as joint, cutaneous and vascular lesions [48]. Behcet's disease can be traced back to an abnormal immune response due to the exposure to a particular antigen in individuals with a genetic predisposition. The onset is between 10 and 30 years with a clear prevalence of the male sex 5–10 times more than women [49]. The stories of oral ulcers and enamel defects have been reported in approximately 25% of patients with CD [50]. There are a few studies in the literature that have elucidated a possible association between BD and CD. Caldas et al. evaluated the association between the two diseases in a 40-year-old woman who presented with asymmetric polyarthralgia, loss of weight, anemia, oral recurrent aphthas (>3/year) and genital ulcerations, inflammatory lower back pain, bowel bleeding and abdominal colic. The biopsy confirmed the diagnosis of CD and a GFD was applied with clinical improvement [51]. Ultimately, it would be desirable for patients with BD to be better investigated for a possible undiagnosed CD.

13. Aphthous Stomatitis

Recurrent aphthous stomatitis (RAS) is a common clinical condition that produces painful ulcerations in the oral cavity. RAS is characterized by multiple recurrent small, round, or ovoid ulcers with circumscribed margins, erythematous haloes typically first presenting in childhood or adolescence. RAS has been recognized for many years as a symptom of CD. A recent meta-analysis showed that celiac patients have greater frequency of RAS (OR = 3.79; 95% CI = 2.67–5.39). RAS patients should be considered at-risk subjects, even in the absence of any gastrointestinal symptoms and should therefore undergo a diagnostic procedure for CD [52]. The etiopathology of RAS is unclear. It is not known whether RAS lesions are directly influenced by the gluten sensitivity disorder, or if they are related to hematinic deficiency with low levels of serum iron, folic acid, and vitamin B12 or trace element deficiencies due to the malabsorption in patients with untreated CD.

14. Oral Lichen Planus

Oral cavity may be involved in CD. The oral manifestations associated to CD are recurrent aphthous stomatitis, glossitis, dental enamel defects, angular cheilitis, burning mouth and oral lichen planus. Oral lichen planus (OLP) is a chronic inflammatory disorder that affects the oral mucosa, gums and tongue with a spectrum of clinical manifestations, including atrophic, erosive, keratotic and ulcerative lesions [53]. OLP, as CD, is characterized by a T-cell autoimmune pathogenesis. Cigic et al. evaluated the prevalence of CD in patients with OLP compared to the controls. In this study, AGA and anti-tTG, were evaluated in 56 OLP patients [54]. CD was diagnosed in eight OLP patients (14.29%) and six OLP patients (10.71%) were positive for IgA Ttg. This confirms the increased frequency of CD in OLP patients [54]. Some erosive, atrophic and ulcerative oral lesions may be caused by underlying haematinic deficiencies associated to the nutrient malabsorption status of CD patients [55].

15. Dermatomyositis

Dermatomyositis (DM) is a rare autoimmune disease that preferentially affects the skin, lungs, muscles and blood vessels and is characterized by proximal and symmetrical muscle weakness with inflammation and damage to the parenchymal cells, causing erythematous and edematous skin manifestations. Usually this is an idiopathic disease. However, it can be associated with other concomitant connective tissue pathologies [56]. It can sometimes occur as a paraneoplastic syndrome associated with gastrointestinal or ovarian malignancies [57]. DM is characterized by the presence of autoantibodies, even if the mechanisms of inflammation and cell damage still remain unclear today [58]. The inflammatory infiltrate in the muscular tissue of DM is represented by T CD4+, B cells and dendritic cells which are preferentially localized around perimysial blood vessels and peripheral areas [59,60]. The inflammation causes damage to the parenchyma and to the blood vessels, so the histological examination shows the presence of a perimysial atrophy, a predominantly perivascular and interfascicular inflammation [59]. The typical histological findings on skin biopsy are vacuolar interface dermatitis with apoptosis, necrotic keratinocytes, and perivascular lymphocytic infiltrate and mucin deposition in the dermis. The inflammatory infiltrate in DM muscle tissue consists of CD4+ T cells, B cells, and dendritic cells that primarily concentrate around perifascicular areas and perimysial blood vessel [58]. Several case reports have highlighted the association between DM and CD [57,61–64].

16. Porphyria

Porphyria, derived from the ancient Greek word "porphura", that is purple, is a group of nine rare diseases: Acute intermittent porphyria (AIP), hereditary coproporphyria (HCP), variegated porphyria (VP), delta-aminolevulinic acid dehydratase deficiency porphyria (ADP), porphyria cutanea tarda (PCT), hepatoerythropoietic porphyria (HEP), congenital erythropoietic porphyria (CEP), erythropoietic protoporphyria (EPP), and X-linked protoporphyria (XLP), characterized by metabolic alterations and caused by malfunctioning of the enzymes involved in the biosynthesis of heme with the accumulation and excretion of porphyrins and their precursors in tissues [65]. The enzyme activity decreases and involves an overproduction of heme precursors, except in XLP [66]. HEP rarely cause clinical manifestations before puberty, as opposed to EPP that manifests symptomatically in the early stages. The precursors of heme of various types accumulate in the liver or bone marrow, which are the most active tissues for the production of heme. All these mechanisms underlie the classification of porphyria as hepatic or erythropoietic. It generally occurs with cutaneous manifestations due to phototoxicity, or with neurological changes such as acute attacks. Based on these differences, the porphyrias are classified as acute or cutaneous. Phototoxicity can occur in all porphyrias, except in ADP and AIP [65]. The urine of patients with this condition may be dark or reddish due to the presence of an excess of porphyrins and related substances. These substances are photosensitizing, and their accumulation causes skin fragility, bullae, scars, hirsutism and the characteristic pigmentation on the photo-exposed areas. This is due both to the release of mediators by leukocytes and mast cells and to the activation of the complement, determining the inflammatory response after photoexposure [67]. Some studies, such as Twaddle and collaborators, have shown a random diagnosis of CD in patients with porphyria [68]. In fact, CD is often associated with DH, underlining some common characteristics of the latter with porphyria. In the VP, the accumulation of 5-aminolevulinic acid and of porfobilinogen provokes both gastrointestinal manifestations and an acute neuropsychiatric syndrome. In this regard, it is important to underline how other works have shown, in patients suffering from CD, a reduction of acute attacks of VP during the GFD [69].

17. Alopecia Areata

Alopecia areata (AA) is a complex, polygenic pathology with autoimmune etiology, which results in the transitory, non-scarring hair loss and the preservation of the hair follicle. By prevalence, it represents the second cause of non-scarring alopecia [70,71]. Clinically, hair loss in alopecia areata manifests itself through very different models. The most frequent pattern is characterized by a small annular or irregular lesion (alopecia areata to patches), usually localized on the scalp, being able to progress until total hair loss, and in this case, the discussion is about total alopecia, associated or not with total loss of all body hair [70]. A biopsy performed on the affected skin shows a lymphocyte infiltrates around the bulb or in the lower part of the hair follicle, thus it suggests an immunological etiology like CD. Recent studies focused on chromosome 6 and more specifically, on the HLA region as the most probable region for the genes that regulate susceptibility to AA [72]. Linkage studies based on a genome-wide association study analysis, have identified an association with many chromosomes and show that AA is a very complex polygenic pathology [70,73]. Both in the AA and in the CD, the presence of organ-specific autoantibodies has been demonstrated [70], with infiltration of T lymphocytes on the lesion site [74]. AA can occur at any age, although most patients develop the disease before the age of 40, with an average age of onset between 25 and 36 years. Early onset between 5 and 10 years, presents itself as a more severe subtype, as an alopecia universalis [75]. Hallaji et al. found that the prevalence of anti-gliadin antibodies in patients with AA had a proportion of 18:100 [76]. In several studies [71,76,77], it has been hypothesized the existence of a CD not diagnosed in patients with AA which improves during a GFD. These positive effects of a GFD on AA, have been associated with the normalization of the immune response [76]. The chronic recurrent phases of CD can be observed during the normal clinical course of AA, and it was noted that patients who followed a GFD regimen showed complete regrowth of hair and other body hair, without highlighting a further recurrence of AA during the follow-up [78]. However, in the study by Mokhtari et al., the frequency distribution of all celiac autoantibodies has been analyzed in patients with AA. The results led to the conclusion that the various biological tests used for the research of subclinical CD do not provide sufficient clear evidence to make the diagnosis of gluten intolerance in patients with AA and other diagnostic approaches are needed [79].

18. Rosacea

Rosacea is an inflammatory skin condition, more frequent in women and primarily characterized by persistent or recurrent episodes of centrofacial erythema [80]. The pathophysiology is not completely understood, but the dysregulation of the immune system as well as changes in the nervous and vascular systems have been identified. Rosacea shares genetic risk loci with autoimmune diseases, such as type 1 diabetes mellitus and CD [81]. One study showed that women with rosacea had a significantly increased risk of CD. In a nationwide cohort study, the prevalence of CD was higher among patients with rosacea when compared to the control subjects (HR = 1.46, 95% CI = 1.11–1.93). However, the pathogenic link is not known. Gastrointestinal symptoms in patients affected by this dermatological condition should warrant clinical suspicion of CD [82].

19. Acquired Hypertrichosis Lanuginosa

Acquired hypertrichosis lanuginose (AHL) is a rare cutaneous manifestation that often underlies the presence of neoplastic pathologies, particularly in the elderly. It is considered as a paraneoplastic manifestation of organic tumor forms, such as a tumor of the gastrointestinal tract, of the lung, of the uterus, of the breast, and often it is indicator of a poor prognosis. It can also be associated with lymphomas. [83]. The etiology is not clear. Corazza and coworkers observed a case of hypertrichosis in a patient suffering from CD [84]. The patient developed a tumor shortly after the diagnosis of CD, confirming that the ACL could represent the unknown tumor spy [84]. However, due to the insufficient data present in the literature, it is not possible to establish a certain correlation.

20. Pyoderma Gangrenosum

Pyoderma gangrenosum (PG) is a rare ulcero-necrotising and neutrophilic dermatosis, whose pathogenesis is unknown. Generally, the main manifestation is a sterile pustule, that rapidly develops into a painful ulcer from the erythematous border [85]. The diagnosis is often a challenge for the clinician and it is often achieved by exclusion. In the literature, many studies have shown the association between inflammatory bowel diseases and in particular, Crohn's disease and ulcerative colitis, and skin manifestations including PG [86]. Weizman et al. have described one of the largest case series of PG among patients with inflammatory bowel disease (IBD) [87]. Moreover, it was observed that the female sex and young age at diagnosis of IBD are predictive factors involved in the development of main cutaneous manifestations [88]. Furthermore, refractory CD resistant to steroids and immunosuppressive drugs has been reported to be associated to PG [89]. The appearance of a pustule transforming to an ulcer in a patient with CD should always arise the suspect for PG [87].

21. Ichthyosiform Dermatoses

Ichthyosiform dermatoses are a group of a skin disorders characterized by clinically evident thickening of the stratum corneum, dry skin and often erythroderma. The term ichthyosis derives from the Greek "ichthys" that means fish, referring to the cutaneous scaling characteristic of these disorders, which is said to resemble the scales of a fish. The attention for this pathology is quite recent. In fact, the first international ichthyosis conference classification was approved in 2009 [90]. The first case report associating the ichthyosis with CD was observed by Menni and co-workers. They reported the clinical history of a twenty-nine year-old woman, who presented ichthyosiform skin manifestations [91]. After just over 10 years, another case that showed this association was reported. In this case, the patient was younger than the first case, but also affected by osteoporosis and secondary hyperparathyroidism. Although the GFD did not allow a complete disappearance of the cutaneous manifestations, it favored an improvement in the quality of life [92].

22. Pellagra

Pellagra is a rare disease caused by niacin deficiency and characterized by a classical triad: Dermatitis, dementia and diarrhea, known as "3D" [93]. The skin signs are the first to appear in over 80% of cases. Initially, itchy and erythematous lesions appear on the area of photo-exposed skin and generally, they are bilateral and symmetrical lesions localized on the dorsum of the hands, arms, face and neck. Subsequently, the gastrointestinal and neurological symptoms occur [93]. In 1937, a case was published of a 15-month-old child with skin manifestations compatible with a non-classical form of pellagra and the simultaneous presence of gastrointestinal disorders related to CD [94]. More than 60 years later, Schattner described another case of a 70-years-old man with a pellagra-like syndrome due to CD [95]. No other cases have been reported, determining a weak association between the two conditions.

23. Generalized Acquired Cutis Laxa

Cutis laxa (CL), also called elastolysis or dermatomegaly, includes a heterogenous group of disorders that affects the elastic tissue and it is characterized by the presence of loose and redundant skin, caused by a reduced number and abnormal properties of elastic fibers in the derma [96]. The etiopathogenesis is still not fully known; it can be congenital or acquired [97]. Only one case in the literature shows the coexistence of acquired CL and CD. In this case, the clinical suspicion of CL was confirmed histologically and analyzed through direct immunofluorescence. The latter has highlighted the presence of IgA deposits in the papillary dermis. It is possible to hypothesize that the IgA deposit constitutes the base of the pathophysiological link between the two diseases [71,98].

24. Skin Malignancies

The variations of the incidence of the skin malignancies in patients affected by CD is a very interesting topic. A study by Ilus et al. studied a population of 32,439 adult celiac patients to evaluate the relative risk for each kind of malignancies [99]. Among cutaneous cancer, a major incidence was registered for basal cell carcinoma and a slightly minor incidence for melanoma [99]. There is instead a known association between CD and lymphomas [99], and cutaneous lymphomas seem also associated to CD. Various case reports show this association, the last one being reported in 2016. The association of cutaneous lymphoma with CD may be determined by a lymphocytic stimulation carried out by the presence of a constant antigen, such as gluten, in the gastrointestinal tract. Some researchers [100] suggested that in predisposed individuals, the resulting dysplastic T cells may migrate into cutis, causing cutaneous T cell lymphoma. The adherence to a GFD decreases the risk for malignancy.

25. Conclusions

CD is an autoimmune enteropathy associated with several extra-intestinal diseases, including various skin manifestations. Different hypotheses have been proposed to explain the possible mechanisms involved in every association between CD and cutaneous manifestations. An abnormal small intestinal permeability seems to be implicated in various dermatological manifestations. The inability of the small intestine to operate as a barrier may allow a major penetration of exogenous antigens with a consequent immunological response that leads to vascular alterations and to malabsorption with secondary vitamin and amino acidic deficiency. However, on the basis of the revision of the literature by the levels of evidence, it can be concluded that only a few associations are very strong and in particular, DH and psoriasis. The other associations between CD and skin diseases are based on case-reports and case series, with very few multicentric controlled studies. In this way, to better assess the involvement of the cutaneous district in CD, large multicentric controlled studies are required. Nevertheless, screening for CD in patients suffering from chronic cutaneous diseases seems to be justified considering that a GFD can significantly improve both gastrointestinal and systemic symptoms.

Author Contributions: Conceptualization, L.A.; methodology, L.A., S.D. and L.B. (Luigi Bennardo); resources, L.B. (Luigi Bennardo), M.P. and M.S.; data curation, S.D.; writing—original draft preparation, L.A. and L.B. (Luigi Boccuto); writing—review and editing L.A., S.D., I.P. and L.B. (Luigi Bennardo); visualization, F.L. and C.P.; supervision, S.P.N.

References

1. Lebwohl, B.; Sanders, D.S.; Green, P.H.R. Coeliac disease. *Lancet* **2018**, *391*, 70–81. [CrossRef]
2. Leonard, M.M.; Sapone, A.; Catassi, C.; Fasano, A. Celiac disease and nonceliac gluten sensitivity: A review. *JAMA* **2017**, *318*, 647–656. [CrossRef] [PubMed]
3. Abenavoli, L.; Proietti, I.; Zaccone, V. Celiac disease: From gluten to skin. *Expert. Rev. Clin. Immunol.* **2009**, *5*, 789–800. [CrossRef] [PubMed]
4. Abenavoli, L.; Proietti, I.; Leggio, L. Cutaneous manifestations in celiac disease. *World J. Gastroenterol.* **2006**, *12*, 843–852. [CrossRef]
5. Hujoel, I.A.; Reilly, N.R.; Rubio-Tapia, A. Celiac disease: Clinical features and diagnosis. *Gastroenterol. Clin. North Am.* **2019**, *48*, 19–37. [CrossRef] [PubMed]
6. OCEBM Levels of Evidence. Available online: https://www.cebm.net/?o=1025 (accessed on 31 May 2019).
7. Palleria, C.; Bennardo, L.; Dastoli, S.; Iannone, L.F.; Silvestri, M.; Manti, A.; Nisticò, S.P.; Russo, E.; De Sarro, G. Angiotensin-converting-enzyme inhibitors and angiotensin II receptor blockers induced pemphigus: A case series and literature review. *Dermatol. Ther.* **2018**, *32*, e12748. [CrossRef]
8. Labidi, A.; Serghini, M.; Karoui, S.; Ben Mustapha, N.; Boubaker, J.; Filali, A. Epilepsy, pemphigus and celiac disease: An exceptional association. *Tunis Med.* **2014**, *92*, 585–586.
9. Drago, F.; Cacciapuoti, M.; Basso, M.; Parodi, A.; Rebora, A. Pemphigus improving with gluten-free diet. *Acta Derm. Venereol.* **2005**, *85*, 84–85. [CrossRef]
10. Antiga, E.; Caproni, M. The diagnosis and treatment of dermatitis herpetiformis. *Clin. Cosmet. Investig. Dermatol.* **2015**, *13*, 257–265. [CrossRef]
11. Salmi, T.T.; Hervonen, K.; Kurppa, K.; Collin, P.; Kaukinen, K.; Reunala, T. Celiac disease evolving into dermatitis herpetiformis in patients adhering to normal or gluten-free diet. *Scand. J. Gastroenterol.* **2015**, *50*, 387–392. [CrossRef]
12. Hull, C.M.; Liddle, M.; Hansen, N. Elevation of IgA anti-epidermal transglutaminase antibodies in dermatitis herpetiformis. *Br. J. Dermatol.* **2008**, *159*, 120–124. [CrossRef] [PubMed]

13. Reunala, T.; Salmi, T.T.; Hervonen, K.; Kaukinen, K.; Collin, P. Dermatitis herpetiformis: A common extraintestinal manifestation of coeliac disease. *Nutrients* **2018**, *12*, 10. [CrossRef] [PubMed]

14. Husby, S.; Koletzko, S.; Korponay-Szabó, I.R.; Mearin, M.L.; Phillips, A.; Shamir, R.; Troncone, R.; Giersiepen, K.; Branski, D.; Catassi, C.; et al. European society for pediatric gastroenterology, hepatology, and nutrition guidelines for the diagnosis of coeliac disease. *J. Pediatr. Gastroenterol. Nutr.* **2012**, *54*, 136–160. [CrossRef] [PubMed]

15. Mendes, F.B.; Hissa-Elian, A.; Abreu, M.A.; Gonçalves, V.S. Review: Dermatitis herpetiformis. *Ann. Bras. Dermatol.* **2013**, *88*, 594–599. [CrossRef] [PubMed]

16. Egan, C.A.; Smith, E.P.; Taylor, T.B.; Meyer, L.J.; Samowitz, W.S.; Zone, J.J. Linear IgA bullous dermatosis responsive to a gluten-free diet. *Am. J. Gastroenterol.* **2001**, *96*, 1927–1929. [CrossRef] [PubMed]

17. Ludvigsson, J.F.; Lindelöf, B.; Rashtak, S.; Rubio-Tapia, A.; Murray, J.A. Does urticaria risk increase in patients with celiac disease? A large population-based cohort study. *Eur. J. Dermatol.* **2013**, *23*, 681–687. [CrossRef] [PubMed]

18. O'Donnell, B.; O'Neill, C.; Francis, D.; Niimi, N.; Barr, R.; Barlow, R.; Kobza, B.A.; Welsh, K.; Greaves, M. Human leucocyte antigen class II associations in chronic idiopathic urticaria. *Br. J. Dermatol.* **1999**, *140*, 853–858. [CrossRef] [PubMed]

19. Rodrigo, L.; Beteta-Gorriti, V.; Alvarez, N.; De Castro, C.G.; De Dios, A.; Palacios, L.; Santos-Juanes, J. Cutaneous and mucosal manifestations associated with celiac disease. *Nutrients* **2018**, *21*, 10. [CrossRef] [PubMed]

20. Davis, A.E., 3rd. Oedema: A current state-of-the-art review, III: Mechanisms of hereditary angioedema. *Ann. Allergy Asthma Immunol.* **2008**, *100*, S7–S12. [CrossRef]

21. Farkas, H.; Visy, B.; Fekete, B.; Karádi, I.; Kovács, J.B.; Kovács, I.B.; Kalmár, L.; Tordai, A.; Varga, L. Association of celiac disease and hereditary angioneurotic edema. *Am. J. Gastroenterol.* **2002**, *97*, 2682–2683. [CrossRef]

22. Henao, M.P.; Kraschnewski, J.L.; Kelbel, T.; Craig, T.J. Diagnosis and screening of patients with hereditary angioedema in primary care. *Ther. Clin. Risk Manag.* **2016**, *12*, 701–711. [CrossRef] [PubMed]

23. Boothe, D.W.; Tarbox, J.A.; Tarbox, M.B. Atopic dermatitis: Pathophysiology. *Adv. Exp. Med. Biol.* **2017**, *1027*, 21–37.

24. Ress, K.; Annus, T.; Putnik, U.; Luts, K.; Uibo, R.; Uibo, O. Celiac disease in children with atopic dermatitis. *Pediatr. Dermatol.* **2014**, *31*, 483–488. [CrossRef] [PubMed]

25. Chen, K.R.; Carlson, J.A. Clinical approach to cutaneous vasculitis. *Am. J. Clin. Dermatol.* **2008**, *9*, 71–92. [CrossRef] [PubMed]

26. Baigrie, D.; Crane, J.S. *Leukocytoclastic Vasculitis (Hypersensitivity Vasculitis)*; StatPearls Publishing: Treasure Island, FL, USA, 2018.

27. Meyers, S.; Dikman, S.; Spiera, H.; Schultz, N.; Janowitz, H. Cutaneous vasculitis complicating coeliac disease. *Gut* **1981**, *22*, 61–64. [CrossRef] [PubMed]

28. Caproni, M.; Bonciolini, V.; D'Errico, A.; Antiga, E.; Fabbri, P. Celiac disease and dermatologic manifestations: Many skin clue to unfold gluten-sensitive enteropathy. *Gastroenterol. Res. Pract.* **2012**, *2012*, 952753. [CrossRef]

29. Spagnuolo, R.; Dastoli, S.; Silvestri, M. Anti interleukin 12/23 in the treatment of erythema nodosum and Crohn disease: A case report. *Dermatol. Ther.* **2019**, *32*, e12811. [CrossRef]

30. Fretzayas, A.; Moustaki, M.; Liapi, O.; Nicolaidou, P. Erythema nodosum in a child with celiac disease. *Case Rep. Pediatr.* **2011**, *2011*, 935153. [CrossRef]

31. Papadopoulos, K.I.; Sjoberg, K.; Lindgren, S.; Hallengren, B. Evidence of gastrointestinal immunoreactivity in patients with sarcoidosis. *J. Int. Med.* **1999**, *245*, 525–531. [CrossRef]

32. Momen, S.E.; Jorizzo, J.; Al-Niaimi, F. Erythema elevatum diutinum: A review of presentation and treatment. *J. Eur. Acad. Dermatol. Venereol.* **2014** *28*, 1594–1602. [CrossRef]

33. Rodriguez-Serna, M.; Fortea, J.M.; Perez, A.; Febrer, I.; Ribes, C.; Aliaga, A. Erythema elevatum diutinum associated with celiac disease: Response to a gluten-free diet. *Pediatr. Dermatol.* **1993**, *10*, 125–128. [CrossRef] [PubMed]

34. Tasanen, K.; Raudasoja, R.; Kallioinen, M.; Ranki, A. Erythema elevatum diutinum in association with coeliac disease. *Br. J. Dermatol.* **1997**, *136*, 624–627. [CrossRef] [PubMed]

35. Compton, N.L.; Chien, A.J. A rare but revealing sign: Necrolytic migratory erythema. *Am. J. Med.* **2013**, *126*, 387–389. [CrossRef]

36. Tamura, A.; Ogasawara, T.; Fujii, Y.; Kanek, H.; Nakayama, A.; Higuchi, S.; Hashimoto, N.; Miyabayashi, Y.; Fujimoto, M.; Komai, E. Glucagonoma with necrolytic migratory erythema: Metabolic profile and detection of biallelic inactivation of DAXX gene. *J. Clin. Endocrinol. Metab.* **2018**, *103*, 2417–2423. [CrossRef] [PubMed]

37. Bennardo, L.; Del Duca, E.; Dastoli, S.; Schipani, G.; Scali, E.; Silvestri, M.; Nisticò, S.P. Potential applications of topical oxygen therapy in dermatology. *Dermatol. Pract. Concept.* **2018**, *8*, 272–276. [CrossRef] [PubMed]

38. Dattola, A.; Silvestri, M.; Bennardo, L.; Del Duca, E.; Longo, C.; Bianchi, L.; Nisticò, S.P. Update of calcineurin inhibitors to treat inverse psoriasis: A systematic review. *Dermatol. Ther.* **2018**, *31*, e12728. [CrossRef] [PubMed]

39. Wu, J.J.; Nguyen, T.U.; Poon, K.Y.; Herrinton, L.J. The association of psoriasis with autoimmune diseases. *J. Am. Acad. Dermatol.* **2012**, *67*, 924–930. [CrossRef]

40. Bhatia, B.K.; Millsop, J.W.; Debbaneh, M.; Koo, J.; Linos, E.; Liao, W. Diet and psoriasis, part II: Celiac disease and role of a gluten-free diet. *J. Am. Acad. Dermatol.* **2014**, *71*, 350–358. [CrossRef]

41. Tsoi, L.C.; Spain, S.L.; Knight, J.; Ellinghaus, E.; Stuart, P.E.; Capon, F.; Ding, J.; Li, Y.; Tejasvi, T.; Gudjonsson, J.E.; et al. Identification of 15 new psoriasis susceptibility loci highlights the role of innate immunity. *Nat. Genet.* **2012**, *44*, 1341–1348. [CrossRef]

42. Cianci, R.; Cammarota, G.; Frisullo, G.; Pagliari, D.; Ianiro, G.; Martini, M.; Frosali, S.; Plantone, D.; Damato, V.; Casciano, F.; et al. Tissue-infiltrating lymphocytes analysis reveals large modifications of the duodenal "immunological niche" in coeliac disease after gluten-free diet. *Clin. Transl. Gastroenterol.* **2012**, *3*, e28. [CrossRef]

43. De Bastiani, R.; Gabrielli, M.; Lora, L.; Napoli, L.; Tosetti, C.; Pirrotta, E. Association between coeliac disease and psoriasis: Italian primary care multicentre study. *Dermatology* **2015**, *230*, 156–160. [CrossRef] [PubMed]

44. Magna, P.; Elbuluk, N.; Orlow, S.J. Recent advances in understanding vitiligo. *F1000Research* **2016**, *5*, pii:F1000 Faculty Rev-2234.

45. Boissy, R.E.; Manga, P. On the etiology of contact/occupational vitiligo. *Pigment Cell Res.* **2004**, *17*, 208–214. [CrossRef] [PubMed]

46. Ezzedine, K.; Lim, H.W.; Suzuki, T.; Katayama, I.; Hamzavi, I.; Lan, C.C.; Goh, B.K.; Anbar, T.; De Castro, S.C.; Lee, A.Y. Revised classification/nomenclature of vitiligo and related issues: The Vitiligo Global Issues Consensus Conference. *Pigment Cell Melanoma Res.* **2012**, *25*, E1–E13. [CrossRef] [PubMed]

47. Shahmoradi, Z.; Najafian, J.; Naeini, F.F.; Fahimipour, F. Vitiligo and autoantibodies of celiac disease. *Int. J. Prev. Med.* **2013**, *4*, 200–203. [PubMed]

48. Abenavoli, L. Behçet's disease and celiac disease: A rare association or a possible link? *Rheumatol. Int.* **2010**, *30*, 1405–1406. [CrossRef] [PubMed]

49. Abenavoli, L.; Proietti, I.; Vonghia, L.; Leggio, L.; Ferrulli, A.; Capizzi, R.; Mirijello, A.; Cardone, S.; Malandrino, N.; Leso, V.; et al. Intestinal malabsorption and skin diseases. *Dig. Dis.* **2008**, *26*, 167–174. [CrossRef] [PubMed]

50. Cheng, J.; Malahias, T.; Brar, P.; Minaya, M.T.; Green, P.H. The association between celiac disease, dental enamel defects, and aphthous ulcers in a United States cohort. *J. Clin. Gastroenterol.* **2010**, *44*, 191–194. [CrossRef] [PubMed]

51. Caldas, C.A.M.; Verderame, L.L.; De Carvalho, J.F. Behçet's disease associated with celiac disease: A very rare association. *Rheumatol. Int.* **2010**, *30*, 523–525. [CrossRef] [PubMed]

52. Nieri, M.; Tofani, E.; Defraia, E.; Giuntini, V.; Franchi, L. Enamel defects and aphthous stomatitis in celiac and healthy subjects: Systematic review and meta-analysis of controlled studies. *J. Dent.* **2017**, *65*, 1–10. [CrossRef] [PubMed]

53. Pastore, L.; Carroccio, A.; Compilato, D.; Panzarella, V.; Serpico, R.; Lo Muzio, L. Oral manifestations of celiac disease. *J. Clin. Gastroenterol.* **2008**, *42*, 224–232. [CrossRef] [PubMed]

54. Cigic, L.; Gavic, L.; Simunic, M.; Ardalic, Z.; Biocina-Lukenda, D. Increased prevalence of celiac disease in patients with oral lichen planus. *Clin. Oral Investig.* **2015**, *19*, 627–635. [CrossRef] [PubMed]

55. Compilato, D.; Carroccio, A.; Campisi, G. Hidden coeliac disease in patients suffering from oral lichen planus. *J. Eur. Acad. Dermatol. Venereol.* **2012**, *26*, 390–391. [CrossRef] [PubMed]

56. Fernandez, A.P. Connective tissue disease: Current Concepts. *Dermatol. Clin.* **2019**, *37*, 37–48. [CrossRef] [PubMed]

57. Song, M.S.; Farber, D.; Bitton, A.; Jass, J.; Singer, M.; Karpati, G. Dermatomyositis associated with celiac disease: Response to a gluten-free diet. *Can. J. Gastroenterol.* **2006**, *20*, 433–435. [CrossRef] [PubMed]

58. Kao, L.; Chung, L.; Fiorentino, D.F. Pathogenesis of dermatomyositis: Role of cytokines and interferon. *Curr. Rheumatol. Rep.* **2011**, *13*, 225–232. [CrossRef] [PubMed]

59. Dalakas, M.C.; Hohlfeld, R. Polymyositis and dermatomyositis. *Lancet* **2003**, *362*, 971–982. [CrossRef]

60. Caproni, M.; Torchia, D.; Cardinali, C.; Volpi, W.; Del Bianco, E.; D'Agata, A.; Fabbri, P. Infiltrating cells, related cytokines and chemokine receptors in lesional skin of patients with dermatomyositis. *Br. J. Dermatol.* **2004**, *151*, 784–791. [CrossRef] [PubMed]

61. De Paepe, B.; Creus, K.K.; De Bleecker, J.L. Role of cytokines and chemokines in idiopathic inflammatory myopathies. *Curr. Opin. Rheumatol.* **2009**, *21*, 610–616. [CrossRef]

62. Molnár, K.; Torma, K.; Siklós, K.; Csanády, K.; Korponay-Szabó, I.; Szalai, Z. Juvenile dermatomyositis and celiac disease. A rare association. *Eur. J. Pediatr. Dermatol.* **2006**, *16*, 153–157.

63. Marie, I.; Lecomte, F.; Hachulla, E. An uncommon association: Celiac disease and dermatomyositis in adults. *Clin. Exp. Rheumatol.* **2001**, *19*, 201–203. [PubMed]

64. Iannone, F.; Lapadula, G. Dermatomyositis and celiac disease association: A further case. *Clin. Exp. Rheumatol.* **2001**, *19*, 757–758. [PubMed]

65. Ramanujam, V.M.; Anderson, K.E. Porphyria diagnostics-part 1: A brief overview of the porphyrias. *Curr. Protoc. Hum. Genet.* **2015**, *86*, 1–26.

66. Ducamp, S.; Schneider-Yin, X.; De Rooij, F.; Clayton, J.; Fratz, E.J.; Rudd, A.; Ostapowicz, G.; Varigos, G.; Lefebvre, T.; Deybach, J.C.; et al. Molecular and functional analysis of the C-terminal region of human erythroid-specific 5-aminolevulinic synthase associated with X-linked dominant protoporphyria (XLDPP). *Hum. Mol. Genet.* **2013**, *22*, 1280–1288. [CrossRef]

67. Anderson, K.E. *Handbook of Porphyrin Science with Applications in Chemistry, Physics, Materials Science, Engineering, Biology, and Medicine, Vol. 29: Porphyrias and Sideroblastic Anemias*; World Scientific Publishing Co.: Hackensack, NJ, USA, 2014; pp. 370–406.

68. Twaddle, S.; Wassif, W.S.; Deacon, A.C.; Peters, T.J. Celiac disease in patients with variegate porphyria. *Dig. Dis. Sci.* **2001**, *46*, 1506–1508. [CrossRef] [PubMed]

69. Urban-Kowalczyk, M.; Œmigielski, J.; Gmitrowicz, A. Neuropsychiatric symptoms and celiac disease. *Neuropsychiatr. Dis. Treat.* **2014**, *10*, 1961–1964. [CrossRef] [PubMed]

70. Pratt, H.; King, L.; Messenger, A.; Christiano, A.; Sundberg, J. Alopecia areata. *Nat. Rev. Dis. Primers.* **2017**, *3*, 17011. [CrossRef] [PubMed]

71. Hietikko, M.; Hervonen, K.; Salmi, T.; Ilus, T.; Zone, J.J.; Kaukinen, K.; Reunala, T.; Lindfors, K. Disappearance of epidermal transglutaminase and IgA deposits from the papillary dermis of patients with dermatitis herpetiformis after a long-term gluten-free diet. *Br. J. Dermatol.* **2018**, *178*, e198–e201. [CrossRef] [PubMed]

72. Barahmani, N.; De Andrade, M.; Slusser, J.P.; Wei, Q.; Hordinsky, M.; Prezzo, V.H.; Christiano, A.; Norris, D.; Reveille, J.; Duvic, M. Human leukocyte antigen class II alleles are associated with risk of alopecia areata. *J. Invest. Dermatol.* **2008**, *128*, 240–243. [CrossRef]

73. Betz, R.C.; Petukhova, L.; Ripke, S. Genome-wide meta-analysis in alopecia areata resolves HLA associations and reveals two new susceptibility loci. *Nature Commun.* **2015**, *6*, 5966. [CrossRef]

74. Carroll, J.; McElwee, K.J.; King, L.E.; Byrne, M.C.; Sundberg, J.P. Gene array profiling and immunomodulation studies define a cell mediated immune response underlying the pathogenesis of alopecia areata in a mouse model and humans. *J. Invest. Dermatol.* **2002**, *119*, 392–402. [CrossRef] [PubMed]

75. Fricke, A.C.V.; Miteva, M. Epidemiology and burden of alopecia areata: A systematic review. *Clin. Cosmet. Investig. Dermatol.* **2015**, *8*, 397–403.

76. Hallaji, Z.; Akhyani, M.; Ehsani, A.H.; Noormohammadpour, P.; Gholamali, F.; Bagheri, M.; Jahromi, J. Prevalence of anti-gliadin antibody in patients with alopecia areata: A case-control study. *Tehran Univ. Med. J.* **2011**, *68*, 738–742.

77. Collin, P.; Reunala, T. Recognition and management of the cutaneous manifestations of Celiac disease. *Am J. Clin. Dermatol.* **2003**, *4*, 13–20. [CrossRef]

78. Naveh, Y.; Rosenthal, E.; Ben-Arieh, Y.; Etzioni, A. Celiac disease-associated alopecia in childhood. *J. Pediatr.* **1999**, *134*, 362–364. [CrossRef]

79. Mokhtari, F.; Panjehpour, T.; Naeini, F.; Hosseini, S.; Nilforoushzadeh, M.; Matin, M. The frequency distribution of celiac autoantibodies in alopecia areata. *Int. J Prev. Med.* **2016**, *7*, 109. [CrossRef] [PubMed]

80. Van Zuuren, E.J. Rosacea. *Nat. Engl. J. Med.* **2017**, *377*, 1754–1764. [CrossRef] [PubMed]

81. Chang, A.L.S.; Raber, I.; Xu, J.; Li, R.; Spitale, R.; Chen, J.; Kiefer, A.K.; Tian, C.; Eriksson, N.K.; Hinds, D.A.; et al. Assessment of the genetic basis of rosacea by genome-wide association study. *J. Invest. Dermatol.* **2015**, *135*, 1548–1555. [CrossRef]

82. Egeberg, A.; Weinstock, L.B.; Thyssen, E.P.; Gislason, G.H.; Thyssen, J.P. Rosacea and gastrointestinal disorders: A population-based cohort study. *Br. J. Dermatol.* **2017**, *176*, 100–106. [CrossRef]

83. Sánchez-Estella, J.; Yuste, M.; Santos, J.C.; Alonso, M.T. Acquired paraneoplastic hypertrichosis lanuginose. *Actas Dermosifiliogr.* **2005**, *96*, 459–461. [CrossRef]

84. Corazza, G.R.; Masina, M.; Passarini, B.; Neri, I.; Varotti, C. Ipertricosi lanuginosa acquisita associata a sindrome celiaca. *G. Ital. Dermatol. Venereol.* **1988**, *123*, 611–612. [PubMed]

85. Braswell, S.F.; Kostopoulos, T.C.; Ortega-Loayza, A.G. Pathophysiology of pyoderma gangrenosum (PG): An updated review. *J. Am. Acad. Dermatol.* **2015**, *73*, 691–698. [CrossRef] [PubMed]

86. Hindryckx, P.; Novak, G.; Costanzo, A.; Danese, S. Disease-related and drug-induced skin manifestations in inflammatory bowel disease. *Expert Rev. Gastroenterol. Hepatol.* **2017**, *11*, 203–214. [CrossRef] [PubMed]

87. Weizman, A.V.; Huang, B.; Targan, S.; Dubinsky, M.; Fleshner, P.; Kaur, M.; Ippoliti, A.; Panikkath, D.; Vasiliauskas, E.; Shih, D.; et al. Pyoderma gangrenosum among patients with inflammatory bowel disease: A descriptive cohort study. *J. Cutan. Med. Surg.* **2014**, *19*, 125–131. [CrossRef] [PubMed]

88. Ampuero, J.; Rojas-Feria, M.; Castro-Fernández, M.; Cano, C.; Romero-Gómez, M. Predictive factors for erythema nodosum and pyoderma gangrenosum in inflammatory bowel disease. *J. Gastroenterol. Hepatol.* **2014**, *29*, 291–295. [CrossRef] [PubMed]

89. Sedda, S.; Caruso, R.; Marafini, I. Pyoderma gangrenosum in refractory celiac disease: A case report. *BMC Gastroenterol.* **2013**, *13*, 162. [CrossRef] [PubMed]

90. Oji, V. Clinical presentation and etiology of ichthyoses. Overview of the new nomenclature and classification. *Hautarzt* **2010**, *61*, 891–902. [CrossRef] [PubMed]

91. Menni, S.; Boccardi, D.; Brusasco, A. Ichthyosis revealing coeliac disease. *Eur. J. Dermatol.* **2000**, *10*, 398–399.

92. Nenna, R.; D'Eufemia, P.; Celli, M.; Mennini, M.; Petrarca, L.; Zambrano, A.; Montuori, M.; La Pietra, M.; Bonamico, M. Celiac disease and lamellar ichthyosis. Case study analysis and review of the literature. *Acta Dermatovenerol. Croat.* **2011**, *19*, 268–270.

93. De Oliveira, A.A.; Bortolato, T.; Bernardes, F.F. Pellagra. *J. Emerg. Med.* **2018**, *54*, 238–240. [CrossRef]

94. Lightwood, R.; Smallpeice, V. Coeliac disease with a conditioned vitamin deficiency resembling, but not typical of Pellagra. *Proc. R. Soc. Med.* **1937**, *31*, 71–73. [CrossRef] [PubMed]

95. Schattner, A. 70-year-old man with isolated weight loss and a pellagra-like syndrome due to celiac disease. *Yale J. Biol. Med.* **1999**, *72*, 15–18. [PubMed]

96. Paulsen, I.F.; Bredgaard, R.; Hesse, B.; Steiniche, T.; Henriksen, T.F. Acquired cutis laxa: Diagnostic and therapeutic considerations. *J. Plast. Reconstr. Aesthet. Surg.* **2014**, *67*, e242–e243. [CrossRef] [PubMed]

97. Berk, D.R.; Bentley, D.D.; Bayliss, S.J.; Lind, A.; Urban, Z. Cutis laxa: A review. *J. Am. Acad. Dermatol.* **2012**, *66*, 842-e1–842-e17. [CrossRef] [PubMed]

98. García-Patos, V.; Pujol, R.M.; Barnadas, M.A.; Pérez, M.; Moreno, A.; Condomines, J.; Gelpi, C.; Rodríguez, J.L.; De Moragas, J.M. Generalized acquired cutis laxa ssociated with coeliac disease: Evidence of immunoglobulin A deposits on the dermal elastic fibers. *Br. J. Dermatol.* **1996**, *135*, 130–134. [CrossRef] [PubMed]

99. Ilus, T.; Kaukinen, K.; Virta, L.J.; Pukkala, E.; Collin, P. Incidence of malignancies in diagnosed celiac patients: A population-based estimate. *Am. J. Gastroenterol.* **2014**, *109*, 1471–1477. [CrossRef] [PubMed]

100. Porter, W.M.; Dawe, S.A.; Bunker, C.B. Dermatitis herpetiformis and cutaneous T-cell lymphoma. *Clin. Exp. Dermatol.* **2001**, *26*, 304–305. [CrossRef] [PubMed]

12

Headache Associated with Coeliac Disease

Panagiotis Zis [1,*], Thomas Julian [2] and Marios Hadjivassiliou [1]

[1] Academic Department of Neurosciences, Sheffield Teaching Hospitals NHS Foundation Trust, Sheffield S10 2JF, UK; m.hadjivassiliou@sheffield.ac.uk

[2] Medical School, University of Sheffield, Sheffield S10 2TN, UK; thjulian07@gmail.com

*   Correspondence: takiszis@gmail.com

Abstract: Objective: The aim of this systematic review was to explore the relationship between coeliac disease (CD) and headache. The objectives were to establish the prevalence of each entity amongst the other, to explore the role of gluten free diet (GFD), and to describe the imaging findings in those affected by headaches associated with CD. Methodology: A systematic computer-based literature search was conducted on the PubMed database. Information regarding study type, population size, the age group included, prevalence of CD amongst those with headache and vice versa, imaging results, the nature of headache, and response to GFD. Results: In total, 40 articles published between 1987 and 2017 qualified for inclusion in this review. The mean pooled prevalence of headache amongst those with CD was 26% (95% CI 19.5–33.9%) in adult populations and 18.3% (95% CI 10.4–30.2%) in paediatric populations. The headaches are most often migraine-like. In children with idiopathic headache, the prevalence of CD is 2.4% (95% CI 1.5–3.7%), whereas data for adult populations is presently unavailable. Brain imaging can be normal, although, cerebral calcifications on CT, white matter abnormalities on MRI and deranged regional cerebral blood flow on SPECT can be present. GFD appears to be an effective management for headache in the context of CD, leading to total resolution of headaches in up to 75% of patients. Conclusions: There is an increased prevalence of CD amongst idiopathic headache and vice versa. Therefore, patients with headache of unknown origin should be screened for CD, as such patients may symptomatically benefit from a GFD.

Keywords: gluten sensitivity; coeliac disease; gluten free diet; migraine; headache

1. Introduction

Gluten-related disorders (GRDs) represent a diverse spectrum of clinical entities for which the ingestion of gluten is a common trigger.

Coeliac disease (CD) is the best-recognised GRD and it is characterized by a small bowel enteropathy occurring in genetically susceptible individuals whilst exposed to the protein gliadin [1]. Non-coeliac gluten sensitivity (NCGS) is a term that is used by gastroenterologists to describe patients with primarily gastrointestinal (GI) symptoms that are related to the ingestion of wheat, barley, and rye, who do not have enteropathy, but do symptomatically benefit from a gluten free diet (GFD) [2] However, in the context of neurological manifestations, patients might have serological evidence of gluten sensitivity (GS); usually anti-gliadin IgG and/or IgA (AGA), with or without transglutaminase (TG) or endomysial antibodies (EMA), but no histological changes on biopsy of the bowel to suggest CD [3]. Such patients might still benefit neurologically from a strict GFD.

Although the gastrointestinal manifestations of GRDs are the most prevalent, a range of debilitating neurological manifestations are increasingly being recognised in clinical practice, often preceding or in the absence of GI symptoms. The most well-known neurological GRDs are cerebellar ataxia [4] and peripheral neuropathy [5], however clear links between GS/CD and epilepsy [3], various movement disorders [6], and headaches [7] have also been described.

The aim of this paper is to systematically review the current literature in order to establish the relationship between headache and CD.

2. Methods

2.1. Literature Search Strategy

This study is reported in accordance with the Preferred Reporting Items for Systematic Reviews and Meta-Analysis (PRISMA) guidelines [8]. A systematic search was performed on the 29 August 2018 using the PubMed database. For the search, two medical subject headings (MeSH terms) were used and they were restricted to title/abstract fields. Term A was "coeliac" or "celiac" or "gluten". Term B was "headache" or "migraine". English language was applied as a filter. The reference lists of included articles were examined in order to identify further relevant articles.

2.2. Inclusion and Exclusion Criteria

Articles to be included in the review were required to meet the following criteria:

1. The study subjects were diagnosed with idiopathic headache and gluten sensitivity or coeliac disease.
2. The study subjects were human.
3. The study contained original data.
4. The study was available as a full-text, English language article, or contained utilisable information in an English language abstract.
5. For randomised control trials, a JADAD score [9] of above 3 to ensure good quality and to reduce any potential bias.

Details of the inclusion process are detailed in the PRISMA chart, Figure 1.

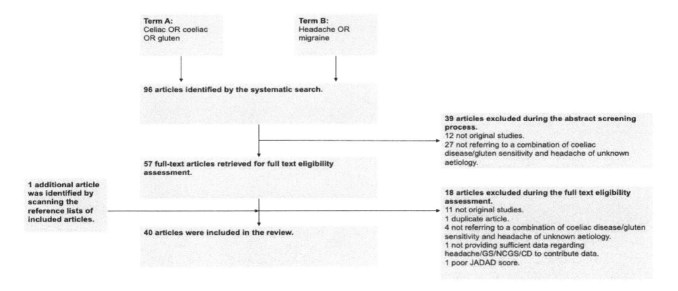

Figure 1. Preferred Reporting Items for Systematic Reviews and Meta-Analysis (PRISMA) chart.

2.3. Statistical Analyses

A database was developed using IBM SPSS Statistics (version 23.0 for Mac, IBM. New York, United States). Data were extracted from each study and included: study type; population size; the age group included; prevalence of GRD/headache; imaging results; the nature of headache; and, response to GFD. Frequencies and descriptive statistics were examined for each variable. The outcomes of interest were the proportion of patients with CD or GS suffering from headache and the proportion of patients suffering from idiopathic headache that had CD or GS.

Meta-analysis of the pooled proportions was conducted in R language [10] while using the default settings of the "meta" package using the "metaprop" function. The meta-analysis of odds ratios was conducted using the RevMan program [11], as suggested by the Cochrane Collaboration Group. Heterogeneity between studies was assessed using the I2 statistic. Data were analysed using a random effects model.

A value of $p < 0.05$ was considered to be statistically significant.

2.4. Compliance with Ethical Guidelines

This article is based upon previously published studies. The article is in compliance with the journal's ethical guidelines.

3. Results

3.1. Selected Studies

The search strategy identified 96 articles. A total of 57 articles were excluded during the eligibility assessment. After perusing the reference lists of included studies, one additional article meeting our inclusion criteria was identified, which had not already been discovered in the aforementioned search strategy. Therefore, in total 40 articles published between 1987 and 2017 qualified for inclusion in this review, studying a total of 42,388 individuals with either headache or GRD (mean number of patients per citation 1059.7 ± 4626.5). The characteristics of the included papers are summarised in Table 1. Figure 1 illustrates the study selection process.

Table 1. Descriptive of studies included in the review.

Parameter	Value
Number of papers	40
Population (%)	
Adult	18 (45.0)
Children	18 (45.0)
Mixed	4 (10.0)
Type of study	
Case report	9 (22.5)
Cohort/Case series	16 (40.0)
Case-controlled study	11 (27.5)
Population-based	2 (5.0)
Survey	2 (5.0)
Gluten-related disorder	
Coeliac disease	36 (90.0)
Mixed group: CD/GS	1 (2.5)
Mixed group: NCGS/GS	3 (7.5)
Type of headache reported	
Migraine	16 (40.0)
All types	6 (15.0)
Not specified	14 (35.0)
Idiopathic intracranial hypertension–related	2 (5.0)
Encephalopathy syndrome	2 (5.0)
Imaging *	
MRI	8 (20.0)
CT	7 (17.5)
SPECT	2 (5.0)
No imaging data	24 (60.0)

Table 1. *Cont.*

Parameter	Value
Year of publication (%)	
Until 2000	5 (12.5)
2000–2009	15 (37.5)
2010–2018	20 (50.0)

* Some citations had data on more than one imaging types.

3.2. Prevalence of Headache in Patients with CD

Only one population based epidemiological study, inclusive of all ages, has been conducted to date [12]. In this population-based retrospective cohort study that was conducted in Sweden, Lebwohl et al. reported that among 28,638 patients with CD and 143,126 controls, headache-related visits occurred in 4.7% and 2.9% of each group, respectively, suggesting a hazard ratio of 1.7 (95% CI 1.6–1.8; $p < 0.0001$). However, in this study, there was no information provided regarding the criteria for headache diagnosis used and if diagnosed, its exact type.

Information about prevalence of headache in adults was available through five cohort [13–17] and four case-controlled studies [18–21]. As shown in Figure 2, the pooled mean prevalence of headache in adults with CD was 26% (95% CI 19.5–33.9%). The meta-analysis of the four case-controlled studies is summarized in Figure 3; the odds of having a headache were significantly higher in the CD groups when compared to controls (OR 2.7, 95% CI 1.7–4.3, $p < 0.0001$).

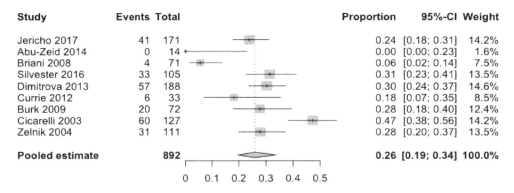

Figure 2. Pooled mean prevalence of headache in adults with coeliac disease.

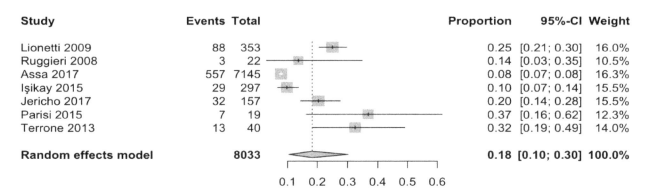

Figure 3. Meta-analysis results as illustrated in the forest plot regarding the odds of having headache in adults with coeliac disease compared to controls.

Information about prevalence of headache in children and adolescents, was available through five cohort [17,22–25], one case-controlled [26], and one population-based study [27]. As shown in Figure 4, the pooled mean prevalence of headache in children and adolescents with CD was 18.3% (95% CI 10.4–30.2%). A cross-sectional, population-based study that was conducted by Assa et al. [27] investigated the association between CD and various comorbidities, demonstrating that the odds of suffering from headache were significantly higher in children and adolescents with CD when compared to controls (OR 2.3, 95% CI 2.1–2.5, $p < 0.0001$).

Study	Events	Total		Proportion	95%-CI	Weight
Lionetti 2009	88	353		0.25	[0.21; 0.30]	16.0%
Ruggieri 2008	3	22		0.14	[0.03; 0.35]	10.5%
Assa 2017	557	7145		0.08	[0.07; 0.08]	16.3%
Işikay 2015	29	297		0.10	[0.07; 0.14]	15.5%
Jericho 2017	32	157		0.20	[0.14; 0.28]	15.5%
Parisi 2015	7	19		0.37	[0.16; 0.62]	12.3%
Terrone 2013	13	40		0.32	[0.19; 0.49]	14.0%
Random effects model		**8033**		**0.18**	**[0.10; 0.30]**	**100.0%**

Figure 4. Pooled mean prevalence of headache in children with coeliac disease.

3.3. Prevalence of CD in Patients with Idiopathic Headache

Headache, usually migraine, has been reported as the first manifestation of CD in several case reports [28–36].

In a case-controlled study, Gabrielli et al. [37] investigated the prevalence of CD amongst 90 adults with idiopathic migraine when compared to blood donor controls. Of them, 4.4% were found to have CD against 0.4% of controls ($p < 0.05$).

Information about prevalence of CD in children with headache was available through two case-control [38,39] and two cohort studies [26,40]. As demonstrated in Figure 5, the pooled mean prevalence of CD in children with idiopathic headache is 2.4% (95% CI 1.5–3.7%), which is significantly higher as compared to the prevalence of CD in the general population in the same age group. Although in one of these studies the authors conclude that that the prevalence of CD was not higher in patients with migraine relative to the control group [38], the other three studies concluded that the odds of a child with headache having CD is significantly higher than in children without headaches, with OR ranging from 1.7 to 8.3 [26,39,40].

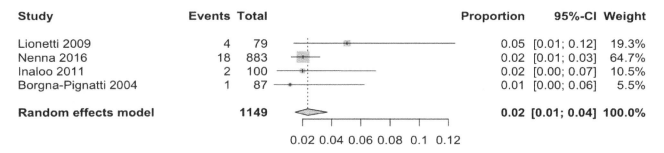

Figure 5. Pooled mean prevalence of coeliac disease in children with idiopathic headache.

3.4. Imaging Findings

Sixteen papers provided information regarding imaging findings [7,14,22,26,28–31,33–37,41–43].

3.4.1. Computed Tomography (CT)

Although brain CT scans in patients with CD and headache are usually normal, there have been cases described of migraine-like headaches with occipital [29,30] or parieto-occipital [33,35] calcifications in both adult and children patients. The two patients with headache and parieto-occipital calcifications being described in the literature were adults, with no evidence of epilepsy or epileptiform activity on EEG. By contrast, all three patients with headache and occipital calcifications were children, of which two also had epilepsy. Cerebral calcifications in the context of CD have been associated with epilepsy [3], which is most commonly known as "epilepsy and cerebral calcification (CEC) syndrome". However, although the available evidence is limited, there are cases with calcifications and migraine-like headaches in the absence of epilepsy. Therefore, patients who present with idiopathic headache in the presence of calcifications in the occipital or parieto-occipital areas of the brain should be screened for CD.

3.4.2. Magnetic Resonance Imaging (MRI)

MRI findings have been reported in isolated case reports and small case series. In a consecutive cohort of 33 adult patients with CD who were referred for a neurological opinion, Currie et al. reported that 12 patients (36%) had white matter abnormalities (WMA) on MRI [14]. When looking specifically into patients with headache, four out of six (67%) had WMA on MRI. In children, one out of six patients with headaches and CD that have been reported to date [22,42,43] was found to have WMA on MRI.

Hadjivassiliou et al. has presented the largest series of patients with CD or GS and WMA on MRI to date [7]. Among 40 adult patients with symptoms and signs of central nervous system dysfunction, most of which had cerebellar ataxia, ten patients (four with CD and six with GS) were found to have WMA. All patients had episodic migraine-like headache. In children with GS the available evidence is limited, however Alehan et al. reported that WMA were present in one out of four TG positive patients [41]. Therefore, patients of all ages who present with idiopathic headache and have non-specific WMA on MRI should be screened for CD and GS.

3.4.3. Single Photon Emission Computed Tomography (SPECT)

Gabrielli et al. conducted a case-controlled study of four adult patients with migraine and newly diagnosed CD and five control patients with migraine, but no CD who underwent a brain SPECT study, which was performed by the administration of 740 MBq of ^{99m}Tc hexemethyl-propylene-amineoxime using a brain-dedicated tomograph [37]. All SPECT studies were performed in the headache free period. All four patients that were affected by both migraine and CD showed evident abnormalities in regional cerebral blood flow. In all cases, a circumscribed area of cortical hypoperfusion was present, whereas there were no interhemispheric asymmetries of cortical regional blood flow in the five migraine patients without evidence of CD.

3.4.4. Positron Emission Tomography (PET)

Lionetti et al. studied the cerebral perfusion in four children headaches and CD with an eight-ring whole-body PET scanner using 2-[18F]-fluoro-2-deoxy-D-glucose, without identifying any abnormalities [26]. This could be because of a selection bias, as the patients that underwent PET had normal standard cerebral imaging, or it might suggest that cerebral hypoperfusion is not present in children with headaches and CD.

3.5. Effect of Gluten-Free Diet

The effect of a gluten-free diet (GFD) has been reported in numerous cohort studies [7,15,17,20,24–26,28,37,40]. In adults, a positive response, defined as a significant reduction in headache frequency, varies from 51.6% [20] to 100% [7,37] of the patients who embarked on a GFD. In up to 75% of adult patients [15] with CD, GFD led to the total resolution of headache. In children, the response rates range between 69.2% [24] and 100% [25,28,40]. In up to 71.3% of paediatric patients [25] with CD, GFD resulted in headache resolution.

As well as direct clinical improvement, it has been demonstrated that a GFD can normalize the cortical hypoperfusion abnormalities that are seen in SPECT [37]. Although, WMA and brain calcifications are not reversible when present, patients on a strict GFD have a lower incidence of WMA [14].

In a survey of pediatric patients with CD that was conducted by Rashid et al., it was reported that up to 13% of patients experience headache after accidental gluten ingestion [44]. In a similar survey of predominantly adults (patients > 16 years old) with CD, Zarkadas et al. found that 23% of patients experienced a headache when they knowingly consumed gluten [45]. In their study, Faulkner-Hogg et al. reported that dietary analysis of patients with persistent symptoms, including headaches, showed that up to 56% of patient still consume traces of gluten. When such patients switched to a strict GFD their symptoms improved [46]. Therefore, specialist dietician advice should always be offered to patients with CD and headaches, and their compliance with the diet should be routinely checked (i.e., AGA titre monitoring).

3.6. Gluten-Related Intracranial Hypertension

Some case reports describe patients who presented with headache secondary to increased intracranial pressure and CD. Dotan et al. reported two cases of boys (three and four years old) who presented with idiopathic intracranial hypertension (IIH). Diagnostic work-up revealed low serum vitamin A titres and further diagnostic work-up led to a diagnosis of CD [43]. A therapeutic regimen of vitamin A supplements, GFD, and acetazolamide proved very effective. Rani et al. reported a single case of a 14-year-old girl with IIH, whose diagnostic work-up revealed CD [42]. Despite the fact that the patient was overweight (BMI 30) a GFD proved to be beneficial, even before the patient started to lose weight and without requiring administration of acetazolamide. Although these data are limited and the evidence is currently weak, the potential link between CD and intracranial hypertension should be investigated further.

3.7. Gluten–Encephalopathy

Gluten encephalopathy is a term that is used to describe a combination of frequent, often intractable, headaches, and cognitive complaints (which patients sometimes describe as a "foggy brain"). Crosato et al. were the first to describe a case of a nine-year-old boy with a history of seizures, headaches, episodes of drowsiness and cerebral calcification on CT who, because of his very low folate levels, was eventually diagnosed with CD [29]. Kakoraç et al. reported a case of a 48-year old man who presented with two episodes of headache, confusion, and seizures and normal MRI, and because of carnitine deficiency, was eventually diagnosed with CD [34].

3.8. NCGS/GS and Headache

A link between headache and NCGS or GS has been also demonstrated in a smaller number of studies.

Information about prevalence of GS in children with headache (all reporting migraine), was available through three case-controlled studies [41,47,48]. As shown in Figure 6, the pooled mean prevalence of GS in children with idiopathic migraine is 6.2% (95% CI 2.6–14.1%). Figure 7 demonstrates that the odds of having migraine are higher (trend for statistical significance) in children with CD as compared to controls (OR 2.8, 95% CI 0.9–8.6, $p = 0.06$).

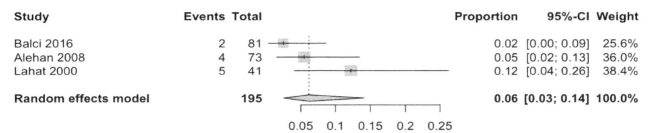

Figure 6. Pooled mean prevalence of serologically confirmed gluten sensitivity in children with idiopathic migraine.

Information about the prevalence of headache in patients with NCGS was available through two studies [49,50]. In a cohort of 486 patients (children and adults), 54% presented with headaches [50]. In a cohort of 78 children with NCGS, 32% presented with headaches, when not on a GFD [49]. It is of interest that 56% of patients with NCGS, when not on a GFD, have positive AGA. This highlights the need to test patients for AGA, the only currently available biomarker of GS.

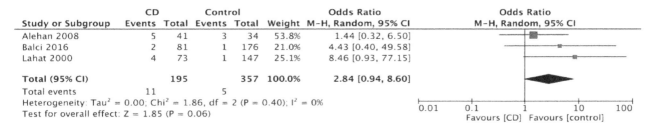

Figure 7. Meta-analysis results as illustrated in the forest plot regarding the odds of having migraine in children with coeliac disease compared to controls.

4. Conclusions and Future Directions

This systematic review, highlights the following key points:

1. There is an increased prevalence of headache amongst patients with CD and an increased prevalence of CD amongst those with idiopathic headache. Such an increased prevalence is evident in both child and adult populations; however, the figures are higher in the latter.

2.   Headaches that are associated with CD are predominantly migraines. However, many studies that were used in this report tended to report headaches without specifying the exact type (i.e., tension, cluster, migraine, etc.) making the interpretation of the findings more difficult.

3.   CT calcifications and WMA are frequent in patients with headaches that are related to CD, and therefore patients with such imaging findings in in the context of idiopathic headache require further testing for CD.

4.   GFD is a very effective treatment for headaches associated with CD and should therefore be offered as soon as possible. This is highly consistent with other neurological GRD, such as the observation that GFD is associated with a significant reduction of pain in patients with gluten neuropathy and an improvement of their quality of life [51,52]. Specialist dietary advise should always be offered, as often patients consume gluten, whilst believe that they are on a strict GFD. Serological testing (i.e., AGA titre) can help in monitoring compliance with diet.

5.   Further studies of the prevalence of GS in patients with idiopathic headache are needed. Currently, to our knowledge, no such studies in adults exist.

6.   Although there is some evidence that brain hypoperfusion and perivascular inflammation might play a role in the pathogenesis of GS-related headaches more studies on the likely pathogenetic mechanisms are needed.

7.   Serum positivity for TG6 antibodies has been identified as a sensitive measure of neurological involvement in GS [53,54] Therefore, a study of the prevalence of TG6 antibodies in patients with headaches that are related to CD and GS should be conducted.

Author Contributions: This work was carried out in collaboration between the authors. P.Z and M.H conceived and designed the study. P.Z and T.J performed the search and collected the data. P.Zdrafted the main part of the manuscript and it was edited by P.Z, T.J and M.H. All authors read and have approved the final manuscript and take full responsibility for its content.

Acknowledgments: This is a summary of independent research carried out at the NIHR Sheffield Biomedical Research Centre (Translational Neuroscience). The views expressed are those of the authors and not necessarily those of the NHS, the NIHR or the Department of Health. Zis is sincerely thankful to the Ryder Briggs Fund. We are sincerely thankful to the Statistical Services Unit, University of Sheffield, for their valuable help with the statistical analysis.

References

1.   Fasano, A.; Catassi, C. Current approaches to diagnosis and treatment of celiac disease: An evolving spectrum. *Gastroenterology* **2001**, *120*, 636–651. [CrossRef] [PubMed]

2.   Sapone, A.; Bai, J.C.; Ciacci, C.; Dolinsek, J.; Green, P.H.R.; Hadjivassiliou, M.; Kaukinen, K.; Rostami, K.; Sanders, D.S.; Schumann, M.; et al. Spectrum of gluten-related disorders: Consensus on new nomenclature and classification. *BMC Med.* **2012**, *10*, 13. [CrossRef] [PubMed]

3.   Julian, T.; Hadjivassiliou, M.; Zis, P. Gluten sensitivity and epilepsy: A systematic review. *J. Neurol.* **2018**. Epub ahead of print. [CrossRef] [PubMed]

4.   Hadjivassiliou, M.; Grünewald, R.A.; Chattopadhyay, A.K.; Davies-Jones, G.A.; Gibson, A.; Jarratt, J.A.; Kandler, R.H.; Lobo, A.; Powell, T.; Smith, C.M.L. Clinical, radiological, neurophysiological, and neuropathological characteristics of gluten ataxia. *Lancet* **1998**, *352*, 1582–1585. [CrossRef]

5.   Hadjivassiliou, M.; Grünewald, R.A.; Kandler, R.H.; Chattopadhyay, A.K.; Jarratt, J.A.; Sanders, D.S.; Sharrack, B.; Wharton, S.B.; Davies-Jones, G.A.B. Neuropathy associated with gluten sensitivity. *J. Neurol. Neurosurg. Psychiatry* **2006**, *77*, 1262–1266. [CrossRef] [PubMed]

6.   Vinagre-Aragón, A.; Zis, P.; Grunewald, R.A.; Hadjivassiliou, M. Movement Disorders Related to Gluten Sensitivity: A Systematic Review. *Nutrients* **2018**, *10*, 1034. [CrossRef] [PubMed]

7.   Hadjivassiliou, M.; Grünewald, R.A.; Lawden, M.; Davies-Jones, G.A.; Powell, T.; Smith, C.M. Headache and CNS white matter abnormalities associated with gluten sensitivity. *Neurology* **2001**, *56*, 385–388. [CrossRef] [PubMed]

8.   Moher, D.; Liberati, A.; Tetzlaff, J.; Altman, D.G.; PRISMA Group. Preferred reporting items for systematic reviews and meta-analyses: The PRISMA statement. *PLoS Med.* **2009**, *6*, e1000097. [CrossRef] [PubMed]

9. Jadad, A.R.; Moore, R.A.; Carroll, D.; Jenkinson, C.; Reynolds, D.J.; Gavaghan, D.J.; McQuay, H.J. Assessing the quality of reports of randomized clinical trials: Is blinding necessary? *Control Clin. Trials* **1996**, *17*, 1–12. [CrossRef]

10. Team, RC. *R: A Language and Environment for Statistical Computing*; R Foundation for Statistical Computing: Vienna, Austria, 2013.

11. The Cochrane Collaboration. *Review Manager*; Version 5.3; The Nordic Cochrane Centre: Copenhagen, Denmark, 2014.

12. Lebwohl, B.; Roy, A.; Alaedini, A.; Green, P.H.R.; Ludvigsson, J.F. Risk of Headache-Related Healthcare Visits in Patients With Celiac Disease: A Population-Based Observational Study. *Headache* **2016**, *56*, 849–858. [CrossRef] [PubMed]

13. Silvester, J.A.; Graff, L.A.; Rigaux, L.; Walker, J.R.; Duerksen, D.R. Symptomatic suspected gluten exposure is common among patients with coeliac disease on a gluten-free diet. *Aliment. Pharmacol. Ther.* **2016**, *44*, 612–619. [CrossRef] [PubMed]

14. Currie, S.; Hadjivassiliou, M.; Clark, M.J.R.; Sanders, D.S.; Wilkinson, I.D.; Griffiths, P.D.; Hoggard, N. Should we be "nervous" about coeliac disease? Brain abnormalities in patients with coeliac disease referred for neurological opinion. *J. Neurol. Neurosurg. Psychiatry* **2012**, *83*, 1216–1221. [CrossRef] [PubMed]

15. Bürk, K.; Farecki, M.-L.; Lamprecht, G.; Roth, G.; Decker, P.; Weller, M.; Rammensee, H.-G.; Oertel, W. Neurological symptoms in patients with biopsy proven celiac disease. *Mov. Disord.* **2009**, *24*, 2358–2362. [CrossRef] [PubMed]

16. Briani, C.; Zara, G.; Alaedini, A.; Grassivaro, F.; Ruggero, S.; Toffanin, E.; Albergoni, M.P.; Luca, M.; Giometto, B.; Ermani, M.; et al. Neurological complications of celiac disease and autoimmune mechanisms: A prospective study. *J. Neuroimmunol.* **2008**, *195*, 171–175. [CrossRef] [PubMed]

17. Jericho, H.; Sansotta, N.; Guandalini, S. Extraintestinal Manifestations of Celiac Disease: Effectiveness of the Gluten-Free Diet. *J. Pediatr. Gastroenterol. Nutr.* **2017**, *65*, 75–79. [CrossRef] [PubMed]

18. Dimitrova, A.K.; Ungaro, R.C.; Lebwohl, B.; Lewis, S.K.; Tennyson, C.A.; Green, M.W.; Babyatsky, M.W.; Green, P.H. Prevalence of migraine in patients with celiac disease and inflammatory bowel disease. *Headache* **2013**, *53*, 344–355. [CrossRef] [PubMed]

19. Cicarelli, G.; Della Rocca, G.; Amboni, M.; Ciacci, C.; Mazzacca, G.; Filla, A.; Barone, P. Clinical and neurological abnormalities in adult celiac disease. *Neurol. Sci.* **2003**, *24*, 311–317. [CrossRef] [PubMed]

20. Zelnik, N.; Pacht, A.; Obeid, R.; Lerner, A. Range of neurologic disorders in patients with celiac disease. *Pediatrics* **2004**, *113*, 1672–1676. [CrossRef] [PubMed]

21. Abu-Zeid, Y.A.; Jasem, W.S.; Lebwohl, B.; Green, P.H.; ElGhazali, G. Seroprevalence of celiac disease among United Arab Emirates healthy adult nationals: A gender disparity. *World J. Gastroenterol.* **2014**, *20*, 15830–15836. [CrossRef] [PubMed]

22. Ruggieri, M.; Incorpora, G.; Polizzi, A.; Parano, E.; Spina, M.; Pavone, P. Low prevalence of neurologic and psychiatric manifestations in children with gluten sensitivity. *J. Pediatr.* **2008**, *152*, 244–249. [CrossRef] [PubMed]

23. Işikay, S.; Kocamaz, H. The neurological face of celiac disease. *Arq. Gastroenterol.* **2015**, *52*, 167–170. [CrossRef] [PubMed]

24. Terrone, G.; Parente, I.; Romano, A.; Auricchio, R.; Greco, L.; Del Giudice, E. The Pediatric Symptom Checklist as screening tool for neurological and psychosocial problems in a paediatric cohort of patients with coeliac disease. *Acta Paediatr.* **2013**, *102*, e325–e328. [CrossRef] [PubMed]

25. Parisi, P.; Pietropaoli, N.; Ferretti, A.; Nenna, R.; Mastrogiorgio, G.; Del Pozzo, M.; Principessa, L.; Bonamico, M.; Villa, M.P. Role of the gluten-free diet on neurological-EEG findings and sleep disordered breathing in children with celiac disease. *Seizure* **2015**, *25*, 181–183. [CrossRef] [PubMed]

26. Lionetti, E.; Francavilla, R.; Maiuri, L.; Ruggieri, M.; Spina, M.; Pavone, P.; Francavilla, T.; Magistà, A.M.; Pavone, L. Headache in Pediatric Patients With Celiac Disease and Its Prevalence as a Diagnostic Clue. *J. Pediatr. Gastroenterol. Nutr.* **2009**, *49*, 202–207. [CrossRef] [PubMed]

27. Assa, A.; Frenkel-Nir, Y.; Tzur, D.; Katz, L.H.; Shamir, R. Large population study shows that adolescents with celiac disease have an increased risk of multiple autoimmune and nonautoimmune comorbidities. *Acta Paediatr.* **2017**, *106*, 967–972. [CrossRef] [PubMed]

28. Diaconu, G.; Burlea, M.; Grigore, I.; Anton, D.T.; Trandafir, L.M. Celiac disease with neurologic manifestations in children. *Rev. Med. Chir. Soc. Med. Nat. Iasi.* **2013**, *117*, 88–94. [PubMed]

29. Crosato, F.; Senter, S. Cerebral occipital calcifications in celiac disease. *Neuropediatrics* **1992**, *23*, 214–217. [CrossRef] [PubMed]

30. Battistella, P.A.; Mattesi, P.; Casara, G.L.; Carollo, C.; Condini, A.; Allegri, F.; Rigon, F. Bilateral cerebral occipital calcifications and migraine-like headache. *Cephalalgia* **1987**, *7*, 125–129. [CrossRef] [PubMed]

31. Serratrice, J.; Disdier, P.; de Roux, C.; Christides, C.; Weiller, P.J. Migraine and coeliac disease. *Headache* **1998**, *38*, 627–628. [CrossRef] [PubMed]

32. Mingomataj, E.Ç.; Gjata, E.; Bakiri, A.; Xhixha, F.; Hyso, E.; Ibranji, A. Gliadin allergy manifested with chronic urticaria, headache and amenorrhea. *BMJ Case Rep.* **2011**, *2011*, bcr1020114907. [CrossRef] [PubMed]

33. La Mantia, L.; Pollo, B.; Savoiardo, M.; Costa, A.; Eoli, M.; Allegranza, A.; Boiardi, A.; Cestari, C. Meningo-cortical calcifying angiomatosis and celiac disease. *Clin. Neurol. Neurosurg.* **1998**, *100*, 209–215. [CrossRef]

34. Karakoç, E.; Erdem, S.; Sökmensüer, C.; Kansu, T. Encephalopathy due to carnitine deficiency in an adult patient with gluten enteropathy. *Clin. Neurol. Neurosurg.* **2006**, *108*, 794–797. [CrossRef] [PubMed]

35. D'Amico, D.; Rigamonti, A.; Spina, L.; Bianchi-Marzoli, S.; Vecchi, M.; Bussone, G. Migraine, celiac disease, and cerebral calcifications: A new case. *Headache* **2005**, *45*, 1263–1267. [CrossRef] [PubMed]

36. Benjilali, L.; Zahlane, M.; Essaadouni, L. A migraine as initial presentation of celiac disease. *Rev. Neurol.* **2012**, *168*, 454–456. [CrossRef] [PubMed]

37. Gabrielli, M.; Cremonini, F.; Fiore, G.; Addolorato, G.; Padalino, C.; Candelli, M.; Gasbarrini, A.; Pola, P.; Gasbarrini, A. Association between migraine and Celiac disease: Results from a preliminary case-control and therapeutic study. *Am. J. Gastroenterol.* **2003**, *98*, 625–629. [CrossRef] [PubMed]

38. Inaloo, S.; Dehghani, S.M.; Farzadi, F.; Haghighat, M.; Imanieh, M.H. A comparative study of celiac disease in children with migraine headache and a normal control group. *Turk. J. Gastroenterol.* **2011**, *22*, 32–35. [CrossRef] [PubMed]

39. Borgna-Pignatti, C.; Fiumana, E.; Milani, M.; Calacoci, M.; Soriani, S. Celiac disease in children with migraine. *Pediatrics* **2004**, *114*, 1371. [CrossRef] [PubMed]

40. Nenna, R.; Petrarca, L.; Verdecchia, P.; Florio, M.; Pietropaoli, N.; Mastrogiorgio, G.; Bavastrelli, M.; Bonamico, M.; Cucchiara, S. Celiac disease in a large cohort of children and adolescents with recurrent headache: A retrospective study. *Dig. Liver Dis.* **2016**, *48*, 495–498. [CrossRef] [PubMed]

41. Alehan, F.; Ozçay, F.; Erol, I.; Canan, O.; Cemil, T. Increased risk for coeliac disease in paediatric patients with migraine. *Cephalalgia* **2008**, *28*, 945–949. [CrossRef] [PubMed]

42. Rani, U.; Imdad, A.; Beg, M. Rare Neurological Manifestation of Celiac Disease. *Case Rep. Gastroenterol.* **2015**, *9*, 200–205. [CrossRef] [PubMed]

43. Dotan, G.; Goldstein, M.; Stolovitch, C.; Kesler, A. Pediatric Pseudotumor Cerebri Associated With Low Serum Levels of Vitamin A. *J. Child. Neurol.* **2013**, *28*, 1370–1377. [CrossRef] [PubMed]

44. Rashid, M.; Cranney, A.; Zarkadas, M.; Graham, I.D.; Switzer, C.; Case, S.; Molloy, M.; Warren, R.E.; Burrows, V.; Butzner, J.D. Celiac disease: Evaluation of the diagnosis and dietary compliance in Canadian children. *Pediatrics* **2005**, *116*, e754–e759. [CrossRef] [PubMed]

45. Zarkadas, M.; Cranney, A.; Case, S.; Molloy, M.; Switzer, C.; Graham, I.D.; Butzner, J.D.; Rashid, M.; Warren, R.E.; Burrows, V. The impact of a gluten-free diet on adults with coeliac disease: Results of a national survey. *J. Hum. Nutr. Diet.* **2006**, *19*, 41–49. [CrossRef] [PubMed]

46. Faulkner-Hogg, K.B.; Selby, W.S.; Loblay, R.H. Dietary analysis in symptomatic patients with coeliac disease on a gluten-free diet: The role of trace amounts of gluten and non-gluten food intolerances. *Scand. J. Gastroenterol.* **1999**, *34*, 784–789. [CrossRef] [PubMed]

47. Lahat, E.; Broide, E.; Leshem, M.; Evans, S.; Scapa, E. Prevalence of celiac antibodies in children with neurologic disorders. *Pediatr. Neurol.* **2000**, *22*, 393–396. [CrossRef]

48. Balcı, O.; Yılmaz, D.; Sezer, T.; Hızlı, Ş. Is Celiac Disease an Etiological Factor in Children With Migraine? *J. Child. Neurol.* **2016**, *31*, 929–931. [CrossRef] [PubMed]

49. Volta, U.; Tovoli, F.; Cicola, R.; Parisi, C.; Fabbri, A.; Piscaglia, M.; Fiorini, E.; Caio, G. Serological tests in gluten sensitivity (nonceliac gluten intolerance). *J. Clin. Gastroenterol.* **2012**, *46*, 680–685. [CrossRef] [PubMed]

50. Volta, U.; Bardella, M.T.; Calabrò, A.; Troncone, R.; Corazza, G.R.; Study Group for Non-Celiac Gluten Sensitivity. An Italian prospective multicenter survey on patients suspected of having non-celiac gluten sensitivity. *BMC Med.* **2014**, *12*, 85. [CrossRef] [PubMed]

51. Zis, P.; Sarrigiannis, P.G.; Rao, D.G.; Hadjivassiliou, M. Gluten neuropathy: Prevalence of neuropathic pain and the role of gluten-free diet. *J. Neurol.* **2018**, *265*, 2231–2236. [CrossRef] [PubMed]

52. Zis, P.; Sarrigiannis, P.G.; Rao, D.G.; Hadjivassiliou, M. Quality of Life in Patients with Gluten Neuropathy: A Case-Controlled Study. *Nutrients* **2018**, *10*, 662. [CrossRef] [PubMed]

53. Zis, P.; Rao, D.G.; Sarrigiannis, P.G.; Aeschlimann, P.; Aeschlimann, D.P.; Sanders, D.; Grünewald, R.A.; Hadjivassiliou, M. Transglutaminase 6 antibodies in gluten neuropathy. *Dig. Liver Dis.* **2017**, *49*, 1196–1200. [CrossRef] [PubMed]

54. Hadjivassiliou, M.; Aeschlimann, P.; Sanders, D.S.; Mäki, M.; Kaukinen, K.; Grünewald, R.A.; Bandmann, O.; Woodroofe, N.; Haddock, G.; Aeschlimann, D.P. Transglutaminase 6 antibodies in the diagnosis of gluten ataxia. *Neurology* **2013**, *80*, 1740–1745. [CrossRef] [PubMed]

13

Hematologic Manifestations in Celiac Disease—A Practical Review

Daniel Vasile Balaban [1,2,*]**, Alina Popp** [1,3,4]**, Florentina Ionita Radu** [2,5] **and Mariana Jinga** [1,2]

[1] "Carol Davila" University of Medicine and Pharmacy, 020021 Bucharest, Romania

[2] Gastroenterology Department, "Dr. Carol Davila" Central Military Emergency University Hospital, 010825 Bucharest, Romania

[3] Pediatrics Department, "Alessandrescu-Rusescu" National Institute for Mother and Child Health, 020395 Bucharest, Romania

[4] Faculty of Medicine and Health Technology, Tampere University and Tampere University Hospital, 33100 Tampere, Finland

[5] Faculty of Medicine, Titu Maiorescu University, 004051 Bucharest, Romania

* Correspondence: vasile.balaban@umfcd.ro

Abstract: Celiac disease (CD) is a systemic autoimmune disease driven by gluten-ingestion in genetically predisposed individuals. Although it primarily affects the small bowel, CD can also involve other organs and manifest as an extraintestinal disease. Among the extraintestinal features of CD, hematologic ones are rather frequent and consist of anemia, thrombocytosis (thrombocytopenia also, but rare), thrombotic or hemorrhagic events, IgA deficiency, hyposplenism, and lymphoma. These hematologic alterations can be the sole manifestation of the disease and should prompt for CD testing in a suggestive clinical scenario. Recognition of these atypical, extraintestinal presentations, including hematologic ones, could represent a great opportunity to increase the diagnostic rate of CD, which is currently one of the most underdiagnosed chronic digestive disorders worldwide. In this review, we summarize recent evidence regarding the hematological manifestations of CD, with focus on practical recommendations for clinicians.

Keywords: celiac disease; anemia; lymphoma; IgA deficiency

1. Introduction

Celiac disease (CD) is a chronic, autoimmune condition triggered by gluten ingestion in genetically susceptible individuals. It can develop at any time throughout the life of individuals carrying the predisposing DQ2/DQ8 haplotype, leading to a gluten-dependent small-bowel inflammation consisting of villous atrophy and crypt hyperplasia. As gluten is the culprit in driving the autoimmune-mediated villous atrophy, its removal from the diet of CD patients leads to symptom relief, restoring of small bowel mucosa, and avoidance of complications. CD has an overall prevalence of about 1% worldwide, with higher rates reported in Northern European countries [1,2].

CD is nowadays widely recognized as a systemic disorder and not only a disease of the small bowel, as many of the adults diagnosed with CD present with extraintestinal manifestations. In fact, the typical presentation with malabsorption syndrome is seen mostly in children and quite rare in adults, who often present with mild, intermittent, and low-intensity digestive symptoms and a wide spectrum of extraintestinal manifestations [3–6].

The extraintestinal features of CD include a wide range of rheumatologic, neurologic, hematologic, endocrine, metabolic, and dermatologic manifestations [6–9]. Among them, hematologic findings are one of the most frequent presentations, and sometimes, they can represent the sole manifestation of the disease [10]. In this setting, a high index of suspicion for CD is needed in patients with unexplained, isolated hematological abnormalities, and this depends on better awareness among physicians of general medicine-related specialties [11].

The hematological features of CD include a variety of conditions—anemia, platelet alterations (thrombocytopenia/thrombocytosis), hemorrhagic or thrombotic events, IgA deficiency, hyposplenism, and the fearful lymphoma (Table 1) [12,13].

A high frequency of hematologic alterations (84%) has been reported in CD patients ever since decades ago [14]. Still, there is a high burden of missed CD cases and significant diagnostic delay in frequent clinical situations, such as chronic, unresponsive iron-deficiency anemia. Better recognition of the hematologic findings could be a window of opportunity to increase the diagnostic rate of CD, which is known to be severely underdiagnosed [15]. Although currently available guidelines from the American College of Gastroenterology (ACG), British Society of Gastroenterology (BSG), European Society for Pediatric Gastroenterology, Hepatology, and Nutrition (ESPGHAN), and European Society for the Study of Coeliac Disease (ESsCD) [16–19] approach some of these hematological features of CD, others are not very well reported.

Our aim was to perform a review of recent literature data regarding hematologic manifestations of CD and their management. For this purpose, we performed a literature search on two databases—PubMed and Embase—from 2010 onwards, using the MESH term "celiac disease" and several keywords referring to the associated hematological features: "hematology", "anemia", "thrombocytosis", "thrombocytopenia", "hemorrhage", "thrombosis", "coagulation", "IgA deficiency", "spleen", and "lymphoma". Articles identified from this search strategy were checked for access to abstract in English and then further evaluated for relevance to the topic. Clinically significant full-text articles were selected for inclusion in this review; also, references of selected articles were further checked for additional possible meaningful articles, which were not identified by the initial search.

In this review, updated knowledge regarding hematologic manifestations of CD is summarized in accordance with recent data published in the literature.

Table 1. Hematologic manifestations of celiac disease (CD).

Hematologic Feature	Frequency	Proposed Mechanism
Anemia	Common	Most frequently iron-deficiency, but may be also due to folate, B12 or copper deficiency
Thrombocytopenia	Rare	Autoimmunity
Thrombocytosis	Relatively common	Iron-deficiency, hyposplenism
Hemorrhagic events	Rare	Vitamin K deficiency
Thrombotic events	Rare	Hyperhomocystinemia, elevated levels of other procoagulants, protein C/S deficiency
Hyposplenism	Common	Autoimmunity
IgA deficiency	Relatively common	Associated conditions
Lymphoma	Rare	Refractory CD

2. Anemia

Anemia in CD patients is multifactorial in etiology; however, iron-deficiency anemia (IDA) is the most common reported [20]. Laboratory workup for IDA can reveal anemia, low mean corpuscular volume, low serum iron, low serum ferritin or anisocytosis (increased red blood cell distribution width) [21]. The main mechanism for IDA in CD is related to malabsorption, as the site of iron absorption—the proximal duodenum—is almost always involved [12]. Severity of iron malabsorption seems to be related to the extent of atrophy along the small bowel, as recent data on ultra-short CD (CD limited to the duodenal bulb) have reported lower proportion of ferritin deficiency in this group compared to extensive CD, both in children and adults [22,23]. Interestingly, anemia in CD is not only related to gluten-driven damage of the bowel mucosa, as it was also reported in patients with positive serology before development of atrophy [24]; this reinforces the need for CD testing in IDA patients and early recommendation of a gluten-free diet in these potential CD patients (the so called "celiac trait") with extraintestinal manifestations [25].

IDA is one of the most frequent extraintestinal presentations of CD and, according to current guidelines, is an indication for CD screening. According to a recent systematic review and meta-analysis, 3.2% of patients with IDA have biopsy-proven CD [26]. Conversely, up to half of newly diagnosed CD patients, both children and adults, have anemia [10,27–29]. In this setting, some authors have even proposed routine duodenal biopsies in IDA patients as a case finding strategy for CD, but this has not proven cost-effective [30–32]. As such, the first step in evaluating the suspicion of CD in IDA patients remains serological testing [33], as it is currently recommended in guidelines [34].

One of the characteristics of IDA in CD is refractoriness to oral iron supplements [35]. If symptomatic, correction of anemia can be done by intravenous iron; otherwise, it usually restores in parallel with the histological recovery of atrophic mucosa on gluten-free diet [36]. Lack of anemia correction on follow-up visits should prompt for search of other causes (colonoscopy, capsule endoscopy) and evaluation for refractory CD [37].

Sharing the same site of absorption as iron, folate deficiency can also occur in CD, leading to macrocytic (or normocytic when deficits are combined) anemia; additionally, we should take into account that normocytic anemia does not rule out IDA, as up to 40% of patients with IDA have normal mean corpuscular volume [38]. Studies have reported up to one fifth of patients having low folate levels [27].

Vitamin B12 deficiency was considered theoretically to be less common in CD, as its absorption takes place in the terminal ileum, which is infrequently involved. However, studies have reported significant proportions for B12 deficiency also [20,27].

Anemia of chronic disease, defined by anemia with high ferritin levels and inflammatory syndrome, has been also described in CD [39,40]. Associated aplastic anemia has also been reported in isolated cases [41–43].

3. Hemorrhagic and Thrombotic Events

Hemorrhagic events can be the presenting feature of CD, including cases of celiac crisis with profound malabsorption and coagulation deficits [44]. A recent review of the literature has found only case reports of hemorrhagic events, comprising otorhinolaryngology, digestive, urology, muscular and alveolar bleeding (the latter defining the Lane Hamilton syndrome) [45]. The mechanism behind hemorrhagic diathesis in CD is mainly represented by vitamin K deficiency, while some studies have also theorized mimicry between factor XIII and tissue transglutaminase [45,46]. Management of hemorrhage consists of intravenous vitamin K and GFD, along with specific measures according to bleeding site.

With respect to thrombotic events, they can also be the prime manifestation of CD. Most cases report on venous thrombosis (deep venous thrombosis, pulmonary embolism, cerebral venous thrombosis, intraabdominal thrombosis), while arterial events have been rarely described [12,47–50]. In addition to case reports, an increased risk of venous thromboembolism has been shown in large cohort studies [51]. Among the proposed mechanisms, hyperhomocystinemia, protein C/S deficiency, high titers of anti-phospholipid antibodies, and platelet abnormalities have been quoted [52,53].

Although rarer than anemia, hemorrhagic/thrombotic events as a manifestation of CD should be acknowledged accordingly, as they can be of significant clinical impact.

4. Lymphoma

CD patients are known to be at increased risk for developing malignancies [54]. Among them, lymphoma is the most fearful complication of CD, as it has a dismal prognosis. In a large population-based case-control study, the odds ratio for developing T-cell lymphoma after a prior diagnosis of CD was 35.8 (95% CI 27.1–47.4) [55]. Patients at risk for lymphoma are those with persistent villous atrophy, meaning those with refractory CD. The absolute risk of lymphoma, while increased, remains low—among 1000 patients with CD followed for 10 years, 7 out of 1000 will develop lymphoma, while the risk is 10/1000 in those with persistent villous atrophy and 4/1000 in healing (similar to that of general population) [56]. Management of lymphoma is multimodal oncologic treatment, but prognosis is often poor.

5. Hyposplenism and Susceptibility to Infections

Spleen dysfunction with hyposplenism has also been reported in CD patients. Its underlying mechanism seems to be related to antibody deposits in the spleen [57]. On a peripheral blood smear, one can find some characteristic changes of hyposplenism such as Howell–Jolly bodies, acanthocytes, and target cells [13].

Measuring spleen size is of interest in case of suspected/confirmed CD, as some small-sampled studies have linked splenic hypotrophy with CD and other have shown an association of small spleen volume with refractory CD [58–60].

Along with the changes in size, functional hyposplenism is of importance in CD patients, as it can lead to thrombocytosis and susceptibility to infections, especially encapsulated bacteria (*Streptococcus pneumoniae, Haemophilus influenzae, Neisseria meningitidis*) [13]. Immunization against these bacteria should be recommended in CD patients [61,62].

Susceptibility to infections is not only related to hyposplenism, as other factors may also contribute—malnutrition, vitamin D deficiency, altered mucosal permeability and gut microbiota. Increased rates of infections in CD patients have been reported for influenza, herpes zoster, pneumonia, tuberculosis, and Clostridium difficile [63–66]. However, the risk of infections requiring hospitalization does not seem to be influenced by mucosal healing [67].

6. IgA Deficiency

There is a strong association between CD and IgA deficiency, meaning that 2%–3% of CD patients have IgA deficiency and about 8% of individuals with IgA deficiency have CD [13]. Several clinical consequences arise: First, there is the susceptibility to develop other small-bowel diseases such as inflammatory bowel disease or parasite infections (Giardiasis for example, which can histologically mimic CD), then there is the issue regarding diagnosis of CD in these patients, as IgA-based serology can lead to false-negative results (for this reason testing for suspicion of CD includes total serum IgA dosing or both IgA and IgG-based serology), and last, there is a risk of serious transfusion reactions in patients with anti-IgA antibodies [68,69].

7. Conclusions

While classical presentations of CD with typical malabsorption syndrome are becoming exceptional, extraintestinal forms are now considered the predominant ones. Among the wide range of extraintestinal features, hematologic-related ones are quite frequent, and they can be the sole manifestation of the disease. IDA is the most frequent hematologic feature of CD, and screening for CD should not be missed in patients with unexplained and refractory to iron-supplementation IDA. Earlier markers of iron-deficiency (alteration in hematological indices of red blood cells) and also changes in platelet numbers should also prompt for testing in a suggestive clinical setting. Hemorrhagic or thrombotic events, otherwise unexplained, can also be the presenting feature of CD. Not least, IgA deficiency and evidence of small-bowel lymphoma should prompt for CD testing. A diagnosis of CD should be always kept in mind in front of a patient with unexplained hematologic abnormalities.

Author Contributions: Conceptualization—D.V.B.; Literature search—all co-authors; writing—original draft preparation, D.V.B.; writing—review and editing, A.P., F.I.R. and M.J.; supervision—A.P., F.I.R. and M.J.

References

1.   Gujral, N.; Freeman, H.J.; Thomson, A.B. Celiac disease: Prevalence, diagnosis, pathogenesis and treatment. *World J. Gastroenterol.* **2012**, *18*, 6036–6059. [CrossRef] [PubMed]

2.   Singh, P.; Arora, A.; Strand, T.A.; Leffler, D.A.; Catassi, C.; Green, P.H.; Kelly, C.P.; Ahuja, V.; Makharia, G.K. Global prevalence of celiac disease: Systematic review and meta-analysis. *Clin. Gastroenterol. Hepatol.* **2018**, *16*, 823–836.e2. [CrossRef] [PubMed]

3.   Leffler, D.A.; Green, P.H.; Fasano, A. Extraintestinal manifestations of coeliac disease. *Nat. Rev. Gastroenterol. Hepatol.* **2015**, *12*, 561–571. [CrossRef] [PubMed]

4.   Reunala, T.; Salmi, T.T.; Hervonen, K.; Kaukinen, K.; Collin, P. Dermatitis Herpetiformis: A Common Extraintestinal Manifestation of Coeliac Disease. *Nutrients* **2018**, *10*, 602. [CrossRef] [PubMed]

5.   Pinto-Sanchez, M.I.; Bercik, P.; Verdu, E.F.; Bai, J.C. Extraintestinal manifestations of celiac disease. *Dig. Dis.* **2015**, *33*, 147–154. [CrossRef] [PubMed]

6.   Rodrigo, L.; Beteta-Gorriti, V.; Alvarez, N.; Gómez de Castro, C.; de Dios, A.; Palacios, L.; Santos-Juanes, J. Cutaneous and mucosal manifestations associated with celiac disease. *Nutrients* **2018**, *10*, 800. [CrossRef]

7.   Dima, A.; Jurcut, C.; Jinga, M. Rheumatologic manifestations in celiac disease. *Rom. J. Intern. Med.* **2019**, *57*, 3–5.

8.   Casella, G.; Bordo, B.M.; Shaclling, R.; Villanacci, V.; Salemme, M.; Di Bella, C.; Bassotti, G. Neurological disorders and celiac disease. *Minerva Gastroenterol. Dietol.* **2016**, *62*, 197–206.

9.   Abenavoli, L.; Luigiano, C.; Larussa, T.; Milic, N.; De Lorenzo, A.; Stelitano, L.; Morace, C.; Consolo, P.; Miraglia, S.; Fagoonee, S.; et al. Liver steatosis in celiac disease: The open door. *Minerva Gastroenterol. Dietol.* **2013**, *59*, 89–95.

10. Catal, F.; Topal, E.; Ermistekin, H.; Acar, N.Y.; Sinanoğlu, M.S.; Karabiber, H.; Selimoğlu, M.A. The hematologic manifestations of pediatric celiac disease at the time of diagnosis and efficiency of gluten free diet. *Turk. J. Med. Sci.* **2015**, *45*, 663–667. [CrossRef]

11. Jinga, M.; Popp, A.; Balaban, D.V.; Dima, A.; Jurcut, C. Physicians' attitude and perception regarding celiac disease: A questionnaire-based study. *Turk. J. Gastroenterol.* **2018**, *29*, 419–426. [CrossRef] [PubMed]

12. Baydoun, A.; Maakaron, J.E.; Halawi, H.; Abou Rahal, J.; Taher, A.T. Hematological manifestations of celiac disease. *Scand. J. Gastroenterol.* **2012**, *47*, 1401–1411. [CrossRef] [PubMed]

13. Halfdanarson, T.R.; Litzow, M.R.; Murray, J.A. Hematologic manifestations of celiac disease. *Blood* **2007**, *109*, 412–421. [CrossRef] [PubMed]

14. Croese, J.; Harris, O.; Bain, B. Coeliac disease. Haematological features, and delay in diagnosis. *Med. J. Aust.* **1979**, *2*, 335–338. [PubMed]

15. Green, P.H. Where are all those patients with Celiac disease? *Am. J. Gastroenterol.* **2007**, *102*, 1461–1463. [CrossRef] [PubMed]

16. Rubio-Tapia, A.; Hill, I.D.; Kelly, C.P.; Calderwood, A.H.; Murray, J.A. American College of Gastroenterology. ACG clinical guidelines: Diagnosis and management of celiac disease. *Am. J. Gastroenterol.* **2013**, *108*, 656–676. [CrossRef] [PubMed]

17. Ludvigsson, J.F.; Bai, J.C.; Biagi, F.; Card, T.R.; Ciacci, C.; Ciclitira, P.J.; Green, H.R.; Hadjivassiliou, M.; Holdoway, A.; Van Hee, D.A.; et al. BSG Coeliac Disease Guidelines Development Group; British Society of Gastroenterology. Diagnosis and management of adult coeliac disease: Guidelines from the British Society of Gastroenterology. *Gut* **2014**, *63*, 1210–1228. [CrossRef] [PubMed]

18. Husby, S.; Koletzko, S.; Korponay-Szabó, I.R.; Mearin, M.L.; Phillips, A.; Shamir, R.; Troncone, R.; Giersiepen, K.; Branski, D.; Catassi, C.; et al. ESPGHAN Working Group on Coeliac Disease Diagnosis; ESPGHAN Gastroenterology Committee; European Society for Pediatric Gastroenterology, Hepatology, and Nutrition guidelines for the diagnosis of coeliac disease. *J. Pediatr. Gastroenterol. Nutr.* **2012**, *54*, 136–160. [CrossRef]

19. Al-Toma, A.; Volta, U.; Auricchio, R.; Castillejo, G.; Sanders, D.S.; Cellier, C.; Mulder, C.J.; Lundin, K.E.A. European Society for the Study of Coeliac Disease (ESsCD) guideline for coeliac disease and other gluten-related disorders. *UEG J.* **2019**, *7*, 583–613. [CrossRef]

20. Berry, N.; Basha, J.; Varma, N.; Varma, S.; Prasad, K.K.; Vaiphei, K.; Vaiphei, N.; Sinha, S.K.; Kochhar, R. Anemia in celiac disease is multifactorial in etiology: A prospective study from India. *JGH Open* **2018**, *2*, 196–200. [CrossRef]

21. Balaban, D.V.; Popp, A.; Beata, A.; Vasilescu, F.; Jinga, M. Diagnostic accuracy of red blood cell distribution width-to-lymphocyte ratio for celiac disease. *Rev. Romana Med. Lab.* **2018**, *26*, 45–50. [CrossRef]

22. Mooney, P.D.; Kurien, M.; Evans, K.E.; Rosario, E.; Cross, S.S.; Vergani, P.; Hadjivassiliou, M.; Murray, J.A.; Sanders, D.S. Clinical and immunologic features of ultra-short celiac disease. *Gastroenterology* **2016**, *150*, 1125–1134. [CrossRef] [PubMed]

23. Doyev, R.; Cohen, S.; Ben-Tov, A.; Weintraub, Y.; Amir, A.; GalaiHadar, T.; Moran-Lev, H.; Yerushalmy-Feler, A. Ultra-short celiac disease is a distinct and milder phenotype of the disease in children. *Dig. Dis. Sci.* **2019**, *64*, 167–172. [CrossRef] [PubMed]

24. Repo, M.; Lindfors, K.; Mäki, M.; Heini, H.; Kaija, L.; Marja-Leena, L.; Päivi, S.; Katri, S.; Kalle, K. Anemia and Iron Deficiency in Children with Potential Celiac Disease. *J. Pediatr. Gastroenterol. Nutr.* **2017**, *64*, 56–62. [CrossRef] [PubMed]

25. Popp, A.; Maki, M. Gluten-induced extra-intestinal manifestations in potential celiac disease-celiac trait. *Nutrients* **2019**, *11*, 320. [CrossRef] [PubMed]

26. Mahadev, S.; Laszkowska, M.; Sundstrom, J.; Björkholm, M.; Lebwohl, B.; Green, P.H.R.; Ludvigsson, J.F. Prevalence of celiac disease in patients with iron deficiency anemia—A systematic review and meta-analysis. *Gastroenterology* **2018**, *155*, 374–382. [CrossRef] [PubMed]

27. Wierdsma, N.J.; van Bokhorst-de van der Scheuren, M.A.; Berkenpas, M.; Mulder, C.J.J.; Van Bodegraven, A.A. Vitamin and mineral deficiencies are highly prevalent in newly diagnosed celiac disease patients. *Nutrients* **2013**, *5*, 3975–3992. [CrossRef]

28. Deora, V.; Aylward, N.; Sokoro, A.; El-Matary, W. Serum vitamins and minerals at diagnosis and follow-up in children with celiac disease. *J. Ped. Gastroenterol. Nutr.* **2017**, *65*, 185–189. [CrossRef]

29. Laurikka, P.; Nurminen, S.; Kivelä, L.; Kurppa, K. Extraintestinal manifestations of celiac disease: Early detection for better long-term outcomes. *Nutrients* **2018**, *10*, 1015. [CrossRef]

30. Herrod, P.J.J.; Lund, J.N. Random duodenal biopsy to exclude coeliac disease as a cause of anaemia is not cost-effective and should be replaced with universally performed pre-endoscopy serology in patients on a suspected cancer pathway. *Tech. Coloproctol.* **2018**, *22*, 121–124. [CrossRef]

31. Grisolano, S.W.; Oxentenko, A.S.; Murray, J.A.; Burgart, L.J.; Dierkhising, R.A.; Alexander, J.A. The usefulness of routine small bowel biopsies in evaluation of iron deficiency anemia. *J. Clin. Gastroenterol.* **2004**, *38*, 756–760. [CrossRef] [PubMed]

32. Mandal, A.K.; Mehdi, I.; Munshi, S.K.; Lo, T.C. Value of routine duodenal biopsy in diagnosing coeliac disease in patients with iron deficiency anaemia. *Postgrad. Med. J.* **2004**, *80*, 475–477. [CrossRef] [PubMed]

33. Lau, M.S.; Mooney, P.; White, W.; Appleby, V.; Moreea, S.; Haythem, I.; Elias, J.E.; Bundhoo, K.; Corbett, G.D.; Wong, L.; et al. Pre-endoscopy point of care test (Simtomax- IgA/IgG-Deamidated Gliadin Peptide) for coeliac disease in iron deficiency anaemia: Diagnostic accuracy and a cost saving economic model. *BMC Gastroenterol.* **2016**, *16*, 115.

34. Goddard, A.F.; James, M.W.; McIntyre, A.S.; Scott, B.B. British Society of Gastroenterology. Guidelines for the management of iron deficiency anaemia. *Gut* **2011**, *60*, 1309–1316. [CrossRef] [PubMed]

35. Hershko, C.; Patz, J. Ironing out the mechanism of anemia in celiac disease. *Hematologica* **2008**, *93*, 1761–1765. [CrossRef] [PubMed]

36. Jericho, H.; Sansotta, N.; Guandalini, S. Extraintestinal Manifestations of Celiac Disease: Effectiveness of the Gluten-Free Diet. *J. Pediatr. Gastroenterol. Nutr.* **2017**, *65*, 75–79. [CrossRef]

37. Hopper, A.D.; Leeds, J.S.; Hurlstone, D.P.; Hadjivassiliou, M.; Drew, K.; Sanders, D.S. Are lower gastrointestinal investigations necessary in patients with coeliac disease? *Eur. J. Gastroenterol. Hepatol.* **2005**, *17*, 617–621. [CrossRef]

38. Johnson-Wimbley, T.D.; Graham, D.Y. Diagnosis and management of iron deficiency anemia in the 21st century. *Adv. Gastroenterol.* **2011**, *4*, 177–184. [CrossRef]

39. Harper, J.W.; Holleran, S.F.; Ramakrishnan, R.; Bhagat, G.; Green, P.H. Anemia in celiac disease is multifactorial in etiology. *Am. J. Hematol.* **2007**, *82*, 996–1000. [CrossRef]

40. Bergamaschi, G.; Markopoulos, K.; Albertini, R.; Sabatino, A.D.; Biag, F.; Ciccocioppo, R.; Arbustini, E.; Corazza, G.R. Anemia of chronic disease and defective erythropoetin production in patients with celiac disease. *Hematologica* **2008**, *93*, 1785–1791. [CrossRef]

41. Badyal, R.K.; Sachdeva, M.U.; Varma, N.; Thapa, B.R. A rare association of celiac disease and aplastic anemia: Case report of a child a review of the literature. *Pediatr. Dev. Pathol.* **2014**, *17*, 470–473. [CrossRef] [PubMed]

42. Basu, A.; Ray, Y.; Bowmik, P.; Rahman, M.; Dikshit, N.; Goswami, R.P. Rare association of coeliac disease with aplastic anemia. report of a case from India. *Indian J. Hematol. Blood Transfus.* **2014**, *30*, 208–211. [CrossRef] [PubMed]

43. Chatterjee, S.; Dey, P.K.; Roy, P.; Sinha, M.K. Celiac disease with pure red cell aplasia: An unusual hematologic association in pediatric age group. *Indian J. Hematol. Blood Transfus.* **2014**, *30*, 383–385. [CrossRef] [PubMed]

44. Balaban, D.V.; Dima, A.; Jurcut, C.; Popp, A.; Jinga, M. Celiac crisis, a rare occurrence in adult celiac disease: A systematic review. *World J. Clin. Cases* **2019**, *7*, 311–319. [CrossRef] [PubMed]

45. Dima, A.; Jurcut, C.; Manolache, A.; Balaban, D.V.; Popp, A.; Jinga, M. Hemorrhagic Events in Adult Celiac Disease Patients. Case Report and Review of the Literature. *J. Gastrointestin. Liver Dis.* **2018**, *27*, 93–99. [PubMed]

46. Sjöber, K.; Eriksson, S.; Tenngart, B.; Roth, E.B.; Leffler, H.; Stenberg, P. Factor XIII and tissue transglutaminase antibodies in coeliac and inflammatory bowel disease. *Autoimmunity* **2002**, *35*, 357–364. [CrossRef] [PubMed]

47. Dumic, I.; Martin, S.; Salfiti, N.; Watson, R.; Alempijevic, T. Deep Venous Thrombosis and Bilateral Pulmonary Embolism Revealing Silent Celiac Disease: Case Report and Review of the Literature. *Case Rep. Gastrointest. Med.* **2017**, *2017*, 5236918. [CrossRef] [PubMed]

48. Ciaccio, E.J.; Lewis, S.K.; Biviano, A.; Iyer, V.; Garan, H.; Green, P.H. Cardiovascular involvement in celiac disease. *World J. Cardiol.* **2017**, *9*, 652–666. [CrossRef] [PubMed]

49. Beyrouti, R.; Mansour, M.; Kacem, A.; Derbali, H.; Mrissa, R. Recurrent cerebral venous thrombosis revealing celiac disease: An exceptional case report. *Acta Neurol. Belg.* **2017**, *117*, 341–343. [CrossRef]

50. Meena, D.S.; Sonwal, V.S.; Bohra, G.K. Celiac disease with Budd-Chiari syndrome: A rare association. *SAGE Open Med. Case Rep.* **2019**, *7*, 1–3. [CrossRef]

51. Ludvigsson, J.F.; Welander, A.; Lassila, R.; Ekbom, A.; Montgomery, S.M. Risk of thromboembolism in 14,000 individuals with coeliac disease. *Br. J. Haematol.* **2007**, *139*, 121–127. [CrossRef] [PubMed]

52. Lerner, A.; Blank, M. Hypercoagulability in celiac disease—An update. *Autoimmun. Rev.* **2014**, *13*, 1138–1141. [CrossRef] [PubMed]

53. Laine, O.; Pitkanen, K.; Lindfors, K.; Huhtala, H.; Niemela, O.; Collin, P.; Kurppa, K.; Kaukinen, K. Elevated serum antiphospholipid antibodies in adults with celiac disease. *Dig. Liver Dis.* **2018**, *50*, 457–461. [CrossRef] [PubMed]

54. Han, Y.; Chen, W.; Li, P.; Ye, J. Association between coeliac disease and risk of any malignancy and gastrointestinal malignancy: A meta-analysis. *Medicine (Baltimore)* **2015**, *94*, e1612. [CrossRef] [PubMed]

55. Van Gils, T.; Nijeboer, P.; Overbeek, L.I.; Castelijn, D.A.; Bouma, G.; Mulder, C.J.; van Leeuwen, F.E.; de Jong, D. Risk of lymphomas and gastrointestinal carcinomas after a diagnosis of celiac disease based on a nationwide population-based case-control. study. *United Eur. Gastroenterol. J.* **2017**, *5* (Suppl. 1), A50. [CrossRef]

56. Lebwohl, B.; Granath, F.; Ekbom, A.; Smedby, K.E.; Murray, J.A.; Neugut, A.I.; Green, P.H.R.; Ludvigsson, J.F. Mucosal healing and risk for lymphoproliferative malignancy in celiac disease: A population-based cohort study. *Ann. Intern. Med.* **2013**, *159*, 169–175. [CrossRef] [PubMed]

57. Korponay-Szabó, I.R.; Halttunen, T.; Szalai, Z.; Laurila, K.; Király, R.; Kovács, J.B.; Fésüs, L.; Mäki, M. In vivo targeting of intestinal and extraintestinal transglutaminase 2 by coeliac autoantibodies. *Gut* **2004**, *53*, 641–648. [CrossRef] [PubMed]

58. Van Gils, T.; Nijeboer, P.; van Waesberghe, J.H.T.; Coupé, V.M.; Janssen, K.; Zegers, J.A.; Nurmohamed, S.A.; Kraal, G.; Jiskoot, S.C.; Bouma, G. Splenic volume differentiates complicated and non-complicated celiac disease. *UEG J.* **2017**, *5*, 374–379. [CrossRef] [PubMed]

59. Di Sabatino, A.; Brunetti, L.; Carnevale Maffè, G.; Giuffrida, P.; Corazza, G.R. Is it worth investigating splenic function in patients with celiac disease. *World J. Gastroenterol.* **2013**, *19*, 2313–2318. [CrossRef]

60. Balaban, D.V.; Popp, A.; Lungu, A.M.; Costache, R.S.; Anca, I.A.; Jinga, M. Ratio of spleen diameter to red blood cell distribution width: A novel indicator for celiac disease. Medicine (Baltimore). *Medicine* **2015**, *94*, e726. [CrossRef]

61. Canova, C.; Ludvigsson, J.; Baldo, V.; Amidei, C.B.; Zanier, A.; Zingone, F. Risk of bacterial pneumonia and pneymococcal infection in youths with celiac disease-A population-based study. *Dig. Liver Dis.* **2019**. [CrossRef] [PubMed]

62. Simons, M.; Scott-Sheldon, L.A.J.; Risech-Neyman, Y.; Moss, S.F.; Ludvigsson, J.F.; Green, P.H.R. Celiac disease and increased risk of pneumococcal infection: A systematic review and meta-analysis. *Am. J. Med.* **2018**, *131*, 83–89. [CrossRef] [PubMed]

63. Ludvigsson, J.; Choung, R.S.; Marietta, E.V.; Murray, J.A.; Emilsson, E. Increased risk of herpes zoster in patients with coeliac disease-nationwide cohort study. *Scand. J. Public Health* **2018**, *46*, 859–866. [CrossRef] [PubMed]

64. Lebwohl, B.; Nobel, Y.R.; Green, P.H.R.; Blaser, M.J.; Ludvigsson, J.F. Risk of Clostridium difficile Infection in Patients with Celiac Disease: A Population-Based Study. *Am. J. Gastroenterol.* **2017**, *112*, 1878–1884. [CrossRef] [PubMed]

65. Walters, J.R.; Bamford, K.B.; Ghosh, S. Coeliac disease and the risk of infections. *Gut* **2008**, *57*, 1034–1035. [CrossRef] [PubMed]

66. Ludvigsson, J.F.; Sanders, D.S.; Maeurer, M.; Jonsson, J.; Grunewald, J.; Wahlstrom, J. Risk of tuberculosis in a large sample of patients with celiac disease-a nationwide cohort study. *Aliment. Pharm.* **2011**, *33*, 689–696. [CrossRef] [PubMed]

67. Emilsson, L.; Lebwohl, B.; Green, P.H.; Murray, J.A.; Mårild, K.; Ludvigsson, J.F. Mucosal healing and the risk of serious infections in patients with celiac disease. *United Eur. Gastroenterol. J.* **2018**, *6*, 55–62. [CrossRef]

68. Wang, N.; Truedsson, L.; Elvin, K.; Andersson, B.A.; Rönnelid, J.; Mincheva-Nilsson, L.; Lindkvist, A.; Ludvigsson, J.F.; Hammarström, L.; Dahle, C. Serological assessment for celiac disease in IgA deficient adults. *PLoS ONE* **2014**, *9*, e93180. [CrossRef]

69. Vassallo, R.R. Review: IgA anaphylactic transfusion reactions, part I: Laboratory diagnosis, incidence, and supply of IgA-deficient products. *Immunohematology* **2004**, *20*, 226–233.

14

The Significance of Low Titre Antigliadin Antibodies in the Diagnosis of Gluten Ataxia

Marios Hadjivassiliou [1,*], Richard A Grünewald [1], David S Sanders [2], Panagiotis Zis [1], Iain Croall [1], Priya D Shanmugarajah [1], Ptolemaios G Sarrigiannis [1], Nick Trott [3], Graeme Wild [4] and Nigel Hoggard [2]

[1] Academic Departments of Neurosciences and Neuroradiology, Sheffield Teaching Hospitals NHS Trust, Sheffield S10 2JF, UK; r.a.grunewald@sheffield.ac.uk (R.A.G.); takiszis@gmail.com (P.Z.); i.croall@sheffield.ac.uk (I.C.); p.d.shanmugarajah@sheffield.ac.uk (P.D.S.); p.sarrigiannis@sheffield.ac.uk (P.G.S.); n.hoggard@sheffield.ac.uk (N.H.)

[2] Departments of Gastroenterology, Sheffield Teaching Hospitals NHS Trust, Sheffield S10 2JF, UK; David.Sanders@sth.nhs.uk (D.S.S.)

[3] Departments of Dietetics, Sheffield Teaching Hospitals NHS Trust, Sheffield S10 2JF, UK; Nick.Trott@sth.nhs.uk (N.T.)

[4] Departments of Immunology, Sheffield Teaching Hospitals NHS Trust, Sheffield S10 2JF, UK; Graeme.Wild@sth.nhs.uk (G.W)

* Correspondence: m.hadjivassiliou@sheffield.ac.uk

Abstract: Background: Patients with gluten ataxia (GA) without enteropathy have lower levels of antigliadin antibodies (AGA) compared to patients with coeliac disease (CD). Magnetic Resonance Spectroscopy (NAA/Cr area ratio) of the cerebellum improves in patients with GA following a strict gluten-free diet (GFD). This is associated with clinical improvement. We present our experience of the effect of a GFD in patients with ataxia and low levels of AGA antibodies measured by a commercial assay. Methods: Consecutive patients with ataxia and serum AGA levels below the positive cut-off for CD but above a re-defined cut-off in the context of GA underwent MR spectroscopy at baseline and after a GFD. Results: Twenty-one consecutive patients with GA were included. Ten were on a strict GFD with elimination of AGA, 5 were on a GFD but continued to have AGA, and 6 patients did not go on a GFD. The NAA/Cr area ratio from the cerebellar vermis increased in all patients on a strict GFD, increased in only 1 out of 5 (20%) patients on a GFD with persisting circulating AGA, and decreased in all patients not on a GFD. Conclusion: Patients with ataxia and low titres of AGA benefit from a strict GFD. The results suggest an urgent need to redefine the serological cut-off for circulating AGA in diagnosing GA.

Keywords: Gluten ataxia; antigliadin antibodies; coeliac disease; MR spectroscopy; gluten sensitive enteropathy; antigliadin antibody titre

1. Introduction

Gluten ataxia (GA) is defined as otherwise idiopathic sporadic ataxia with serological evidence of gluten sensitivity in the absence of an alternative cause [1]. The presence or absence of an enteropathy is not a prerequisite for its diagnosis [2]. Indeed, up to 50% of patients with GA do not have an enteropathy, yet they still benefit from a gluten-free diet (GFD) [2]. For this reason, IgG and IgA native antigliadin antibodies (AGA) are currently the most sensitive marker for GA when compared to endomysium (EMA) and transglutaminase 2 antibodies (TG2), both of which are specific for the presence of enteropathy (Coeliac Disease-CD) [2]. Despite this, the majority of immunology laboratories in the UK and other countries have abandoned the use of native AGA assays in the diagnosis of CD because of poor specificity. Estimation of specificity, however, is based on the presence of a gold standard, in this case the presence of enteropathy (CD). It is now widely accepted that sensitivity to gluten can be present without enteropathy [3]. The only current serological biomarker helpful in diagnosing gluten sensitivity without enteropathy is AGA [4].

Patients with CD often have high titres of circulating AGA, whereas patients with GA and no enteropathy tend to have low titres. The serological cut-off for significant titre in commercially available AGA assays is calculated to maximize diagnostic specificity using data from patients with CD. This would not necessarily be applicable to those patients with gluten sensitivity who do not have enteropathy and those patients with extraintestinal manifestations.

Having previously demonstrated the beneficial effect of a GFD in patients with GA using MR spectroscopy of the cerebellum, in this report we present our experience of the effect of a GFD in patients with ataxia and AGA levels that are below what is considered positive, as defined by the manufacturer, but above a newly defined cut-off AGA level based on our extensive experience in managing patients with GA and the re-evaluation of over 500 patients with GA.

2. Methods

This report is based on prospective observational case series of patients regularly attending the gluten sensitivity/neurology clinic run by one of the authors (M.H.). The South Yorkshire Research Ethics Committee has confirmed that no ethical approval is indicated given that a gluten-free diet is a recognized treatment for suspected patients with GA and that all investigations/interventions were clinically indicated and did not form part of a research study.

2.1. AGA Serological Testing

In January 2015, the immunology lab at Sheffield Teaching Hospitals NHS Trust changed the ELISA AGA (IgG and IgA) assay to Phadia 2500 [5]. The decision was based on the benefits of an automated high throughput process. After consultation with the clinicians using the AGA assay, a decision was made to provide numerical values for the AGA results instead of just positive/negative results.

The manufacturers provided the following information regarding positivity (for both IgA and IgG) of their assay: 0–7 U/mL negative, 7–10 U/mL borderline, >10 U/mL positive.

2.2. Patient Selection and Follow-up

The Sheffield Ataxia Centre cares for over 1800 patients with progressive ataxia, including over 500 patients with GA. All patients with ataxia undergo extensive investigations to try and identify a cause [6]. Such investigations include serological testing for AGA, EMA and TG2. Our previous report on the effect of a GFD on MR spectroscopy in 117 patients with GA was based on those patients with AGA serological positivity (with or without serological positivity for TG2 and EMA antibodies and/or enteropathy) using previous commercial AGA assays by our immunology lab, or those patients who had a value of over 7 U/mL using the new assay [7]. Fifty percent of our cohort of patients with GA have an enteropathy (CD). As expected in patients with enteropathy, EMA and TTG antibodies are also positive. All patients diagnosed with GA at our centre are routinely advised to adopt a strict GFD and are referred to an experienced dietitian for GFD advice. Strict adherence to a GFD is assumed when there is elimination of all gluten related antibodies. If patients have persistently positive antibodies, they are reviewed by an experienced dietitian (NT) for further advice. Patients who still have persistently positive AGA are assumed not to be strict with a GFD.

In the current report we have included only those consecutive patients with serological results for IgG and/or IgA AGA over 3 U/mL but less than 7 U/mL. The lower cut-off value of 3 U/mL was derived based on our experience in the diagnosis and management of over 500 patients with GA who regularly attend the Sheffield Ataxia Centre and either did not adopt a GFD or were on a partial (non-strict) GFD. All of these patients were repeatedly tested using the new assay, irrespective of their GFD status. The new serological cut-off was also based on AGA estimation in those GA patients already on a strict GFD who had persistently absent circulating AGA, using previous assays and with evidence of improvement of their ataxia clinically and on MR spectroscopy. All of these patients with GA who remained neurologically stable had values below 3 U/mL on the new assay. Patients on partial or no GFD had levels above 3 U/mL but often less than 7 U/mL. We therefore used the cut-off of 3 U/mL, below which we assumed strict adherence to a GFD.

Consecutive patients included in this report attend the Sheffield Ataxia Centre on a 6 monthly basis. All patients had undergone more than one clinical MR spectroscopy scan for the purpose of diagnosis and monitoring of their ataxia since 2015, the year of the introduction of the new AGA assay. Only a third of the patients reported here underwent gastroscopy and duodenal biopsy to establish the presence of enteropathy (triad of villus atrophy, crypt hyperplasia and increased intraepithelial lymphocytes). This was based on patient choice after informing them of their serological results, including the negative serology for TG2 and EMA antibodies. None of these patients had enteropathy as predicted by the negative EMA and TG2 antibodies, but presence or not of enteropathy was not an exclusion criterion. Patients were reviewed by an experienced dietitian (NT) who provided detailed advice on a GFD with further monitoring by telephone or face-to-face consultations. The patients underwent repeat clinical evaluation and further serological testing at approximately 6 monthly intervals. Strict adherence to a GFD was indicated by serological elimination of circulating AGA (<3 U/mL). For the purpose of this report, the patients were divided into 3 groups: those with strict adherence to GFD with AGA levels of <3 U/mL, those with partial adherence to a GFD as evident from the presence of AGA (above 3 U/mL but less that 7 U/mL), and a third group consisting of patients that declined GFD (AGA level above 3 U/mL and less than 7 U/mL).

We also reviewed the AGA results in patients with classical CD presenting to gastroenterology clinics and patients with idiopathic sporadic ataxia. Data on the prevalence of AGA (range between 3–7 U/mL) was also available from healthy volunteers as part of another ongoing study.

2.3. MR Spectroscopy

In addition to volumetric 3T MR imaging, all patients underwent single-voxel H^1 MR spectroscopy of the cerebellum. This imaging protocol is in clinical use as part of the investigation of all patients with cerebellar ataxia attending the Sheffield Ataxia Centre. The brain imaging protocol for structural, volumetric, and spectroscopy studies has been previously described [7]. The main measurement is the NAA/Cr area ratio within the cerebellar vermis. N-acetyl aspartate (NAA) reflects the health of neurons and is a reliable marker of monitoring neuronal energy impairment and dysfunction. Creatine (Cr) is a stable metabolite with little variation between different pathologies. As such, it is typically used as an internal standard in MR spectroscopy from which metabolite ratios can be calculated.

A baseline MR spectroscopy scan was done on all patients and a repeat scan was done after the introduction of the GFD. In common with other immune-mediated ataxias, the cerebellar vermis is primarily involved in GA; therefore, MR spectroscopy results reported here are measurements from the cerebellar vermis.

2.4. Statistical Analysis

Change in mean values between the groups was compared with Student's two-tailed t-test for unpaired samples. A value of $p < 0.05$ was considered significant.

3. Results

A total of 21 consecutive patients with GA were included at the time of writing this report. Detailed clinical characteristics of patients with GA have been described previously. The patients included in this report did not differ in any way from those patients with GA described previously [1,8].

All patients had two MR spectroscopy scans at baseline and the second after a mean interval of 19 months (range 5 months to 36 months). Of the 21 patients, 10 were on a strict GFD with elimination of all antibodies (IgG and/or IgA AGA <3 U/mL), 5 were on a GFD but still had serological evidence of circulating AGA, indicating ongoing exposure to gluten (IgG and/or IgA >3 U/mL), and 6 patients were not on the diet (IgG and/or IgA AGA >3 U/ml and <7 U/mL). There were no significant differences in the duration of ataxia between the 3 groups. The patients on partial GFD were significantly younger that the other 2 groups. There were, however, no significant differences in age between the strict GFD and no GFD groups. Those patients that declined a GFD also had a repeat scan for monitoring purposes. The NAA/Cr area ratio taken from the cerebellar vermis increased in all 10 patients on a strict diet, but in only 1 out of 5 (20%) patients on a partial GFD with persistent circulating AGA. In the remaining 4, the NAA/Cr area ratio decreased. In all of the 6 patients not on a diet, there was a decrease in NAA/Cr area ratio on repeat scanning. These results are illustrated in Figures 1 and 2. A Chi squared contingency table looking at numbers improved on MR spectroscopy on a strict diet compared with no diet was significant $p < 0.0001$. A comparison of the change in MR spectroscopy values from baseline between the 3 groups showed the following: no diet mean change −0.098, Standard error of the Mean (SEM) 0.06, partial diet mean change −0.028, SEM 0.087 and strict diet mean change +0.092, SEM 0.06. Comparison between the strict diet and no diet groups was significant ($p < 0.0001$), as was the comparison between partial diet and no diet ($p = 0.0028$).

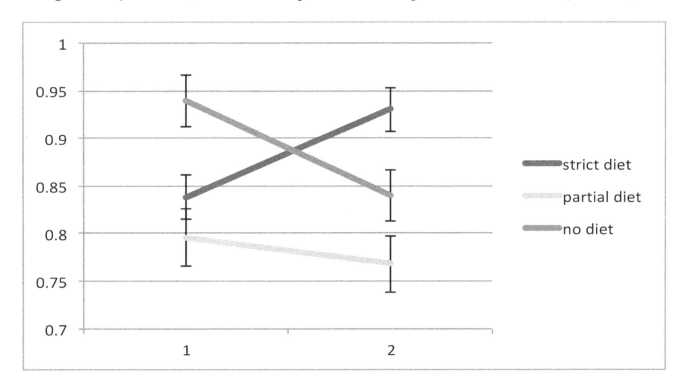

Figure 1. NAA/Cr area ratio in patients with gluten ataxia without enteropathy following the introduction of a gluten-free diet (GFD) in the 2 sub-groups (number of patients on gluten free diet 10, partial diet 5). The third subgroup consisted of 6 patients who declined a GFD. All patients had antigliadin antibodies (AGA) IgG and/or IgA of >3 U/mL and <7 U/mL at baseline. Both the partial diet and no diet groups still had AGA values >3 U/mL at the time of the second scan. All 10 patients on a strict GFD showed improvement of the NAA/Cr area ratio (vertical axis) of the vermis 4 of the 5 patients on partial GFD and all 6 patients not on GFD showed deterioration of the NAA/Cr ratio. A Chi squared contingency table looking at numbers improved on magnetic resonance spectroscopy on a strict diet compared with no diet was significant $p < 0.0001$.

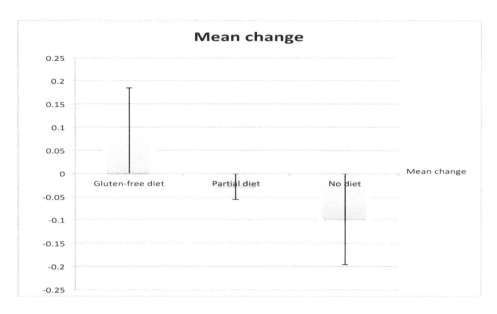

Figure 2. Mean change of the area ratio of NAA/Cr from baseline in the 3 groups.

Using the same serological cut-off for AGA titres of >3 U/mL, the prevalence of AGA positivity amongst 68 patients with classical CD presenting to the gastroenterologists was 100%. The mean baseline value for AGA titre in this classical CD group was 46.5 U/mL. This compares to a mean AGA titre of 4.1 U/mL in the 21 patients reported here. The prevalence amongst 28 healthy controls was 7%, and the prevalence amongst 197 patients with otherwise idiopathic sporadic ataxia was 39%. This group of 197 did not include patients with ataxia who had AGA levels over 7 U/mL or those who also had enteropathy. Table 1 summarises the clinical and serological characteristics of the GA groups.

Table 1. Summary of clinical characteristics and the change in magnetic resonance spectroscopy and antigliadin antibody titre at baseline and at the time of the second scan in the 3 groups. The differences in numbers improved and in the changes in MR spectroscopy between the strict GFD and the not on GFD groups were significant $p < 0.0001$. There were no significant clinical differences between the strict GFD and the partial or not on diet groups. The patients on partial GFD were significantly younger than the other 2 groups. GA = gluten ataxia; NAA/Cr = N Acetyl Aspartate to Creatine ratio; GFD = Gluten Free Diet; AGA = Antigliadin antibodies; SD standard deviation.

Dietary Status in GA Groups	Numb per Group	Mean Age	Mean Duration of Ataxia in Years	Mean MR Spectroscopy Change from Baseline (NAA/Cr Area Ratio)	Numb Improv-ed	Mean AGA Antibody Titre at Baseline (SD)	Mean AGA Antibody Titre at the Time of 2nd Scan (SD)
strict GFD	10	65	6.4	+0.092	10	3.6 (0.46)	1.8 (0.74)
partial GFD	5	50	6.6	−0.028	1	4.5 (1.3)	3.8 (1)
not on diet	6	77	7.3	−0.098	0	4.2 (1.3)	4.2 (1.8)

4. Discussion

We have previously demonstrated clinical and MR spectroscopic improvement in patients with GA after a year of strict adherence to a gluten-free diet [7,9]. The current study demonstrates that in patients with GA with low titres of AGA, NAA/Cr area ratio within the cerebellar vermis improves with strict adherence to a gluten-free diet, worsens with on-going exposure to gluten, and also largely worsens with partial adherence to a gluten-free diet, as indicated by persistently positive circulating AGA. The improvement in MR spectroscopy was accompanied by clinical improvement or stabilisation of the ataxia in the strict GFD group.

The advantage of MR spectroscopy as a monitoring tool is that it can be easily performed as part of routine MR imaging, it is reproducible in an individual on a particular scanner, and relies on objective measurements such as the NAA/Cr area ratio [7,10]. It therefore overcomes the disadvantages of the clinical scales (interrater variability, fluctuation of ataxia symptoms and signs due to fatigue, insensitive scales in disabled patients and ceiling effect). Other groups have also demonstrated good correlation between MR spectroscopy and the clinical status as assessed by ataxia rating scales [11]. This report also demonstrates the importance of strict adherence to the GFD. Amongst those patients on the diet, but not strict, only 20% improved on MR spectroscopy as opposed to 100% in those on a strict GFD. Strict diet with serological evidence of elimination of all antibodies appears to have the potential to stabilise and partially reverse immune mediated damage to the cerebellum.

This report also demonstrates that for extraintestinal manifestations of gluten sensitivity, and in particular for those patients without enteropathy, the level of circulating AGA that is still significant is lower than that seen in the context of enteropathy. This means that the serological cut-off titre for diagnosing GA requires adjustment. This has major implications for the diagnosis of GA. Our data from 197 patients with idiopathic sporadic ataxia collected since 2015 (the year of the introduction of the new assay), excluding those with positive AGA (using the manufacturer's serum cut-off level for positivity) and those with CD, showed that 39% had AGA levels between 3 and 7 U/mL. As we have shown here, these patients also benefited from a strict GFD. Up until now, such patients would have remained undiagnosed and therefore followed a progressive course as a result of ongoing exposure to gluten. Indeed, some of these patients had been under regular follow-up in our ataxia clinic but were negative for AGA on previous assays used by our immunology lab.

We have found MR spectroscopy a reliable and useful tool in the monitoring of patients with GA and other ataxias. Improvement of NAA/Cr in patients adherent to a GFD bolsters the diagnosis of GA and, in our experience, is accompanied by clinical improvement [9]. Such improvement also acts as a motivation for patients to continue with the GFD. The commonest cause for the lack of improvement tends to be poor adherence to the GFD.

Both this report and previous publications from our group have highlighted the importance of using the correct serological markers for the diagnosis of GA. The presence of enteropathy (associated with the presence of positive TG2 and endomysium antibodies) does not influence the response to the GFD, and thus any patient with positive antigliadin antibodies and no other cause of ataxia should be offered a strict gluten-free diet, even in the absence of enteropathy.

In conclusion, using MR spectroscopy data we have demonstrated that patients with ataxia and low titre of AGA improve on a strict GFD. We are therefore proposing a new AGA titre cut-off level that should be used in the diagnosis of GA.

Author Contributions: M.H. runs the Gluten Sensitivity/Neurology Clinic and with P.D.S. runs dedicated ataxia clinics from where all patients were identified. D.S.S. runs the coeliac clinic and was responsible for all the gastroscopies and duodenal biopsies as well as serological testing of patients with CD. P.Z. performed the serological testing of healthy cotrols. N.H. and I.C. were responsible for MR spectroscopy. N.T. provided all the dietetic input. G.W. was responsible for the AGA assay and the provision of numerical data for the AGA results. R.A.G., P.G.S and P.Z. provided all the statistical advice. M.H. produced the first draft with contributions from all authors. The final version was approved by all the authors.

Acknowledgments: This is a summary of independent research supported by BRC and carried out at the National Institute for Health Research (NIHR) Sheffield Clinical Research Facility. The views expressed are those of the authors and not necessarily those of the BRC, NHS, the NIHR, or the Department of Health.

References

1. Hadjivassiliou, M.; Grünewald, R.A.; Chattopadhyay, A.K.; Davies-Jones, G.A.B.; Gibson, A.; Jarratt, J.A.; Kandler, R.H.; Lobo, A.; Powell, T.; Smith, C.M.L. Clinical, radiological, neurophysiological and neuropathological characteristics of gluten ataxia. *Lancet* **1998**, *352*, 1582–1585. [CrossRef]

2.   Hadjivassiliou, M.; Rao, D.G.; Grunewald, R.A.; Aeschlimann, D.P.; Sarrigiannis, P.G.; Hoggard, N.; Aeschlimann, P.; Mooney, P.D.; Sanders, D.S. Neurological dysfunction in Coeliac Disease and Non-Coeliac Gluten Sensitivity. *Am. J. Gastroenterol.* **2016**, *111*, 561–567. [CrossRef] [PubMed]

3.   Aziz, I.; Hadjivassiliou, M.; Sanders, D.S. Does gluten sensitivity in the absence of coeliac disease exist? *BMJ* **2012**, *345*, e7907. [CrossRef] [PubMed]

4.   Aziz, I.; Hadjivassiliou, M.; Sanders, D.S. The spectrum of non-coeliac gluten sensitivity. *Nat. Rev. Gastroenterol. Hepatol.* **2015**, *12*, 516–526. [CrossRef] [PubMed]

5.   Available online: www.phadia.com/da/Products/Phadia-Laboratory-Systems/Phadia-2500/ (accessed on 4 September 2018).

6.   Hadjivassiliou, M.; Martindale, J.; Shanmugarajah, P.; Grunewald, R.A.; Sarrigiannis, P.G.; Beauchamp, N.; Garrard, K.; Warburton, R.; Sanders, D.S.; Friend, D.; et al. Causes of progressive cerebellar ataxia: Prospective evaluation of 1500 patients. *J. Neurol. Neurosurg. Psychiatry* **2016**, *88*, 301–309. [CrossRef] [PubMed]

7.   Hadjivassiliou, M.; Grunewald, R.A.; Sanders, D.S.; Shanmugarajah, P.; Hoggard, N. Effect of gluten-free diet on MR spectroscopy in gluten ataxia. *Neurology* **2017**, *89*, 1–5. [CrossRef] [PubMed]

8.   Hadjivassiliou, M. Advances in Therapies of Cerebellar Disorders: Immune mediated Ataxias. *CNS Neurol. Disord. Drug Targets* **2018**. [CrossRef] [PubMed]

9.   Hadjivassiliou, M.; Davies-Jones, G.A.B.; Sanders, D.S.; Grünewald, R.A. Dietary treatment of gluten ataxia. *J. Neurol. Neurosurg. Psychiatry* **2003**, *74*, 1221–1224. [CrossRef] [PubMed]

10. Currie, S.; Hadjivassiliou, M.; Craven, I.J.; Wilkinson, I.D.; Griffiths, P.D.; Hoggard, N. Magnetic resonance spectroscopy of the brain. *Postgrad. Med. J.*. [CrossRef] [PubMed]

11. Oz, G.; Hutter, D.; Tkac, I.; Clark, H.B.; Gross, M.D.; Jiang, H.; Eberly, L.E.; Bushara, K.O.; Gomez, C.M. Neurochemical alterations in spinocerebellar ataxia type 1 and their correlations with clinical status. *Mov. Disord.* **2010**, *25*, 1253–1261. [CrossRef] [PubMed]

15

Micronutrients Dietary Supplementation Advices for Celiac Patients on Long-Term Gluten-Free Diet with Good Compliance

Mariangela Rondanelli [1,2], **Milena A. Faliva** [3], **Clara Gasparri** [3], **Gabriella Peroni** [3], **Maurizio Naso** [3], **Giulia Picciotto** [3], **Antonella Riva** [4], **Mara Nichetti** [3], **Vittoria Infantino** [5], **Tariq A. Alalwan** [6] **and Simone Perna** [6,*]

[1]   IRCCS Mondino Foundation, 27100 Pavia, Italy
[2]   Department of Public Health, Experimental and Forensic Medicine, University of Pavia, 27100 Pavia, Italy
[3]   Endocrinology and Nutrition Unit, Azienda di Servizi alla Persona "Istituto Santa Margherita", University of Pavia, 27100 Pavia, Italy
[4]   Research and Development Unit, Indena, 20139 Milan, Italy
[5]   University of Bari, Department of Biomedical Science and Human Oncology, 70121 Bari, Italy
[6]   Department of Biology, College of Science, University of Bahrain, Sakhir Campus P. O. Box 32038, Bahrain
*   Correspondence: sperna@uob.edu.bh

Abstract: *Background and objective*: Often micronutrient deficiencies cannot be detected when patient is already following a long-term gluten-free diet with good compliance (LTGFDWGC). The aim of this narrative review is to evaluate the most recent literature that considers blood micronutrient deficiencies in LTGFDWGC subjects, in order to prepare dietary supplementation advice (DSA). *Materials and methods*: A research strategy was planned on PubMed by defining the following keywords: celiac disease, vitamin B12, iron, folic acid, and vitamin D. *Results*: This review included 73 studies. The few studies on micronutrient circulating levels in long-term gluten-free diet (LTGFD) patients over 2 years with good compliance demonstrated that deficiency was detected in up to: 30% of subjects for vitamin B12 (DSA: 1000 mcg/day until level is normal, then 500 mcg), 40% for iron (325 mg/day), 20% for folic acid (1 mg/day for 3 months, followed by 400–800 mcg/day), 25% for vitamin D (1000 UI/day or more-based serum level or 50,000 UI/week if level is <20 ng/mL), 40% for zinc (25–40 mg/day), 3.6% of children for calcium (1000–1500 mg/day), 20% for magnesium (200–300 mg/day); no data is available in adults for magnesium. *Conclusions*: If integration with diet is not enough, starting with supplements may be the correct way, after evaluating the initial blood level to determine the right dosage of supplementation.

Keywords: celiac disease; vitamin B12; iron; folic acid; vitamin D; long-term GFD therapy (LTGFD); LTGFD with good compliance (LTGFDWGC)

1. Introduction

Celiac disease (CD) is an immune-mediated systemic disorder triggered by the ingestion of gluten and prolamines in genetically predisposed individuals. It is characterized by inflammation of the small bowel mucosa—the immune reaction—which occurs after ingestion of gluten that leads to intestinal villous atrophy, crypt hyperplasia, and increased number of intraepithelial lymphocytes [1]. CD is a multifactorial disease and its pathogenesis involves both genetic and environmental factors [2]. Genetic composition for the development of the disease is evident. In fact, more than 90% of celiac patients are human leukocyte antigen (HLA)-DQ2 haplotype positive and almost all of the rest carry HLA-DQ8. These genes are necessary but not sufficient for CD development [3,4]. The predisposing

DQ2 and DQ8 heterodimers are composed of the association of α and β chains. A recent meta-analysis showed that the HLA genotypes coding for DQ2 or DQ8 heterodimers, but also those including only the alleles of the respective β chains (regardless of the concomitant presence of DQ2 or DQ8 α chains) have an increased risk of developing pediatric CD [5]. Recently, another meta-analysis evaluated the predictive values of HLA-DQB1*02 allele, suggesting the major relevance of this specific allele, rather than the expression of the full DQ2 and/or DQ8 heterodimers, in raising the risk to develop pediatric CD [6]. In addition, a risk gradient according to single or double copy of HLA-DQB1*02 has been revealed [6]. Gluten ingestion represents the major environmental factor, contributing to the development of the pathology, but there are several other conditions involved in the etiology of CD, including viral infections, gut microbiota, breastfeeding, early life feeding practice, and smoking [3,4].

CD can occur at any stage of life and with a great variety of signs and symptoms. In fact, it is considered a multisystem immunological disorder rather than a disease restricted only to the gastrointestinal tract. Consequently, it is important to make diagnosis not only in individuals with classic gastrointestinal symptoms, but also in subjects who have a more nuanced or extra-intestinal clinical features, since the consequences can be important in both cases [2]. To date, nutritional therapy has been the only effective treatment for patients with CD that demands a strict compliance with a gluten-free diet (GFD). Non-adherence to the GFD increases the risk of morbidity and mortality, as a result of associated conditions, which include infertility, skeletal disorders and malignancy. Once diagnosed, patients should be tested for micronutrient deficiencies, including iron, folic acid, vitamin B12, and vitamin D [7].

The 2013 American College of Gastroenterology guidelines reported that micronutrient deficiencies (in particular iron, folic acid, vitamins B6 and B12, vitamin D, copper, and zinc) are frequent in celiac patients at the time of celiac diagnosis. Therefore, patients with newly diagnosed celiac disease, micronutrient deficiencies should be found and integrated. These tests should include iron, folic acid, vitamin D, vitamin B12 and more [7].

Following the United Kingdom 2015 National Institute for Health and Care Excellence guidelines, it was reported that some patients with celiac disease may need additional nutritional supplements, mainly in the early stages after diagnosis, suggesting, however, that this should be identified through an appropriate ongoing monitoring and that integration should begin after a full evaluation [8].

These two guidelines are derived from, and in agreement with, the more recent reviews demonstrating that in celiac patients, at time of diagnosis, nutritional deficiencies are often found in vitamins and minerals, such as folic acid, vitamin B12, vitamin D, calcium, magnesium and zinc.

However, at the same time, in subjects undergoing GFD for a long time with good compliance, it has been described that micronutrient deficiencies may persist due to an inadequate full reintegration of the mucous membrane [9]. Some patients with long-term treated CD may still have abnormal small bowel mucosa and persistent villous atrophy on follow-up, with or without ongoing or recurrent symptoms, despite an apparently GFD [4,10]. According to Lanzini et al., the complete recovery of duodenal mucosa with histological normalization, after a median 16 months GFD in patients diagnosed at an adult age occurs only in 8% of cases [11]. The majority of adult patients achieving remission with intraepithelial lymphocytosis (65%) and a substantial proportion showing no-change (26%) or deterioration (1%) of duodenal histology [11]. This condition seems to be more common in adults older than an age of 50 years [12], but occurs even in 19% of children who underwent follow-up biopsy at least 1 year after starting the GFD [13]. When other possible causes of villous atrophy are excluded, refractory celiac disease is diagnosed [4]. Even in the absence of symptoms this condition is not positive, because it may predispose to severe complications, such as osteoporosis and malignancy [14].

Moreover, gluten-free products are usually low in some micronutrients, such as magnesium and folic acid, and gluten-free cereals found in nature have a lower magnesium content compared with gluten-containing ones [9].

This topic is highly debated in the literature. In fact, there is a widespread agreement on the importance of supplementation at the time of diagnosis, but there is still no consensus for when and what additional nutrients are needed in subjects on long-term GFD (LTGFD).

Given this background, the aim of this narrative review is to evaluate the literature that considers blood nutritional deficiencies in celiac subjects on LTGFD therapy with good compliance (LTGFDWGC) in order to prepare dietary supplementation advice for these patients.

2. Materials and Methods

The present narrative review was performed following the steps by Egger et al. [15] as follows:

1. Configuration of a working group: three operators skilled in clinical nutrition (one acting as a methodological operator and two participating as clinical operators).
2. Formulation of the revision question on the basis of considerations made in the abstract: "the state of the art on nutritional deficiencies in celiac subjects on LTGFD therapy with good compliance; "good compliance" was defined as those patients who had been apparently carefully compliant with the GFD for a at least one year based on dietary history, and this was supported by the absence of coeliac antibodies (if present at diagnosis), or having a healed duodenal biopsy if previous coeliac serology was unavailable".
3. Identification of relevant studies: a research strategy was planned on PubMed (Public MedIine run by the National Center of Biotechnology Information (NCBI) of the National Library of Medicine of Bathesda (USA)) as follows: (a) Definition of the keywords (celiac disease; vitamin B12; iron; folic acid; vitamin D; calcium; zinc; magnesium; LTGFD therapy; LTGFDWGC), allowing the definition of the interest field of the documents to be searched, grouped in quotation marks (" ... ") and used separately or in combination; (b) use of: the Boolean (a data type with only two possible values: true or false) AND operator, that allows the establishments of logical relations among concepts; (c) Research modalities: advanced search; (d) Limits: time limits: papers published in the last 20 years; humans; adults; languages: English; (e) Manual search performed by the senior researchers experienced in clinical nutrition through the revision of reviews and individual articles on management of inflammation and oxidative stress by dietary approach in celiac patients published in journals qualified in the Index Medicus.
4. Analysis and presentation of the outcomes: we create paragraphs about different micronutrients, and the data extrapolated from the "revised studies" were collocated in tables; in particular, for each study we specified the author and year of publication and study characteristics.
5. The analysis was carried out in the form of a narrative review of the reports. At the beginning of each section, the keywords considered and the type of studies chosen are reported. We evaluated, as is suitable for the narrative review, studies of any design which considered the nutritional deficiencies in celiac adult subjects on LTGFD therapy with good compliance.

3. Results

This review included 73 eligible studies and the dedicated flowchart is shown in Figure 1.

Table 1 shows the reviews made on nutrient deficiencies in celiac patients at time of diagnosis and after LTGFDWGC.

Table S1 shows the studies concerning circulating levels and supplementation of micronutrients in celiac patients after LTGFDWGC.

The literature shows that nutritional deficiencies, considered by evaluating the blood values of these micronutrients, in celiac subjects on LTGFD with good compliance, relate to vitamin B12, folic acid, vitamin D, calcium, iron, magnesium, zinc, selenium, thiamine, riboflavin, niacin and vitamin K (Table 1).

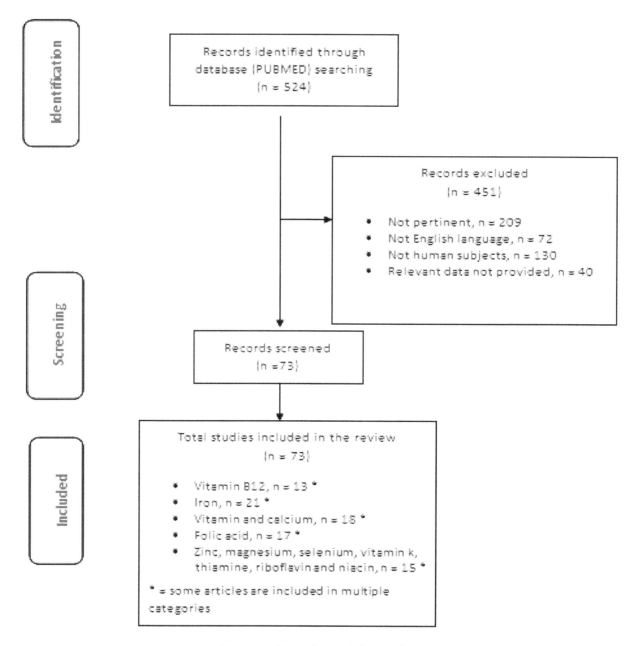

Figure 1. Flowchart of the study.

Table 1. Reviews on nutrient deficiencies in celiac patients at time of diagnosis and after GFD.

Authors	Type of Study	Country and Year	Results
[2]	Review	Italy, 2010	Common nutrient deficiencies in celiac subjects at diagnosis are: iron, calcium, magnesium, vitamin D, zinc, folate, niacin, vitamin B12, riboflavin, calorie/protein, and fiber. Deficiencies in folate, niacin, and vitamin B12 may occur after LTGFD.
[9]	Review	Italy, 2016	Low levels of fibers, folate, vitamin B12, vitamin D, calcium, iron, zinc and magnesium are common at diagnosis stage. In some subsets of treated celiac disease (CD) patients they can persist.

Table 1. *Cont.*

Authors	Type of Study	Country and Year	Results
[16]	Review	USA, 2005	Deficiencies in fiber, iron, calcium, vitamin D, magnesium, zinc, folate, niacin, vitamin B12, and riboflavin can occur at time of diagnosis. Deficiencies in fiber, iron, calcium, vitamin D, and magnesium can persist after following a GFD. Diet and gluten-free products are often low in B vitamins, calcium, vitamin D, iron, zinc, magnesium, and fiber.
[17]	Review	Italy, 2013	Reduced levels of iron, folate, vitamin B12, and vitamin D are common at the time of diagnosis. After GFD low levels of folate, vitamin B12 and vitamin D can persist.
[18]	Review	Italy, 2013	Common deficiencies at diagnosis include: fiber, iron, calcium, vitamin D, magnesium, zinc, folate, niacin, and vitamin B12. Deficiencies of fiber, iron, calcium, vitamin D, magnesium, zinc, folate, niacin, vitamin B12 may persist after following a GFD. Deficiencies of fiber, folate, niacin, vitamin B12, and riboflavin may persist after LTGFD.

3.1. Vitamin B12

This research was carried out based on the keywords "vitamin B12" AND "supplementation" AND "long-term GFD with good compliance" AND "celiac patient" OR "celiac disease". Of the 13 studies that were taken into account, 6 were review-type papers, 3 were prospective studies, 2 were observational studies and 2 were randomized controlled trials.

The absorption of dietary vitamin B12 occurs mainly in the terminal ileum through an active, specific and saturable transport mechanism. Vitamin B12 is released from food proteins after exposure to gastric acid. Vitamin B12 links to a salivary and gastric R protein; then pancreatic proteases destroy the R protein in the duodenum, releasing cobalamin which creates a complex with intrinsic factor (IF) that is secreted by the parietal cells in the stomach. The complex B12-FI migrates up to the terminal ileum aided by intestinal peristalsis, and binds itself through its proteic fraction to a specific cellular receptor. The complex dissociates and cobalamin enters the enterocytes of the small intestine. When the vitamin is administered orally in high doses, a small proportion along the entire intestine is absorbed through a passive diffusion mechanism.

Absorption site remains relatively preserved in patients with CD, so deficiency of vitamin B12 should be unusual. Nevertheless, numerous studies have shown that circulating levels of this vitamin are inadequate in about 5–40% of patients with CD at diagnosis [19–22] and in about 2.9-41% of patients following a GFD [20,21].

A real link exists between CD and vitamin B12 deficiency, but it has not been established. Some studies have shown that GFD and, where required, supplementation with vitamin B12 is effective in resolving neurological complications associated with deficiency of this vitamin. It has been shown that concentration of vitamin B12 tends to normalize in patients with a LTGFD [17,23].

However, there is evidence that supplementation may also be useful in subjects undergoing GFD. Hallert et al. [24] conducted a double-blind study to evaluate the effects of supplementation with B vitamins in adult CD patients for a long time, which involved daily administration of 0.8 mg of folic acid, 0.5 mg of cyanocobalamin, and 3 mg of pyridoxine for a period of 6 months. In these patients, there was improvement of psychiatric symptoms, and a significant return to normal vitamin B12 values with reduction of homocysteine values, which is often elevated in patients with vitamin B12 deficiency. Indeed, the catabolism of homocysteine requires vitamin B12 and folate. Consequently, hyperhomocysteinemia may reflect a deficit of both nutrients [25]. Great attention to the levels of homocysteine is needed in patients with CD. Celiac patients appear to have an increased risk of venous thromboembolism and vascular disorders [26] and high levels of homocysteine is a risk factor for these chronic diseases [27]. Supplementation of vitamin B12 and folate tends to decrease homocysteine values [24], so it could represent a prevention behavior.

In some patients, it is therefore necessary to integrate this element, even when following a strict GFD. In such cases, administration of vitamin B12 can be given via the oral or intramuscular routes.

In a study carried out by Bolaman et al. on general populations with megaloblastic anemia due to deficiency of cobalamin, oral supplementation was as effective as intramuscular treatment. Oral administration seems to be less costly and more tolerable than intramuscular delivery [28]. Furthermore, a review carried out by Vidal-Alaball et al. on general populations showed that in patients with a deficiency of vitamin B12, oral administration of 2000 mcg/day or 1000 mcg/day, followed by 1000 mcg/week and then 1000 mcg/month, can be as effective as intramuscular administration in showing improvement in hematological and neurological levels [29].

In patients with CD, supplementation is recommended for those in which there remains a blood deficiency despite GFD. Hallert et al. have shown how the oral administration of 500 mcg of cyanocobalamin in subjects undergoing GFD is effective in restoring the homocysteine value (which is an indirect measurement of vitamin B12 and folate). It suggests that the absorption after oral administration, especially in subjects undergoing GFD, is effective [24]. Furthermore, Theethira et al. suggested measuring vitamin B12 levels at diagnosis and then every 1–2 years for symptoms, and to treat with 1000 mcg orally until levels normalize, and then considering daily gluten-free multi vitamin/mineral supplementation [30].

In conclusion, considering the site of absorption (terminal ileum) of vitamin B12, which remains relatively preserved in patients with CD, deficiency of this vitamin should be infrequent; however, circulating levels of this vitamin could remain inadequate up to 41% in LTGGFDWGC patients. Given this background, in addition to its pivotal role in preventing hyperomocysteinemia, an annual routine follow-up of blood vitamin B12 level is mandatory in subjects undergoing LTGFD. Regarding dose and route of administration, the literature showed that in celiac patients with vitamin B12 deficiency, oral administration of 1000 mcg of vitamin B12 until levels normalized, followed by daily gluten-free multi-vitamin/mineral supplementation with 500 mcg of vitamin B12 is effective [30].

3.2. Iron

This research was carried out based on the keywords "iron" AND "supplementation" AND "long-term GFD with good compliance" AND "celiac patient" OR "celiac disease". Of the 21 studies that were taken into consideration, 8 were prospective studies, 5 were reviews, 3 were observational case studies, 2 were case control studies, 1 was a randomized controlled trial, 1 was a report and 1 was a guidelines.

Iron deficiency often occurs in celiac patients, and it is followed in many cases by iron deficiency anemia. Studies have shown that the prevalence of this event in patients with newly diagnosed CD seems to be between 10–80%. The prevalence of deficiency after 6 months of GFD is about 70%, after 1 year, it is about 50%, and after 2 years, it is about 40% [17,19,31–37].

Iron is an essential trace element, being part of the heme structure, the non-protein component of numerous iron proteins (such as hemoglobin, myoglobin and cytochromes). Its excretion cannot be controlled, so the amount of iron in the body depends mainly on its absorption, which takes place in the duodenum and proximal jejunum.

Iron deficiency anemia in CD patients mainly arises from malabsorption, although the possibility of intestinal bleeding cannot be excluded and must be considered [38,39].

In the general population, initial treatment of iron deficiency should be continued until hemoglobin and iron stores are normalized. This goal is usually obtained with oral iron administration. Although it is occasionally recommended to take iron supplements before breakfast in order to increase the absorption, this significantly reduces the tolerance. For this reason, it seems reasonable to suggest the administration with food. All ferrous salts, including ferrous fumarate, ferrous lactate, ferrous succinate, ferrous glutamate, and ferrous sulphate, share similar bioavailability. Preparations of iron glycinate represent a valid therapeutic alternative, since they have a good bioavailability and a lower frequency of side effects, such as constipation [40–42].

Treatment with oral iron is, in the general population, slow in reaching its goal, and good compliance is required to be successful. In addition to this, anemia is often severe, and a quick response is necessary. Sometimes the tolerance is poor, and in these situations the use of parenteral iron is fully justified. The efficacy and safety of parenteral iron sucrose use have been demonstrated in several clinical studies and have been confirmed by extensive clinical practice [43]. To supply the quantities required, several doses are needed. Other intravenous drugs such as ferric carboxymaltose have been introduced [44] and would require fewer infusions to provide the required dose. Ferric carboxymaltose is a robust and stable non-dextran intravenous iron formulation with the advantage of having a very low immunogenic potential, and therefore is not predisposed to anaphylactic reactions. Its properties permit the administration of large doses (15 mg/kg; maximum of 1000 mg/infusion) in a single and rapid session (15-min infusion) [45].

Therapy on the general population should start with a low dose and the intake should be constant until the iron deposits are not restored [40]. It is fundamental that treatment of an underlying cause should prevent further iron loss, but all patients should have iron supplementation, both to correct anemia and to replenish body stores. This is achieved most simply and cheaply with oral ferrous sulphate 200 mg twice daily. Lower doses may be as effective and better tolerated, and should be considered in patients not tolerating traditional doses. Other iron compounds (e.g., ferrous fumarate, ferrous gluconate) or formulations (iron suspensions) may also be tolerated better than ferrous sulphate. Oral iron should be continued for 3 months after the iron deficiency has been corrected so that stores are replenished [46].

Regarding celiac patients, in subjects in which iron supplementation is needed, it should be started orally. In the decision on when to start, some authors suggest undertaking supplementation in the moment in which the intestinal lesions are healed [40], while other studies suggest taking the supplement immediately at the time of diagnosis, without waiting for the healing of the mucosa [47]. In most of these patients, GFD is enough to solve the framework of anemia [48], although it may take a long time. In other cases it is necessary to help the patient with supplementation [36]. A study carried out on 25 pediatric patients with CD and iron deficiency showed good efficacy of oral administration of iron, (investigated with ferrous bisglycinate chelate 0.5 mg per kg body weight, reaching a maximum of 28 mg) both in patients with GFD and in those newly diagnosed [47]. A study carried out on celiac pediatric patients showed that the therapeutic dose in pediatric patients with an iron deficiency is 3 mg of elemental iron per kg body weight per day. The prophylactic dose in pediatric patients is 2 mg of elemental iron per kg body weight per day reaching a maximum dosage of 30 mg per day [36].

Since gluten-free products are characterized by a low iron content [49], the intake of foods rich in this mineral, such as meat, should be recommended to patients initiating a GFD.

Theethira et al. suggested measuring serum iron and ferritin at diagnosis, repeating every 3–6 months until ferritin was normal, and then every 1–2 years for symptoms. Moreover, they suggested iron supplements (325 mg), 1–3 tablets based on initial ferritin level until iron stores are restored, and consideration of intravenous (IV) iron for severe symptomatic iron deficiency anemia or intolerance of oral iron.

In conclusion, it seems that when long GFD, including food tips to consume adequate dietary iron, is not enough to restore iron levels (40% of LTGFDWGC subjects are iron-deficient), the right approach could be to start with oral administration of iron.

Based on this background, a semi-annual steady and routine follow-up of blood iron and ferritin levels is mandatory in subjects undergoing LTGFD [30].

3.3. Folic Acid

This research was carried out based on the keywords "folic acid" AND "supplementation" AND "long-term GFD with good compliance" AND "celiac patient" OR "celiac disease". A total of 17 studies were taken into consideration. Among these studies, 7 were prospective studies, 5 were review studies, 2 were observational case studies, 2 were randomized controlled trials, and 1 was a report.

The term "folate" describes the vitamer group B, based on the main structure of folic acid, which shares the same vitamin activity. This group of vitamins is essential for the synthesis and repairing of DNA, and they also act as cofactors for the enzymes involved in several biological reactions. Folate occurs naturally in some foods, and its synthetic form, folic acid, is added to many food products to increase the dietary intake. An example of supplementation is the addition of folic acid to wheat flour, which has been introduced in 52 countries worldwide since 2007 [50].

Folate deficiency was detected in about 10–85% of adult patients with CD at diagnosis, and in about 0-20% of patients following a GFD [17,20,22,51–54]. Usually the folate deficiency in CD occurs in patients with lesions in the ileum [48,55,56].

Tighe et al. compared in the general population the effectiveness of 0.2 mg folic acid per day with that of 0.4 and 0.8 mg/day in lowering homocysteine concentrations over a 6-month period. It has been seen that folic acid significantly reduces the risk of stroke overall by 18%, but to a greater extent by up to 25% in those trials that showed greater homocysteine lowering or in persons with no history of stroke. The lowest dose of folic acid required to achieve effective reductions in homocysteine is controversial but important for food fortification policy given recent concerns about the potential adverse effects of overexposure to this vitamin. This study supports the potential benefit of enhancing folate status and/or lowering homocysteine in the primary prevention of stroke. The authors suggest that a folic acid dose as low as 0.2 mg per day can, if administered for 6 months, effectively lower homocysteine concentrations [57].

Numerous studies have shown that a GFD would be sufficient to normalize folate status [21,48,58], but one other [23] show that in a certain percentage of patients, folate levels remain low despite GFD maintained for over 10 years. A possible explanation for this phenomenon is the reduced content of folate in gluten-free foods as previously described by Thompson [49]. Another hypothesis is that in celiac patients genetic alterations of the proteins involved in absorption and metabolism of folate may be present [17].

Hallert et al. suggested providing patients with good information about folate-rich foods. They also recommended starting supplementation in patients who show blood deficiencies after GFD [17,23].

Dosage should be decided in relation to the initial value of the subject. In a study conducted by Hallert et al. on celiac patients, they administered 0.8 mg of folic acid leading to normalization of homocysteine values [24].

In conclusion, folate deficiency was detected in up to 20% of patients on LTGFDWGC. Given this background, a semi-annual routine follow-up of blood folic acid level is mandatory in these subjects. Dosage of supplementation should be decided in relation to the detected value in the subject. The literature suggests supplementation with 1 mg/day of folic acid for 3 months, followed by a reduction to 400–800 mcg/day [30] or with 0.8 mg of folic acid [24] in order to improve the poor folate status.

3.4. Vitamin D and Calcium

This research was carried out based on the keywords "vitamin D" OR "calcium" AND "long-term GFD with good compliance" AND "supplementation" AND "celiac patient" OR "celiac disease". A total of 18 studies were taken into account. Of these studies, 5 were review studies, 4 were prospective studies, 3 were case reports, 2 were observational studies, 2 were guidelines, 1 was a case-control study and 1 was a meta-analysis study.

3.4.1. Vitamin D

The cholecalciferol, or vitamin D3, can be synthesized in the basal layers of the epidermis starting from cholesterol, by the action of ultraviolet rays of sunlight, and this should be the main source of vitamin D for the body. Another source of vitamin D is food, from which the absorption occurs mainly in the terminal ileum.

Numerous studies have shown low levels of vitamin D in many untreated celiac patients. Vitamin D deficiency, investigated through blood value, was detected in about 8–88% of adult CD patients at diagnosis, and in about 0–25% of patients following a GFD [17].

Nevertheless, certain patients, mainly post-menopausal women, continue to present bone density levels below the normal range [59,60]. This seems to be partly due to lack of vitamin D1.

If GFD is not sufficient to bring the values in the normal range, supplementation of vitamin D and calcium is required [17,61–63]. The Endocrine Society guidelines recommend, for the general population, that serum levels of vitamin D are at least equal to 30 ng/mL, and that it is necessary to decide the dosage of supplementation in relation to the initial value of the subject [64].

A meta-analysis conducted on general populations by Shab-Bidar et al. shows that a significant increase in serum levels of vitamin D in adults is achieved with a dose of $\geq$800 UI/day, at least after 6–12 months of supplementation [65].

Consider that for the celiac patient, a commonly applied strategy in cases of serious vitamin D deficiency is to prescribe a "loading dose" (e.g., 50,000 UI/week for 8 weeks) followed by reduced doses, as shown by Duerksen in a case report study of a woman with CD [66].

In a study aimed at detecting the effects of calcium and vitamin D supplementation in celiac children by Muzzo et al., daily supplementation with 1000 mg of calcium and 400 UI of vitamin D for 24 months was shown to have beneficial effects on the bone mass of celiac patients in whole body and femoral neck measurements; however, these values did not reach the controls [67].

A recent study carried out by Zanchetta et al. suggests an intake of 1000–1500 mg/day of calcium in two or more divided intakes of dairy products and a dose of vitamin D necessary to maintain a blood level of 30 ng/mL [68].

Moreover, Theethira et al. suggested measuring vitamin D levels at diagnosis, repeating every 3 months until levels are normalized, and then every 1–2 years or for symptoms. If necessary, integrate with 1000 (or more-based serum level) UI/day or 50.000 UI weekly if level is <20 ng/mL.

In conclusion, blood vitamin D deficiency was detected in about 0–25% of patients following a LTGFDWGC [69].

3.4.2. Calcium

Calcium deficiency was detected in about 41% of adult patients with CD at the diagnosis [32] and 3.6% of treated children [70]. This seems to be due to malabsorption related to intestinal epithelial damage, but it could also be linked to a reduced expression of a protein regulated by vitamin D that controls the absorption of calcium [17,71]. Calcium absorption is impaired due to mucosal atrophy. Therefore, to avoid hypocalcemia, parathyroid hormone increases substantially (secondary hyperparathyroidism) and stimulates osteoclast-mediated bone degradation. Calcium is then obtained from the skeleton reservoir, but this high remodeling state can lead to osteopenia and osteoporosis, altering bone microstructure and increasing fracture risk [68].

In a study relating to the persistence of calcium deficiency despite a GFD, Kavak et al. undertook the analysis of reduced intake and absorption, rather than the percentage of shortage investigated by blood values in children patients after GFD [70]. The authors reported a reduction in calcium intake in about 76–88% of patients adhering to a GFD [69]. Pazianas et al. described a reduced fractional calcium absorption in adult celiac patients adhering to a GFD despite adequate calcium intake. Taken into account their reduced fractional calcium absorption, the authors concluded that their daily dose should be at least 1200 mg per day [72]. Larussa et al. showed that asymptomatic patients following a GFD for at least 2 years showed normal circulating serum calcium and parathyroid hormone (PTH) levels [73,74]. Zanchetta et al. showed a significant reduction of bone resorption parameters and PTH values, with a significant increase in serum calcium and vitamin D after GFD. Sategna-Guidetti et al.

described significant improvement of bone mineral density values in newly diagnosed CD patients after 1 year of following a GFD [53,68].

Regarding supplementation, Zanchetta et al. suggested 1000–1500 mg/day in two or more divided intakes of dairy products. The authors concluded that calcium supplementation may be an option if the patient is not able or willing to fulfill the required intake through dietary means [68]. Theethira et al. found that more than 50% of patients consume less than the recommended daily intake of calcium. They recommended that CD patients undergo regular assessments with a dietitian and that the recommended intake of calcium, including supplementation should be 1200–1500 mg/day [30].

3.5. Other Micronutrients

This research was carried out based on the keywords "zinc" OR "magnesium" OR "selenium" OR "vitamin K" OR "thiamine" OR "riboflavin" OR "niacin" AND "supplementation" AND "long-term GFD with good compliance" AND "celiac patient" OR "celiac disease". Of the 15 studies that were taken into account, 9 were review studies, 2 were report studies, 2 were prospective studies, 1 was an observational study, and 1 was a case-control study.

3.5.1. Zinc

Zinc deficiency was detected in more than 50% of adult patients with CD at diagnosis, and between 0–40% of patients following a GFD [17]. The lack of this mineral seems to be linked in part to the its reduced absorption, due also to the degree of inflammation of the mucosa.

In the review by Theethira et al., they proposed to measure the serum zinc levels of CD patients at diagnosis and repeat after 3 months until the level is normal, followed by every 1–2 years for symptoms. They also suggested zinc supplementation between 25–40 mg/day until zinc levels were normal [30].

3.5.2. Magnesium

Magnesium deficiency was detected in about 21.4% of adult patients with CD at the diagnosis, and a similar percentage (19.6%) in patients following a GFD [75].

This deficiency can be explained by malabsorption, but GFD may also lead to possible nutrient deficiencies because gluten-free products are usually lower in magnesium, and gluten-free cereals found in nature have a lower magnesium content compared with gluten-containing ones [9].

Furthermore, it has been seen that the resolution of mucosal inflammation may not be sufficient to resolve the shortage of magnesium in celiac patient. The deficiency may also be linked to a reduced intake of this mineral.

Breedon reported that some CD patients need additional magnesium supplement of 200–300 mg/day in the form of magnesium oxide or magnesium chloride, while others can improve magnesium levels through dietary means [76].

3.5.3. Selenium

Selenium deficiency is particularly remarkable because a GFD leads to its absence in cereal foods such as wheat and its derivatives, which are a source of selenium [77]. There are no sufficient literature data to describe a percentage of deficiency investigated through the blood level.

Reduced concentrations of selenium in whole blood, plasma, and leucocytes might develop in several ways. Firstly, GFD might contain a reduced amount of selenium compared with a normal diet, and, secondly, there might be malabsorption of selenium even when the patient is clinically well. Between the extraintestinal symptoms associated with CD, autoimmune thyroid diseases are more evident, underlining that CD-related autoimmune alterations can be modulated not only by gluten but also by various concurrent endogenous (genetic affinity, over-expression of cytokines) and exogenous (environment, nutritional deficiency) factors. The thyroid is particularly sensitive to selenium deficiencies because selenoproteins are significant in biosynthesis and activity of thyroid hormones, while other selenoproteins, including glutathione peroxidase are involved in inhibiting apoptosis. Thus, selenium malabsorption in CD patients can be considered a key factor directly leading to thyroid and intestinal damage [78].

Studies have shown that in celiac patients, selenium supplementation between 120–200 mcg/day is within a safe range. It is important, however, not to exceed the tolerable upper limit of 400 mcg/day for selenium, as this can lead to gastrointestinal upset, hair loss and nerve damage [79].

3.5.4. Vitamin K

Vitamin K deficiency, investigated by markers like PIVKA-II or by prothrombin times, was detected in about 25% of adult patients with CD at the diagnosis, and it seems to return to acceptable levels in almost all patients following a GFD [72,80].

There are limited available data that relate the role of vitamin K and bone health in children and adults with CD. Pazianas et al. examined vitamin K status in children newly diagnosed with CD using prothrombin times as a marker of vitamin K status and found that approximately 35% of children were lacking this marker [72]. However, this may have been an underestimate of the prevalence of vitamin K deficiency as prothrombin time is a very insensitive marker of overall vitamin K status [72]. More sensitive markers of vitamin K status include serum levels of PIVKA-II, which is a vitamin K-dependent protein [80].

In the study carried out by Mager et al., over 25% of children were vitamin K deficient at diagnosis, investigated by PIVKA-II (which is a protein increasing in vitamin K absence), but it resolved in all children after 1 year. This seems to be due in part to improvements in vitamin K intake on the GFD. However, the remaining one-third of children and adolescents continued to have vitamin K intakes considerably lower than the adequate intake on the GFD [80].

Suboptimal dietary intake of vitamin K is common in this population, including when on a GFD. There are no sufficient literature data to recommend a specific dose of supplementation in celiac patient. Therefore, careful consideration should be given to routine supplementation of this nutrient at time of diagnosis of CD.

3.5.5. Niacin, Riboflavin and Thiamin

Deficiency of other micronutrients, like niacin, riboflavin and thiamin have been described in several reviews at the time of diagnosis, although in the literature there is no accurate data on the percentage of celiac patients with such deficiencies [2,16,18]. Deficiencies of niacin and riboflavin may persist after a GFD [2,18]. Regarding thiamin, a study carried out by Shepherd et al. found that the inadequacy of thiamin was more common after GFD implementation than at time of diagnosis [81]. This can be explained by the fact that many gluten-free cereal products do not provide the same levels of thiamin, riboflavin, and/or niacin as enriched wheat flour products. As a result, a GFD that routinely includes gluten-free cereal products could be deficient in one or more of these nutrients, especially if these foods are, in large part, refined and unenriched [82].

Although there is insufficient data in the literature to recommend a dose for supplementation, it is considered useful to carry out control of blood values after diagnosis and after a period of GFD.

4. Discussion

It is evident from the analyzed reviews that there emerges an attention towards nutritional deficiencies that occur in celiac patients after an even longer period of GFD with good compliance. The suggested course of action is a half-yearly routine search in patients on LTGFD nutritional deficiencies, such as low levels of folic acid, vitamin B12, vitamin D, calcium, iron, zinc, selenium and magnesium and the need to establish a personalized supplementation plan, following patients over time, to avoid stopping of integration once the values are returned to their normal range, as shown in Table 2.

Table 2. Supplementation of nutrients in generic state deficiency and in celiac patient.

Nutrient	Route of Administration	Dosage and Sources
Vitamin B12	Oral preferable to intramuscular	• 500 mcg/day ** [24] • 1000 mcg orally until the level is normal and then consider daily gluten-free multi vitamin/mineral supplement ** [30] • 2000 or 1000 mcg/day, then 1000 mcg/week, then 1000 mcg/month * [29]
Iron	Oral preferable to intravenous	• A study on 25 pediatric patients with celiac disease and iron deficiency showed good efficacy of oral administration of iron, (investigated by Bisglycinate Ferrous Chelate) both in patients with gluten-free diet and in those newly diagnosed ** [47] • Therapeutic dose in pediatric patients: 3 mg of elementary iron/kg/day. Prophylactic dose in pediatric patients: 2 mg of elementary iron/kg /day until a maximum dosage of 30 mg/day ** [36] • Iron supplements (325 mg) 1–3 tablets based on initial ferritin level until iron stores are restored. Consider i.v. iron for severe symptomatic iron deficiency anemia or intolerance of oral iron ** [30] • Ferrous sulphate 200 mg 1 or 2/day, (ferrous fumarate, ferrous gluconate) or formulations (iron suspensions) that may also be tolerated better than ferrous sulphate. Oral iron should be continued for 3 months * [46] • Therapy should start with a low dose (one tablet/day of any ferrous sulphate commercially available or any other type of iron), and the intake should be constant until the iron deposits are not restored * [40] • Intravenous ferric carboxymaltose is a stable complex with the advantage of being non-dextran-containing and a very low immunogenic potential and therefore not predisposed to anaphylactic reactions. Its properties permit the administration of large doses (15 mg/kg; maximum of 1000 mg/infusion) in a single and rapid session (15-min infusion) * [45]
Folic acid	Oral preferable to parenteral	• −800 mcg/day ** [24] • 1 mg/day of folic acid for 3 months and once diarrhea improves 400–800 mcg/day ** [30]
Vitamin D—Calcium	Oral preferable to parenteral	• 50.000 U.I./week for 8 weeks, then reduce the dose ** [66] • 1000 mg of calcium and 400 U of vitamin D daily ** [67] • Calcium: 1000–1500 mg/day in two or more divided intakes of dairy products. If the patient is not able or willing to fulfill the required intake through the diet, calcium supplements can be given. Vitamin D: dose necessary to maintain a blood level of 30 ng/mL ** [68] • Vitamin D: 1000 (or more-based serum level) U.I./day or 50.000 U.I. weekly if level is <20 ng/mL. Calcium: recommended intake of calcium, including supplementation, for patients with CD is 1200–1500 mg/day ** [30] • -Vitamin D: ≥800 IU/day, at least for 6/12 months of supplementation * [65]

* Therapy in literature in generic state deficiency ** Therapy in literature in celiac patient.

To help patients reduce deficiencies of minerals (calcium, phosphorus, sodium, potassium, chloride and magnesium) and trace elements (iron, zinc and selenium) it is important to advise them to introduce into their eating habits pseudo-cereals, in which the content of these elements can be twice as high as in other cereals. For example, in teff, iron and calcium contents (11–33 mg/100 g and 100–150 mg/100 g, respectively) are higher than those of wheat, barley, sorghum and rice [18].

It seems important to explain to patients that nutritional education and dietary supplementation should become part of the therapeutic process, which must last a lifetime.

5. Conclusions

In conclusion, if correct GFD is not enough, and the blood levels of micronutrients remain low, it is mandatory to start with personalized supplements. In this case, it would be helpful to evaluate the initial blood level to determine the right dosage of supplementation and repeat the examinations to keep under control values.

In any case, there are a lot of unresolved questions regarding the causes and the mechanisms that lead to these nutritional deficiencies. Further studies are absolutely required for the detailed understanding of this topic.

Author Contributions: Conceptualization, M.R.; methodology, S.P.; data curation, G.P., M.A.F., M.N., A.R., M.N. and C.G.; writing—original draft preparation, M.R.; writing—review and editing, T.A.A., S.P. and G.P.

References

1. Husby, S.; Koletzko, S.; Korponay-Szabó, I.R.; Mearin, M.L.; Phillips, A.; Shamir, R.; Troncone, R.; Giersiepen, K.; Branski, D.; Catassi, C.; et al. European Society for Pediatric Gastroenterology, Hepatology, and Nutrition Guidelines for the Diagnosis of Coeliac Disease. *J. Pediatr. Gastroenterol. Nutr.* **2012**, *54*, 136–160. [CrossRef] [PubMed]

2. Saturni, L.; Ferretti, G.; Bacchetti, T. The Gluten-Free Diet: Safety and Nutritional Quality. *Nutrients* **2010**, *2*, 16–34. [CrossRef] [PubMed]

3. Lindfors, K.; Ciacci, C.; Kurppa, K.; Lundin, K.E.A.; Makharia, G.K.; Mearin, M.L.; Murray, J.A.; Verdu, E.F.; Kaukinen, K. Coeliac Disease. *Nat. Rev. Dis. Primers* **2019**, *5*, 3. [CrossRef] [PubMed]

4. Lebwohl, B.; Sanders, D.S.; Green, P.H.R. Coeliac Disease. *Lancet* **2018**, *391*, 70–81. [CrossRef]

5. De Silvestri, A.; Capittini, C.; Poddighe, D.; Valsecchi, C.; Marseglia, G.; Tagliacarne, S.C.; Scotti, V.; Rebuffi, C.; Pasi, A.; Martinetti, M.; et al. HLA-DQ Genetics in Children with Celiac Disease: A Meta-Analysis Suggesting a Two-Step Genetic Screening Procedure Starting with HLA-DQ β Chains. *Pediatr. Res.* **2018**, *83*, 564–572. [CrossRef] [PubMed]

6. Capittini, C.; De Silvestri, A.; Rebuffi, C.; Tinelli, C.; Poddighe, D.; Capittini, C.; De Silvestri, A.; Rebuffi, C.; Tinelli, C.; Poddighe, D. Relevance of HLA-DQB1*02 Allele in the Genetic Predisposition of Children with Celiac Disease: Additional Cues from a Meta-Analysis. *Medicina (B. Aires)* **2019**, *55*, 190. [CrossRef] [PubMed]

7. Rubio-Tapia, A.; Hill, I.D.; Kelly, C.P.; Calderwood, A.H.; Murray, J.A. ACG Clinical Guidelines: Diagnosis and Management of Celiac Disease. *Am. J. Gastroenterol.* **2013**, *108*, 656–676. [CrossRef]

8. I.C.G.T. *Coeliac Disease*; National Institute for Health and Care Excellence: London, UK, 2015.

9. Vici, G.; Belli, L.; Biondi, M.; Polzonetti, V. Gluten Free Diet and Nutrient Deficiencies: A Review. *Clin. Nutr.* **2016**, *35*, 1236–1241. [CrossRef]

10. Ciacci, C.; Ciclitira, P.; Hadjivassiliou, M.; Kaukinen, K.; Ludvigsson, J.F.; McGough, N.; Sanders, D.S.; Woodward, J.; Leonard, J.N.; Swift, G.L. The Gluten-Free Diet and Its Current Application in Coeliac Disease and Dermatitis Herpetiformis. *United Eur. Gastroenterol. J.* **2015**, *3*, 121–135. [CrossRef]

11. Lanzini, A.; Lanzarotto, F.; Villanacci, V.; Mora, A.; Bertolazzi, S.; Turini, D.; Carella, G.; Malagoli, A.; Ferrante, G.; Cesana, B.M.; et al. Complete Recovery of Intestinal Mucosa Occurs Very Rarely in Adult Coeliac Patients despite Adherence to Gluten-Free Diet. *Aliment. Pharmacol. Ther.* **2009**, *29*, 1299–1308. [CrossRef]

12. Lebwohl, B.; Murray, J.A.; Rubio-Tapia, A.; Green, P.H.R.; Ludvigsson, J.F. Predictors of Persistent Villous Atrophy in Coeliac Disease: A Population-Based Study. *Aliment. Pharmacol. Ther.* **2014**, *39*, 488–495. [CrossRef] [PubMed]

13. Leonard, M.M.; Weir, D.C.; DeGroote, M.; Mitchell, P.D.; Singh, P.; Silvester, J.A.; Leichtner, A.M.; Fasano, A. Value of IgA TTG in Predicting Mucosal Recovery in Children with Celiac Disease on a Gluten-Free Diet. *J. Pediatr. Gastroenterol. Nutr.* **2017**, *64*, 286–291. [CrossRef] [PubMed]

14. Kaukinen, K.; Peraaho, M.; Lindfors, K.; Partanen, J.; Woolley, N.; Pikkarainen, P.; Karvonen, A.-L.; Laasanen, T.; Sievaneh, H.; Maki, M.; et al. Persistent Small Bowel Mucosal Villous Atrophy without Symptoms in Coeliac Disease. *Aliment. Pharmacol. Ther.* **2007**, *25*, 1237–1245. [CrossRef]

15. Egger, M.; Dickersin, K.; Smith, G.D. Problems and Limitations in Conducting Systematic Reviews. In *Systematic Reviews in Health Care*; BMJ Publishing Group: London, UK, 2008; pp. 43–68.

16. Kupper, C. Dietary Guidelines and Implementation for Celiac Disease. *Gastroenterology* **2005**, *128* (Suppl. 1), S121–S127. [CrossRef]

17. Caruso, R.; Pallone, F.; Stasi, E.; Romeo, S.; Monteleone, G. Appropriate Nutrient Supplementation in Celiac Disease. *Ann. Med.* **2013**, *45*, 522–531. [CrossRef]

18. Penagini, F.; Dilillo, D.; Meneghin, F.; Mameli, C.; Fabiano, V.; Zuccotti, G.V. Gluten-Free Diet in Children: An Approach to a Nutritionally Adequate and Balanced Diet. *Nutrients* **2013**, *5*, 4553–4565. [CrossRef]

19. Harper, J.W.; Holleran, S.F.; Ramakrishnan, R.; Bhagat, G.; Green, P.H.R. Anemia in Celiac Disease Is Multifactorial in Etiology. *Am. J. Hematol.* **2007**, *82*, 996–1000. [CrossRef] [PubMed]

20. Dahele, A.; Ghosh, S. Vitamin B12 Deficiency in Untreated Celiac Disease. *Am. J. Gastroenterol.* **2001**, *96*, 745–750. [CrossRef]

21. Dickey, W.; Ward, M.; Whittle, C.R.; Kelly, M.T.; Pentieva, K.; Horigan, G.; Patton, S.; McNulty, H. Homocysteine and Related B-Vitamin Status in Coeliac Disease: Effects of Gluten Exclusion and Histological Recovery. *Scand. J. Gastroenterol.* **2008**, *43*, 682–688. [CrossRef]

22. Halfdanarson, T.R.; Litzow, M.R.; Murray, J.A. Hematologic Manifestations of Celiac Disease. *Blood* **2007**, *109*, 412–421. [CrossRef]

23. Hallert, C.; Grant, C.; Grehn, S.; Grännö, C.; Hultén, S.; Midhagen, G.; Ström, M.; Svensson, H.; Valdimarsson, T. Evidence of Poor Vitamin Status in Coeliac Patients on a Gluten-Free Diet for 10 Years. *Aliment. Pharmacol. Ther.* **2002**, *16*, 1333–1339. [CrossRef] [PubMed]

24. Hallert, C.; Svensson, M.; Tholstrup, J.; Hultberg, B. Clinical Trial: B Vitamins Improve Health in Patients with Coeliac Disease Living on a Gluten-Free Diet. *Aliment. Pharmacol. Ther.* **2009**, *29*, 811–816. [CrossRef] [PubMed]

25. Green, R. Indicators for Assessing Folate and Vitamin B-12 Status and for Monitoring the Efficacy of Intervention Strategies. *Am. J. Clin. Nutr.* **2011**, *94*, 666S–672S. [CrossRef] [PubMed]

26. Ludvigsson, J.F.; Welander, A.; Lassila, R.; Ekbom, A.; Montgomery, S.M. Risk of Thromboembolism in 14,000 Individuals with Coeliac Disease. *Br. J. Haematol.* **2007**, *139*, 121–127. [CrossRef] [PubMed]

27. Eichinger, S. Are B Vitamins a Risk Factor for Venous Thromboembolism? Yes. *J. Thromb. Haemost.* **2006**, *4*, 307–308. [CrossRef] [PubMed]

28. Bolaman, Z.; Kadikoylu, G.; Yukselen, V.; Yavasoglu, I.; Barutca, S.; Senturk, T. Oral versus Intramuscular Cobalamin Treatment in Megaloblastic Anemia: A Single-Center, Prospective, Randomized, Open-Label Study. *Clin Ther.* **2003**, *25*, 3124–3134. [CrossRef]

29. Vidal-Alaball, J.; Butler, C.C.; Cannings-John, R.; Goringe, A.; Hood, K.; McCaddon, A.; McDowell, I.; Papaioannou, A. Oral Vitamin B12 versus Intramuscular Vitamin B12 for Vitamin B12 Deficiency. *Cochrane Database Syst. Rev.* **2005**, *3*. [CrossRef] [PubMed]

30. Theethira, T.G.; Dennis, M.; Leffler, D.A. Nutritional Consequences of Celiac Disease and the Gluten-Free Diet. *Expert Rev. Gastroenterol. Hepatol.* **2014**, *8*, 123–129. [CrossRef]

31. Fasano, A.; Berti, I.; Gerarduzzi, T.; Not, T.; Colletti, R.B.; Drago, S.; Elitsur, Y.; Green, P.H.R.; Guandalini, S.; Hill, I.D.; et al. Prevalence of Celiac Disease in At-Risk and Not-at-Risk Groups in the United States: A Large Multicenter Study. *Arch. Intern. Med.* **2003**, *163*, 286–292. [CrossRef]

32. Malterre, T. Digestive and Nutritional Considerations in Celiac Disease: Could Supplementation Help? *Altern. Med. Rev.* **2009**, *14*, 247–257.

33. Haapalahti, M.; Kulmala, P.; Karttunen, T.J.; Paajanen, L.; Laurila, K.; Mäki, M.; Mykkänen, H.; Kokkonen, J. Nutritional Status in Adolescents and Young Adults with Screen-Detected Celiac Disease. *J. Pediatr. Gastroenterol. Nutr.* **2005**, *40*, 566–570. [CrossRef] [PubMed]

34. Lo, W.; Sano, K.; Lebwohl, B.; Diamond, B.; Green, P.H.R. Changing Presentation of Adult Celiac Disease. *Dig. Dis. Sci.* **2003**, *48*, 395–398. [CrossRef] [PubMed]

35. Kolho, K.L.; Färkkilä, M.A.; Savilahti, E. Undiagnosed Coeliac Disease Is Common in Finnish Adults. *Scand. J. Gastroenterol.* **1998**, *33*, 1280–1283. [PubMed]

36. Kapur, G.; Patwari, A.K.; Narayan, S.; Anand, V.K. Iron Supplementation in Children with Celiac Disease. *Indian J. Pediatr.* **2003**, *70*, 955–958. [CrossRef] [PubMed]

37. Annibale, B.; Severi, C.; Chistolini, A.; Antonelli, G.; Lahner, E.; Marcheggiano, A.; Iannoni, C.; Monarca, B.; Delle Fave, G. Efficacy of Gluten-Free Diet Alone on Recovery from Iron Deficiency Anemia in Adult Celiac Patients. *Am. J. Gastroenterol.* **2001**, *96*, 132–137. [CrossRef]

38. Hopper, A.D.; Leeds, J.S.; Hurlstone, D.P.; Hadjivassiliou, M.; Drew, K.; Sanders, D.S. Are Lower Gastrointestinal Investigations Necessary in Patients with Coeliac Disease? *Eur. J. Gastroenterol. Hepatol.* **2005**, *17*, 617–621. [CrossRef]

39. Oxford, E.C.; Nguyen, D.D.; Sauk, J.; Korzenik, J.R.; Yajnik, V.; Friedman, S.; Ananthakrishnan, A.N. Impact of Coexistent Celiac Disease on Phenotype and Natural History of Inflammatory Bowel Diseases. *Am. J. Gastroenterol.* **2013**, *108*, 1123–1129. [CrossRef]

40. Aspuru, K.; Villa, C.; Bermejo, F.; Herrero, P.; López, S.G. Optimal Management of Iron Deficiency Anemia Due to Poor Dietary Intake. *Int. J. Gen. Med.* **2011**, *4*, 741–750. [CrossRef]

41. Mimura, E.C.M.; Breganó, J.W.; Dichi, J.B.; Gregório, E.P.; Dichi, I. Comparison of Ferrous Sulfate and Ferrous Glycinate Chelate for the Treatment of Iron Deficiency Anemia in Gastrectomized Patients. *Nutrition* **2008**, *24*, 663–668. [CrossRef]

42. Pineda, O.; Ashmead, H.D. Effectiveness of Treatment of Iron-Deficiency Anemia in Infants and Young Children with Ferrous Bis-Glycinate Chelate. *Nutrition* **2001**, *17*, 381–384. [CrossRef]

43. Fishbane, S.; Kowalski, E.A. The Comparative Safety of Intravenous Iron Dextran, Iron Saccharate, and Sodium Ferric Gluconate. *Semin. Dial.* **2000**, *13*, 381–384. [CrossRef] [PubMed]

44. Kulnigg, S.; Stoinov, S.; Simanenkov, V.; Dudar, L.V.; Karnafel, W.; Garcia, L.C.; Sambuelli, A.M.; D'Haens, G.; Gasche, C. A Novel Intravenous Iron Formulation for Treatment of Anemia in Inflammatory Bowel Disease: The Ferric Carboxymaltose (FERINJECT) Randomized Controlled Trial. *Am. J. Gastroenterol.* **2008**, *103*, 1182–1192. [CrossRef] [PubMed]

45. Friedrisch, J.R.; Cançado, R.D. Intravenous Ferric Carboxymaltose for the Treatment of Iron Deficiency Anemia. *Rev. Bras. Hematol. Hemoter.* **2015**, *37*, 400–405. [CrossRef] [PubMed]

46. Goddard, A.F.; McIntyre, A.S.; Scott, B.B. Guidelines for the Management of Iron Deficiency Anaemia. British Society of Gastroenterology. *Gut* **2000**, *46* (Suppl. 3–4), IV1–IV5. [CrossRef] [PubMed]

47. Mazza, G.A.; Marrazzo, S.; Gangemi, P.; Battaglia, E.; Giancotti, L.; Miniero, R. Oral Iron Absorption Test with Ferrous Bisglycinate Chelate in Children with Celiac Disease. *Minerva Pediatr.* **2019**, *71*, 139–143. [CrossRef] [PubMed]

48. Vilppula, A.; Kaukinen, K.; Luostarinen, L.; Krekelä, I.; Patrikainen, H.; Valve, R.; Luostarinen, M.; Laurila, K.; Mäki, M.; Collin, P. Clinical Benefit of Gluten-Free Diet in Screen-Detected Older Celiac Disease Patients. *BMC Gastroenterol.* **2011**, *11*, 136. [CrossRef] [PubMed]

49. Thompson, T. Folate, Iron, and Dietary Fiber Contents of the Gluten-Free Diet. *J. Am. Diet. Assoc.* **2000**, *100*, 1389–1396. [CrossRef]

50. Centers for Disease Control and Prevention (CDC). Trends in Wheat-Flour Fortification with Folic Acid and Iron–Worldwide, 2004 and 2007. *MMWR. Morb. Mortal. Wkly. Rep.* **2008**, *57*, 8–10.

51. Howard, M.R.; Turnbull, A.J.; Morley, P.; Hollier, P.; Webb, R.; Clarke, A. A Prospective Study of the Prevalence of Undiagnosed Coeliac Disease in Laboratory Defined Iron and Folate Deficiency. *J. Clin. Pathol.* **2002**, *55*, 754–757. [CrossRef]

52. Hallert, C.; Tobiasson, P.; Walan, A. Serum Folate Determinations in Tracing Adult Coeliacs. *Scand. J. Gastroenterol.* **1981**, *16*, 263–267. [CrossRef]

53. Sategna-Guidetti, C.; Grosso, S.B.; Grosso, S.; Mengozzi, G.; Aimo, G.; Zaccaria, T.; Di Stefano, M.; Isaia, G.C. The Effects of 1-Year Gluten Withdrawal on Bone Mass, Bone Metabolism and Nutritional Status in Newly-Diagnosed Adult Coeliac Disease Patients. *Aliment. Pharmacol. Ther.* **2000**, *14*, 35–43. [CrossRef]

54. Ponziani, F.R.; Cazzato, I.A.; Danese, S.; Fagiuoli, S.; Gionchetti, P.; Annicchiarico, B.E.; D'Aversa, F.; Gasbarrini, A. Folate in Gastrointestinal Health and Disease. *Eur. Rev. Med. Pharmacol. Sci.* **2012**, *16*, 376–385. [PubMed]

55. Patwari, A.K.; Anand, V.K.; Kapur, G.; Narayan, S. Clinical and Nutritional Profile of Children with Celiac Disease. *Indian Pediatr.* **2003**, *40*, 337–342. [PubMed]

56. Kemppainen, T.A.; Kosma, V.M.; Janatuinen, E.K.; Julkunen, R.J.; Pikkarainen, P.H.; Uusitupa, M.I. Nutritional Status of Newly Diagnosed Celiac Disease Patients before and after the Institution of a Celiac Disease Diet–Association with the Grade of Mucosal Villous Atrophy. *Am. J. Clin. Nutr.* **1998**, *67*, 482–487. [CrossRef] [PubMed]

57.   Tighe, P.; Ward, M.; McNulty, H.; Finnegan, O.; Dunne, A.; Strain, J.; Molloy, A.M.; Duffy, M.; Pentieva, K.; Scott, J.M. A Dose-Finding Trial of the Effect of Long-Term Folic Acid Intervention: Implications for Food Fortification Policy. *Am. J. Clin. Nutr.* **2011**, *93*, 11–18. [CrossRef] [PubMed]

58.   Saibeni, S.; Lecchi, A.; Meucci, G.; Cattaneo, M.; Tagliabue, L.; Rondonotti, E.; Formenti, S.; De Franchis, R.; Vecchi, M. Prevalence of Hyperhomocysteinemia in Adult Gluten-Sensitive Enteropathy at Diagnosis: Role of B12, Folate, and Genetics. *Clin. Gastroenterol. Hepatol.* **2005**, *3*, 574–580. [CrossRef]

59.   Pantaleoni, S.; Luchino, M.; Adriani, A.; Pellicano, R.; Stradella, D.; Ribaldone, D.G.; Sapone, N.; Isaia, G.C.; Di Stefano, M.; Astegiano, M. Bone Mineral Density at Diagnosis of Celiac Disease and after 1 Year of Gluten-Free Diet. *Sci. World J.* **2014**, *2014*, 1–6. [CrossRef]

60.   Szymczak, J.; Bohdanowicz-Pawlak, A.; Waszczuk, E.; Jakubowska, J. Low Bone Mineral Density in Adult Patients with Coeliac Disease. *Endokrynol. Pol.* **2012**, *63*, 270–276. [CrossRef]

61.   García-Porrúa, C.; González-Gay, M.A.; Avila-Alvarenga, S.; Rivas, M.J.; Soilan, J.; Penedo, M. Coeliac Disease and Osteomalacia: An Association Still Present in Western Countries. *Rheumatology* **2000**, *39*, 1435. [CrossRef]

62.   McNicholas, B.A.; Bell, M. Coeliac Disease Causing Symptomatic Hypocalcaemia, Osteomalacia and Coagulapathy. *BMJ Case Rep.* **2010**, *2010*, bcr0920092262. [CrossRef]

63.   Sahebari, M.; Sigari, S.Y.; Heidari, H.; Biglarian, O. Osteomalacia Can Still Be a Point of Attention to Celiac Disease. *Clin. Cases Miner. Bone Metab.* **2011**, *8*, 14–15. [PubMed]

64.   Holick, M.F.; Binkley, N.C.; Bischoff-Ferrari, H.A.; Gordon, C.M.; Hanley, D.A.; Heaney, R.P.; Murad, M.H.; Weaver, C.M.; Endocrine Society. Evaluation, Treatment, and Prevention of Vitamin D Deficiency: An Endocrine Society Clinical Practice Guideline. *J. Clin. Endocrinol. Metab.* **2011**, *96*, 1911–1930. [CrossRef] [PubMed]

65.   Shab-Bidar, S.; Bours, S.; Geusens, P.P.M.M.; Kessels, A.G.H.; van den Bergh, J.P.W. Serum 25(OH)D Response to Vitamin D3 Supplementation: A Meta-Regression Analysis. *Nutrition* **2014**, *30*, 975–985. [CrossRef] [PubMed]

66.   Duerksen, D.R.; Ali, M.; Leslie, W.D. Dramatic Effect of Vitamin D Supplementation and a Gluten-Free Diet on Bone Mineral Density in a Patient with Celiac Disease. *J. Clin. Densitom.* **2012**, *15*, 120–123. [CrossRef]

67.   Muzzo, S.; Burrows, R.; Burgueño, M.; Ríos, G.; Bergenfreid, C.; Chavez, E.; Leiva, L. Effect of Calcium and Vitamin D Supplementation on Bone Mineral Density of Celiac Children. *Nutr. Res.* **2000**, *20*, 1241–1247. [CrossRef]

68.   Zanchetta, M.B.; Longobardi, V.; Bai, J.C. Bone and Celiac Disease. *Curr. Osteoporos. Rep.* **2016**, *14*, 43–48. [CrossRef] [PubMed]

69.   Krupa-Kozak, U. Pathologic Bone Alterations in Celiac Disease: Etiology, Epidemiology, and Treatment. *Nutrition* **2014**, *30*, 16–24. [CrossRef] [PubMed]

70.   Kavak, U.S.; Yüce, A.; Kocak, N.; Demir, H.; Saltik, I.N.; Gürakan, F.; Ozen, H. Bone Mineral Density in Children with Untreated and Treated Celiac Disease. *J. Pediatr. Gastroenterol. Nutr.* **2003**, *37*, 434–436. [CrossRef] [PubMed]

71.   Staun, M.; Jarnum, S. Measurement of the 10,000-Molecular Weight Calcium-Binding Protein in Small-Intestinal Biopsy Specimens from Patients with Malabsorption Syndromes. *Scand. J. Gastroenterol.* **1988**, *23*, 827–832. [CrossRef]

72.   Pazianas, M.; Butcher, G.P.; Subhani, J.M.; Finch, P.J.; Ang, L.; Collins, C.; Heaney, R.P.; Zaidi, M.; Maxwell, J.D. Calcium Absorption and Bone Mineral Density in Celiacs after Long Term Treatment with Gluten-Free Diet and Adequate Calcium Intake. *Osteoporos. Int.* **2005**, *16*, 56–63. [CrossRef]

73.   Larussa, T.; Suraci, E.; Nazionale, I.; Leone, I.; Montalcini, T.; Abenavoli, L.; Imeneo, M.; Pujia, A.; Luzza, F. No Evidence of Circulating Autoantibodies against Osteoprotegerin in Patients with Celiac Disease. *World J. Gastroenterol.* **2012**, *18*, 1622–1627. [CrossRef] [PubMed]

74.   Larussa, T.; Suraci, E.; Imeneo, M.; Marasco, R.; Luzza, F. Normal Bone Mineral Density Associates with Duodenal Mucosa Healing in Adult Patients with Celiac Disease on a Gluten-Free Diet. *Nutrients* **2017**, *9*, 98. [CrossRef] [PubMed]

75.   Rujner, J.; Socha, J.; Syczewska, M.; Wojtasik, A.; Kunachowicz, H.; Stolarczyk, A. Magnesium Status in Children and Adolescents with Coeliac Disease without Malabsorption Symptoms. *Clin. Nutr.* **2004**, *23*, 1074–1079. [CrossRef] [PubMed]

76. Breedon, C. Medical Center Aunt Cathy's Guide to: Thinking About OTHER Nutrition Issues in Celiac Disease. Available online: http://www.mnsna.org/wp-content/uploads/2010/07/Aunt-C-Celiac-Disease-short-OtherNutr-Issues-Sanf-this-12-no-date.pdf (accessed on 3 July 2019).

77. Stazi, A.V.; Trinti, B. Selenium Status and Over-Expression of Interleukin-15 in Celiac Disease and Autoimmune Thyroid Diseases. *Ann. Ist. Super. Sanita* **2010**, *46*, 389–399. [CrossRef] [PubMed]

78. Hinks, L.J.; Inwards, K.D.; Lloyd, B.; Clayton, B.E. Body Content of Selenium in Coeliac Disease. *Br. Med. J.* **1984**, *288*, 1862–1863. [CrossRef]

79. Faerber Emily Community Rotation. Selenium Supplement Information for Your Gluten-Free Patients. 2011. Available online: http://depts.washington.edu/nutr/wordpress/wp-content/uploads/2015/03/Selenium_2012.pdf (accessed on 3 July 2019).

80. Mager, D.R.; Qiao, J.; Turner, J. Vitamin D and K Status Influences Bone Mineral Density and Bone Accrual in Children and Adolescents with Celiac Disease. *Eur. J. Clin. Nutr.* **2012**, *66*, 488–495. [CrossRef]

81. Shepherd, S.J.; Gibson, P.R. Nutritional Inadequacies of the Gluten-Free Diet in Both Recently-Diagnosed and Long-Term Patients with Coeliac Disease. *J. Hum. Nutr. Diet.* **2013**, *26*, 349–358. [CrossRef]

82. Thompson, T. Thiamin, Riboflavin, and Niacin Contents of the Gluten-Free Diet: Is There Cause for Concern? *J. Am. Diet. Assoc.* **1999**, *99*, 858–862. [CrossRef]

16

There is no Association between Coeliac Disease and Autoimmune Pancreatitis

Giulia De Marchi [1], **Giovanna Zanoni** [2], **Maria Cristina Conti Bellocchi** [1], **Elena Betti** [3], **Monica Brentegani** [2], **Paola Capelli** [4], **Valeria Zuliani** [1], **Luca Frulloni** [1], **Catherine Klersy** [5] and **Rachele Ciccocioppo** [1,*]

[1] Gastroenterology Unit, Department of Medicine, AOUI Policlinico G.B. Rossi, University of Verona; Piazzale L.A. Scuro, 10, 37134 Verona, Italy; giuli.dema@yahoo.it (G.D.M.); mcristina.contibellocchi@gmail.com (M.C.C.B.); valeria.zuliani@univr.it (V.Z.); luca.frulloni@univr.it (L.F.)

[2] Immunology Unit, Department of Pathology and Diagnostics, AOUI Policlinico G.B. Rossi, Piazzale L.A. Scuro, 10, 37134 Verona, Italy; giovanna.zanoni@aovr.veneto.it (G.Z.); monica.brentegani@aovr.veneto.it (M.B.)

[3] Clinica Medica I, Department of Internal Medicine, IRCCS Policlinico San Matteo Foundation, Piazzale Golgi, 19, 27100 Pavia, Italy; elena.betti19@gmail.com

[4] Pathology Unit, Department of Pathology and Diagnostics, AOUI Policlinico G.B. Rossi, Piazzale L.A. Scuro, 10, 37134 Verona, Italy; paola.capelli@aovr.veneto.it

[5] Clinical Epidemiology & Biometry Unit, IRCCS Fondazione Policlinico San Matteo; Viale Golgi 19, 27100 Pavia, Italy; klersy@smatteo.pv.it

* Correspondence: rachele.ciccocioppo@univr.it

Abstract: Autoimmune pancreatitis (AIP) is a rare disorder whose association with coeliac disease (CD) has never been investigated, although CD patients display a high prevalence of both endocrine and exocrine pancreatic affections. Therefore, we sought to evaluate the frequency of CD in patients with AIP and in further medical pancreatic disorders. The screening for CD was carried out through the detection of tissue transglutaminase (tTG) autoantibodies in sera of patients retrospectively enrolled and divided in four groups: AIP, chronic pancreatitis, chronic asymptomatic pancreatic hyperenzymemia (CAPH), and control subjects with functional dyspepsia. The search for anti-endomysium autoantibodies was performed in those cases with borderline or positive anti-tTG values. Duodenal biopsy was offered to all cases showing positive results. One patient out of 72 (1.4%) with AIP had already been diagnosed with CD and was following a gluten-free diet, while one case out of 71 (1.4%) with chronic pancreatitis and one out of 92 (1.1%) control subjects were diagnosed with de novo CD. No cases of CD were detected in the CAPH group. By contrast, a high prevalence of cases with ulcerative colitis was found in the AIP group (13.8%). Despite a mutual association between CD and several autoimmune disorders, our data do not support the serologic screening for CD in AIP. Further studies will clarify the usefulness of CD serologic screening in other pancreatic disorders.

Keywords: autoimmune pancreatitis; coeliac disease; pancreatic disorders; screening

1. Introduction

Coeliac disease (CD) is an autoimmune condition affecting the small bowel mucosa of a proportion of subjects carrying the human leukocyte antigen (HLA)-DQ2 or -DQ8 haplotypes upon gluten ingestion [1]. Its prevalence, as assessed by serologic tests, is 0.4% in South America, 0.5% in Africa and North America, 0.6% in Asia, and 0.8% in Europe and Oceania, with higher values in female versus male individuals (0.6% vs. 0.4%; $p < 0.001$) [2]. The intestinal lesions encompass a variable degree of villous atrophy and crypt hyperplasia, with a heavy lymphocytic infiltrate of both the epithelial and lamina propria layers (Figure 1) [3]. The clinical picture is multifaceted, ranging from an overt malabsorption syndrome to apparently asymptomatic forms, with anaemia, isolated fatigue, cryptic hypertransaminasaemia, infertility, peripheral and central neurologic disorders, osteopenia, short stature, and dental enamel defects, being the main findings [1,4]. A gluten-free diet leads to an almost complete recovery of both mucosal lesions and clinical features in the vast majority of cases [1]. Remarkably, owing the same genetic and/or environmental predisposing factors, CD patients are at risk of developing further systemic or organ-specific immune-mediated disorders, with type 1 diabetes being the most prevalent and widely studied association, thus justifying the mutual serologic screening [5]. By contrast, no information about the possible association between CD and autoimmune pancreatitis (AIP), the immune-mediated condition affecting the exocrine component of the pancreas, is available so far.

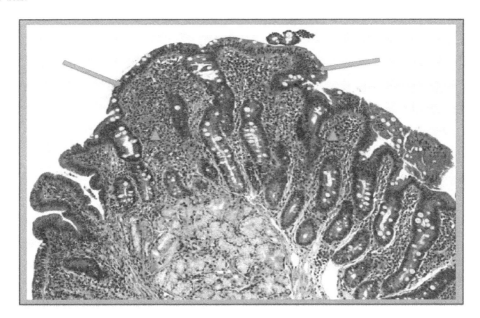

Figure 1. Histological features of duodenal mucosa of active coeliac disease showing subtotal villous atrophy with crypt hyperplasia and heavy lymphocytic inflammatory infiltrate in both the epithelial (arrows) and lamina propria (head arrows) compartments (hematoxylin-eosin, original magnification × 100).

AIP is a rare (estimated prevalence of 0.82:100,000 [6]), chronic fibro-inflammatory condition affecting the whole or a part of the gland, characterized by specific histological, radiological and serological aspects that disappear following a course of steroid therapy [7]. Two different types of AIP (type 1 and type 2) can be distinguished histologically. The first is the so called lymphoplasmacytic sclerosing pancreatitis displaying a dense periductal infiltration of plasma cells, mainly immunoglobulin (Ig)G4 positive, and lymphocytes, peculiar storiform fibrosis, and oblitering venulitis (Figure 2). The second, also called idiopathic duct-centric pancreatitis, is characterized by the presence of intraluminal and intraepithelial neutrophils in medium-sized and small ducts as well as in acini, often leading to destruction and obliteration of the duct lumen. However, the diagnosis of type 1 or type 2 AIP can be made even in the absence of histology by applying a combination of two or more of the following International Consensus Diagnostic Criteria [8]: (1) characteristic imaging features of both the parenchyma and main duct, i.e., a diffuse enlargement with delayed enhancement of the parenchyma with a long or multiple duct strictures without marked upstream dilatation in the typical form, while a segmental/focal enlargement with delayed enhancement of the parenchyma with segmental short duct narrowing in the atypical one; (2) increased level of IgG4; (3) other organ involvement, i.e., biliary duct, retroperitoneum, kidneys, salivary/lachrymal gland, as assessed histologically or radiologically; (4) response to steroid therapy. In those cases where distinctive criteria cannot be identified, the diagnosis of AIP not otherwise specified is given.

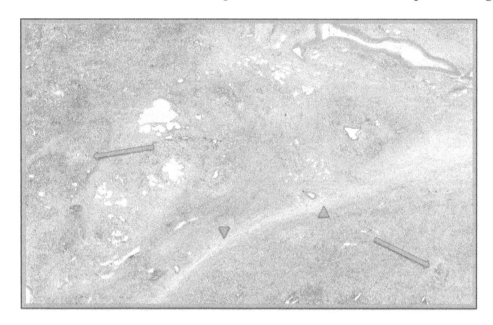

Figure 2. Histological features of autoimmune pancreatitis showing a dense periductal infiltration of plasma cells and lymphocytes leading to obliteration of the affected veins (**arrows**), and peculiar storiform fibrosis (**head arrows**) (hematoxylin-eosin, original magnification × 100).

At variance with AIP, some evidence is available in the literature about the association between CD and non-immune-mediated disorders of the exocrine pancreas. Indeed, CD patients have been found to be at increased risk of developing both acute and chronic pancreatitis in comparison to the general population [9,10]. In addition, patients with villous atrophy, including CD, may carry an exocrine pancreatic insufficiency [11]. Finally, asymptomatic pancreatic hyperamylasemia, which usually precedes the diagnosis of CD and often disappears following a gluten-free diet, has been also described [12]. Similarly, macroamylasemia, a benign condition caused by circulating complexes of pancreatic or salivary amylases bound to plasma proteins that cannot be cleared by the renal glomeruli, has also been described in adulthood CD, but it possibly decreases or resolves after a strict gluten-free diet [13].

The aim of this study, therefore, was to establish the prevalence of CD in patients suffering from AIP by using the sera collected in the Biobank of a Tertiary Italian referral centre for pancreatic diseases. This gave us the unique opportunity to include also patients with non-immune-mediated pancreatic disorders, i.e., chronic pancreatitis and chronic asymptomatic pancreatic hyperenzymemia (CAPH), as control diseased groups, other than control subjects.

2. Patients and Methods

2.1. Study Population

Four groups of adult patients not taking steroids or immunosuppressive therapy at the time of blood sample harvest were enrolled in this study, as detailed below:

Group 1 (AIP). The sera of 72 out of 259 patients diagnosed with AIP (type 1 n = 43, type 2 n = 16, not otherwise specified n = 13) according to the International Consensus Diagnostic Criteria [8] were collected at the Pancreas Institute of the Policlinico G.B. Rossi (AOUI and University of Verona, Italy), from January 2003 through December 2017. Specifically, 40 out of 43 with type 1 AIP (93%), 2 out of 16 with type 2 AIP (12.5%), and 0 out of 13 with not otherwise specified AIP (0%) displayed IgG4 positivity.

Group 2 (chronic pancreatitis). A cohort of 71 out of 492 patients diagnosed with chronic pancreatitis from January 2012 to December 2017 was included in the study. The diagnostic criteria, as adapted following our experience, included at least one of the following criteria: (1) presence of pancreatic-type pain, history of acute/recurrent pancreatitis, presence of steatorrhea or diabetes, weight loss; (2) imaging findings of pancreatic parenchyma atrophy, main pancreatic duct dilation >6 mm and/or presence of irregularities, secondary ducts dilation, presence of pancreatic calcifications; (3) laboratory findings of decreased level of faecal elastase-1 (<100 μg/g of stool), glycated haemoglobin >6.5%; (4) histological features of chronic pancreatitis (loss of acinar cells, presence of interlobular fibrosis, infiltration of inflammatory cells and relative conservation of intralobular ducts and islets) in surgical specimens [14].

Group 3 (CAPH). This group comprised 32 out of 160 patients who were found with CAPH from January 2012 to December 2017. The diagnosis was made when the serum levels of lipases and/or pancreatic amylases were found above the upper normal limits (>10%) for at least three consecutive times lasting for more than six months in the absence of pancreatic-type pain [15]. Moreover, in all cases no lesions of the parenchyma and/or the ductal system were evident at the magnetic resonance of the abdomen with cholangiopancreatography sequences.

Group 4 (control subjects). The serum samples of a cohort of 92 patients suffering from functional dyspepsia, as assessed following the Rome III criteria [16], were collected from June 2012 to December 2016. The presence of relevant co-morbidities, such as primary immunodeficiencies, cancer, active infections or organ failure, was considered an exclusion criterion.

The demographic and clinical features of the study groups are listed in Table 1.

Table 1. Demographic and clinical features of the study population.

	Autoimmune Pancreatitis	Chronic Pancreatitis	Chronic Pancreatic Hyperenzymemia	Control Subjects
Number of cases	72	71	32	92
Male/female ratio	55/17	57/14	18/14	48/44
Mean age in years (SD)	56.5 (16.9)	55.1 (13.2)	52.7 (14.6)	45.7 (18.3)
Body mass index: kg/m^2 (mean ± SD)	25.1 ± 4.1	23.2 ± 5.7	24.9 ± 4.4	22.7 ± 5.2
Time from diagnosis in months (mean ± SD)	25.4 ± 29.3	81 ± 37.5	n.a.	n.a.
Concomitant autoimmune disorders: IBD	13 (10 UC)	1 (Crohn)	0	1 (UC)
Thyroiditis	5	1	1	2
Psoriasis	3	0	0	1
Asthma	1	2	0	2
Coeliac disease	1 *	0	0	0
Rheumatic diseases	2	1	0	3
Thrombocytopenia	1	0	0	0

Abbreviation: SD: Standard Deviation; IBD: inflammatory bowel disease; n.a.: not applicable; UC: ulcerative colitis.
* case already diagnosed with coeliac disease.

The Biobank of the Pancreas Institute, Policlinico G.B. Rossi, AOUI and University of Verona, Italy had been previously approved by the local Ethics Committee (Protocol number 5604, 2 February 2012). This study was approved by the local Ethics Committee (Protocol number 49061, 7 July 2018) and each enrolled patient gave written informed consent.

2.2. Screening for Coeliac Disease

Detection of tissue transglutaminase (tTG) IgA antibody was performed by using a commercial Elisa test (Eu-tTG®IgA kit, Eurospital, Trieste, Italy; cut-off levels: negative < 9 U/mL, borderline 9–15 U/mL, positive > 15 U/mL). Patients with borderline or positive tTG IgA results underwent investigation for IgA anti-endomysium antibodies (EMA-IgA), which was performed by indirect immunofluorescent technique (Eurospital), according to the manufacturer's instructions. Sera with low tTG IgA levels (<1 U/mL) were also evaluated by tTG IgG antibody determination (Eu-tTG®IgG kit, Eurospital, Trieste, Italy; cut-off levels: negative < 20 U/mL, positive ≥ 20 U/mL).

Duodenal mucosal sampling was offered to all cases with positive tTG-IgA and/or EMA-IgA. Four biopsies from the second part of the duodenum and two from the bulb were taken during upper endoscopy for the histological examination according to the Corazza–Villanacci classification [3].

2.3. Statistical Analysis

Continuous variables were expressed as the mean and standard deviation (SD). Discrete data were tabulated as numbers and percentages. The prevalence of CD was computed, together with its 95% exact binomial confidence intervals (95% CI) overall, for pancreatic disorders as a whole and by diagnostic group. Stata 15 (StataCorp, College Station, TX, USA) was used for computation.

3. Results

A total of 267 serum samples harvested from 178 males and 89 females (mean age: 51.8 years, range: 18–85) were included in this study, with 175 being from patients with pancreatic disorders and 92 from control subjects with functional dyspepsia. Worth of note, a large prevalence of males was found in both AIP and chronic pancreatitis groups, accordingly with literature data [7,17], whereas a similar proportion of both genders was observed in the other two groups. As shown in Table 1, one case out of 72 patients of group 1 (1.4%), who was diagnosed with type 1 AIP, had already received the diagnosis of CD two years earlier because of unexplained hypertransaminasemia and weight loss. Since then, he was following a strict gluten-free diet with full recovery of laboratory and clinical features. Therefore, his CD serology resulted negative, and a normal mucosal architecture was found at histology (see Table 2). The radiological findings that led to the diagnosis of AIP type 1, together with a high level of IgG4, are shown in Figure 3. The serologic screening did not detect any further case of CD among patients affected by AIP. However, in two cases a search for tTG-IgG was carried out because of a very low level of tTG-IgA (less than 1.0 U/mL), giving negative results (4.34 and 6.25 U/mL). Remarkably, a consistent number of patients with AIP (13 out 72, 20.8%, of whom three had type 1 and 10 had type 2 AIP) was also affected by inflammatory bowel disease, mostly ulcerative colitis (10 out of 13 cases, while two had indeterminate colitis and one had Crohn's disease). Specifically, one case was diagnosed with ulcerative colitis and AIP simultaneously, whereas the diagnosis of ulcerative colitis preceded that of AIP by a median interval of 28 months (range, 3 to 67 months) in the remaining patients. The vast majority of ulcerative colitis patients (eight out of 10) were not taking systemic corticosteroids at the time of diagnosis of AIP, although they had previously undergone this therapy; only a small proportion of them (three out of 10) was under biological agents (anti-tumour necrosis factor monoclonal antibody). Also, one patient amongst the 71 with chronic pancreatitis (1.4%) showed a positive value of both tTG-IgA antibodies, although at low titre (15,875 U/mL), and EMA-IgA at 1:5 dilution. The histologic examination of the duodenal biopsies showed the characteristic lesions, thus confirming the diagnosis of CD (see Table 2), and the patient was willing to start a gluten-free diet. When collecting his clinical history, aphthous stomatitis appeared evident. One further case was found within the group of patients with functional dyspepsia (1.1%), displaying positivity for both tTG-IgA (value 123 U/mL) and EMA-IgA at 1:16 dilution, thus leading to a definitive diagnosis of CD upon the demonstration of the characteristic lesions at histologic examination of the duodenal biopsies (see Table 2). Interestingly, she complained of infertility. An additional two cases in this group showed borderline values of tTG-IgA (12.44 and 13.47 U/mL) but was negative for the EMA test; hence, they did not undergo endoscopy, whereas in four cases a search for tTG-IgG was carried out because of a very low level of tTG-IgA (less than 1.0 U/mL), giving negative results (5.42, 5.73, 5.8, 8.15 U/mL). By contrast, no cases of positive CD serology were detected among the 32 patients with CAPH (mean value of tTG-IgA: 2.93 U/mL, range 1.276–7.537 U/mL). Therefore, as shown in

Table 2, a total of three cases were identified to suffer from CD (two active and one treated) in the study population; that prevalence was similar in patients with pancreatic disorders and control subjects (overall prevalence 1.1%). Confidence intervals were consistent and ranged from 0% to about 10% in the single diagnostic groups and up to 4% in aggregated diagnoses.

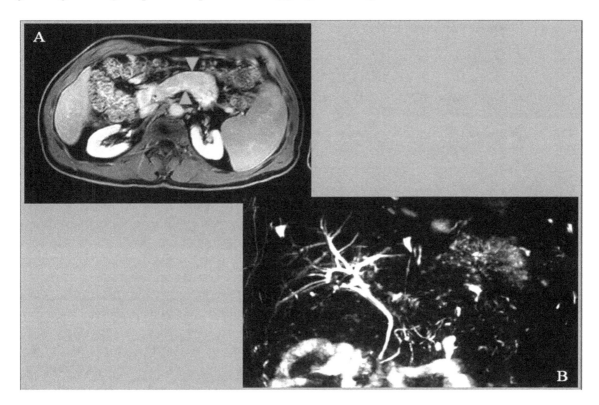

Figure 3. Abdominal magnetic resonance scan showing a diffuse enlargement of the body of the pancreas, with a "sausage-like" aspect (**A**), and multiple long stenosis of the main pancreatic duct at the cholangiopancreatography sequences (**B**).

Table 2. Cases with positive results at the serological screening with their histological findings.

	N	tTG IgA	tTg IgG	EMA	Histology [§]	Prevalence (95% CI)
Group 1	72	0	0	0	Grade A lesions *	1.4% (0.0–7.5)
Group 2	71	1	0	1	Grade B1 lesions	2.4% (0.0–7.6)
Group 3	32	0	0	0	Not performed	0% (0.0–10.9)
Group 4	92	1 + 2 borderline	0	1	Grade B2 lesions	1.1% (0.0–5.9)
Pancreatic disorders	175	1	0	1	–	1.1% (0.1–4.1)
Total	267	2	0	2	3	1.1% (0.2–3.2)

Abbreviations. EMA: anti-endomysium autoantibody; IgA: class A immunoglobulin; IgG: class G immunoglobulin; N: number of cases; tTG: tissue transglutaminase. [§] Following the Corazza–Villanacci classification [3]. * case already diagnosed with coeliac disease.

4. Discussion

Limited information is available about the occurrence of exocrine pancreatic disorders during the course of CD [18], while strong evidence demonstrates an association between CD and type 1 diabetes [5,19]. In fact, approximately 90% of patients with type 1 diabetes carry either HLA-DQ2 or -DQ8 haplotypes as compared to 30% of the general population [20], with those diabetic cases homozygous for DR3-DQ2 having a 33% risk for the presence of tTG autoantibodies [21]. This is why the heterodimers encoded by these HLA haplotypes efficiently bind negatively charged peptides derived from gliadin upon tTG deamidation, thus eliciting a T- and B-cell mediated immune response [22]. This, in turn, leads to an upregulation of key pro-inflammatory molecules, such as interferon-γ [23] and interleukin (IL)-21 [24], responsible for tissue damage. It has also been suggested that dietary gluten could be involved in the pathogenesis of type 1 diabetes [25]. Conversely, a gluten-free diet largely prevented diabetes onset in non-obese diabetic mice, possibly through a modification of the gut microbiota [26].

However, autoimmune attack against the pancreas may involve not only the endocrine component, but also the exocrine one, giving rise to AIP. This is the pancreatic manifestation of the IgG4-related disease, whose genetic susceptibility and pathogenic mechanisms are still poorly understood [7]. Nonetheless, almost all of the candidate genes are directly or indirectly implicated in the regulation of the immune response [7]. A further aspect supporting an autoimmune background is the large proportion of AIP patients displaying autoantibodies, mostly against enzymes, such as lactoferrin, carbonic anhydrases, pancreatic secretory trypsin inhibitor, and trypsinogens [27,28]. Even CD is characterized by the presence of autoantibodies against a ubiquitous enzyme, tTG2, which, besides being the main autoantigen and target of the anti-endomysium autoantibodies [29], catalyses a specific and ordered deamidation of gliadin peptides, giving rise to immunodominant epitopes [22]. In addition, tTG2 seems to play a crucial role in the development of secondary autoimmunity through a post-translational modification of additional proteins, leading to the generation of neoantigens [30]. Also of note, transgenic HLA-DQ8 mice, grown in germ-free conditions and fed a gluten-free diet, developed acute pancreatitis after intra-peritoneal injection of cerulein, a cholecystokinin analogue that causes hyperstimulation of the exocrine component [31]. Whether or not gliadin was then introduced in the diet of these mice, an increased level of IgG1 (homologous of human IgG4) was observed, together with a histological pattern resembling that of human AIP [31]. Moreover, an increased level of serum IgG4 was documented in patients suffering from both CD and pancreatic exocrine insufficiency [32], while an increased number of IgG4+ cells was occasionally found at the mucosal levels of CD patients [33]. Finally, it is conceivable that the mucosal dysbiosis found in CD patients [34] might also contribute to an autoimmune attack in close organs, like the pancreas.

Despite these hypotheses, only one case suffering from both CD and AIP has been reported so far [35], thus we sought to investigate a putative association between these two immune-mediated conditions, taking advantage of the sera collected at the Biobank of a Tertiary Referral centre for pancreatic diseases. We found one patient among the 72 AIP patients who had already received the diagnosis of CD two years earlier. Therefore, the same prevalence of CD in AIP as that of the general population [2] was evident (1.4%). This also suggests that a gluten-free diet does not protect against the development of AIP. One possible explanation may lie in the different genetic predisposition since, at least in the Japanese population, an association of the DRB1*0405-DQB1*0401 haplotype with AIP was found [36], whereas CD is associated with the HLA-DQ2 and -DQ8 ones [1,5]. Moreover, unlike classic autoimmune diseases in which T-cells with regulatory effect are defective in number and/or function, they are likely activated in AIP. Indeed, an increased rate of transcription factor Forkhead box P3+CD4+CD25+ T-cells in both pancreatic tissue [37] and peripheral blood [38] was found in AIP patients, together with upregulation of two cytokines with modulatory functions, i.e., IL-10 and transforming growth factor-β [7]. These seem to be key molecules since the former contributes to IgG4 class switching [39], while the latter is involved in the development of fibrosis [40].

At variance with CD, a strong association between AIP and IBD (18.0% of cases), mostly ulcerative colitis (13.9%), has been found in our cohort of Caucasian patients, thus confirming previous reports [41,42]. However, the prevalence was higher than that found in either an American [41] or an Asiatic [42] study, where a frequency of 5.6% and 5.8%, respectively, was found. Likewise, both have a retrospective design and a similar sample size (71 and 104 AIP cases, respectively) [41,42].

However, the tools applied for the diagnosis of AIP were different, since the HISORt criteria for AIP [43] were used in the former, whereas the Asian Diagnostic Criteria for AIP [44] were used in the latter, thus possibly affecting the final results. The discrepancy may also be partly related to ethnic differences and to the relatively small number of patients recruited. Interestingly, the course of ulcerative colitis was worst in those suffering from both diseases since, during the follow-up period of 10 years, 33.3% of patients underwent a colectomy versus none of those suffering from ulcerative colitis alone [42]. Finally, although Berkson's bias (patients with two uncommon diseases are more likely to be referred to a tertiary medical centre than patients with just one such disease) [45] could have inflated the magnitude of this association, our data strongly suggest that the AIP and ulcerative colitis are related to some degree whose extent deserves further investigation.

As far as the non-immune-mediated pancreatic disorders are concerned, it is widely acknowledged that both functional and anatomical changes of the gland may be caused by or coexist with CD [18]. A Swedish register study, indeed, found an increased risk of both acute and chronic pancreatitis in patients with adulthood CD during the observational period of 1964 to 2003 [9]. Furthermore, it was estimated that over 20% of patients with CD have defective exocrine pancreatic function [10]. This seems to be related to an impaired secretion of cholecystokinin pancreozymin secondary to enteropathy and/or malnutrition, since normalization of both intestinal mucosa and nutritional status restores the secretion of digestive hormones and enzymes [46]. Nevertheless, no information on the prevalence of CD in non-immune-mediated pancreatic disorders is available so far. We found one case in the chronic pancreatitis group (1.4%) and one in the control subject group (1.1%), again overlapping with the prevalence in the general population [2]. Thus, despite a relationship between CD and pancreatic disorders having been demonstrated, the opposite does not seem true. Accordingly, we did not find any positivity at the serologic screening for CD in the CAPH group, even though an abnormal elevation of serum amylase and/or lipase was found in CD patients but disappeared upon a course of gluten-free diet [12].

Obviously, our study has strengths and weaknesses. A point of strength is that this is the first study investigating the prevalence of CD in patients suffering from pancreatic disorders, whereas the studies published so far did the opposite. Moreover, if we consider that AIP is a rare and difficult-to-diagnose condition, the large sample size available, together with the appropriateness of the diagnosis, put us in a privileged situation where the putative higher prevalence of CD in this clinical setting might have been demonstrated, if there was any. The limitations include the retrospective design and the small sample size (and thus the relatively large confidence intervals) of the CAPH and chronic pancreatitis groups in comparison with the overall institutional cohorts due to the low level of willingness to give serum samples for future unknown studies, whereas the lack of sex and age matching among AIP and chronic pancreatitis patients with CAPH and control cases was largely expected [7,47]. In addition, serum IgG or IgG4 levels were not available in non-AIP groups because they are not routinely measured. Despite these limitations, our cohort of 72 patients with AIP represents one of the largest single-centre experiments to date.

5. Conclusions

In summary, our findings suggest that there is a low probability of there being an association of CD with AIP, thus serological screening for CD is not recommended in patients with AIP. By contrast, a strong association between AIP and ulcerative colitis appears evident. AIP is a relatively "new" diagnostic entity, thus further prospective and multicentre studies are needed to confirm the conclusions of this study.

Author Contributions: Conceptualization, R.C.; data curation, G.D.M. and E.B.; formal analysis, C.K., V.Z. and L.F.; funding acquisition, R.C.; investigation, R.C.; methodology, G.Z. and M.B.; project administration, M.C.C.B.; resources, P.C.; supervision, L.F.; validation, R.C.; writing—original draft, G.D.M.; writing—review & editing, C.K. and R.C.

Abbreviations

AIP	autoimmune pancreatitis
CD	coeliac disease
CAPH	chronic asymptomatic pancreatic hyperenzymemia
CI	confidence interval
EMA	anti-endomysium antibodies
HLA	human leukocyte antigen
Ig	immunoglobulin
SD	standard deviation
tTG	tissue transglutaminase

References

1. Lebwohl, B.; Sanders, D.S.; Green, P.H.R. Coeliac disease. *Lancet* **2018**, *391*, 70–81. [CrossRef]
2. Singh, P.; Arora, A.; Strand, T.A.; Leffler, D.A.; Catassi, C.; Green, P.H.; Kelly, C.P.; Ahuja, V.; Makharia, G.K. Global prevalence of celiac disease: Systematic review and meta-analysis. *Clin. Gastroenterol. Hepatol.* **2018**, *16*, 823–836. [CrossRef] [PubMed]
3. Corazza, G.R.; Villanacci, V.; Zambelli, C.; Milione, M.; Luinetti, O.; Vindigni, C.; Chioda, C.; Albarello, L.; Bartolini, D.; Donato, F. Comparison of the interobserver reproducibility with different histologic criteria used in celiac disease. *Clin. Gastroenterol. Hepatol.* **2007**, *5*, 838–843. [CrossRef] [PubMed]
4. Leffler, D.A.; Green, P.H.R.; Fasano, A. Extraintestinal manifestations of coeliac disease. *Nat. Rev. Gastroenterol Hepatol.* **2015**, *12*, 561–571. [CrossRef] [PubMed]
5. Lundin, K.E.A.; Wijmenga, C. Coeliac disease and autoimmune disease—Genetic overlap and screening. *Nat. Rev. Gastroenterol. Hepatol.* **2015**, *12*, 507–515. [CrossRef] [PubMed]
6. Uchida, K.; Masamune, A.; Shimosegawa, T.; Okazaki, K. Prevalence of IgG4-related disease in Japan based on nationwide survey in 2009. *Int. J. Rheumatol.* **2012**, *2012*, 358371. [CrossRef] [PubMed]
7. Hart, P.A.; Zen, Y.; Chari, S.T. Recent advances in autoimmune pancreatitis. *Gastroenterology* **2015**, *149*, 39–51. [CrossRef] [PubMed]
8. Shimosegawa, T.; Chari, S.T.; Frulloni, L.; Kamisawa, T.; Kawa, S.; Mino-Kenudson, M.; Kim, M.H.; Kloppel, G.; Lerch, M.M.; Lohr, M.; et al. International consensus diagnostic criteria for autoimmune pancreatitis: Guidelines of the International Association of Pancreatology. *Pancreas* **2011**, *40*, 352–358. [CrossRef] [PubMed]
9. Ludvigsson, J.F.; Montgomery, S.M.; Ekbom, A. Risk of pancreatitis in 14,000 individuals with celiac disease. *Clin. Gastroenterol. Hepatol.* **2007**, *5*, 1347–1353. [CrossRef] [PubMed]
10. Sadr-Azodi, O.; Sanders, D.S.; Murray, J.A.; Ludvigsson, J.F. Patients with celiac disease have an increased risk for pancreatitis. *Clin. Gastroenterol. Hepatol.* **2012**, *10*, 1136–1142. [CrossRef] [PubMed]
11. Walkowiak, J.; Herzig, K.H. Fecal elastase-1 is decreased in villous atrophy regardless of the underlying disease. *Eur. J. Clin. Investig.* **2001**, *31*, 425–430. [CrossRef]
12. Carroccio, A.; Di Prima, L.; Scalici, C.; Soresi, M.; Cefalù, A.B.; Noto, D.; Averna, M.R.; Montalto, G.; Iacono, G. Unexplained elevated serum pancreatic enzymes: A reason to suspect celiac disease. *Clin. Gastroenterol. Hepatol.* **2006**, *4*, 455–459. [CrossRef] [PubMed]
13. Rajvanshi, P.; Chowdhury, J.R.; Gupta, S. Celiac sprue and macroamylasaemia: Potential clinical and pathophysiological implications. Case study. *J. Clin. Gastroenterol.* **1995**, *20*, 304–306. [CrossRef] [PubMed]
14. Duggan, S.N.; Nì Chonchubhair, H.M.; Lawal, O.; O'Connor, D.B.; Conlon, K.C. Chronic pancreatitis: A diagnostic dilemma. *World J. Gastroenterol.* **2016**, *22*, 2304–2313. [CrossRef] [PubMed]
15. Amodio, A.; Manfredi, R.; Katsotourchi, A.M.; Gabbrielli, A.; Benini, L.; Mucelli, R.P.; Vantini, I.; Frulloni, L. Prospective evaluation of subjects with chronic asymptomatic pancreatic hyperenzymemia. *Am. J. Gastroenterol.* **2012**, *107*, 1089–1095. [CrossRef] [PubMed]
16. Longstreth, G.F.; Thompson, W.G.; Chey, W.D.; Houghton, L.A.; Mearin, F.; Spiller, R.C. Functional bowel disorders. *Gastroenterology* **2006**, *130*, 1480–1491. [CrossRef] [PubMed]
17. Yadav, D.; Lowenfels, A.B. The epidemiology of pancreatitis and pancreatic cancer. *Gastroenterology* **2013**, *144*, 1252–1261. [CrossRef] [PubMed]

18. Pezzilli, R. Exocrine pancreas involvement in celiac disease: A review. *Recent. Pat. Inflamm. Allergy Drug Discov.* **2014**, *8*, 167–172. [CrossRef] [PubMed]

19. Weiss, B.; Pinhas-Hamiel, O. Celiac disease and diabetes: When to test and treat. *J. Pediatr. Gastroenterol. Nutr.* **2017**, *64*, 175–179. [CrossRef] [PubMed]

20. Smyth, D.J.; Plagnol, V.; Walker, N.M.; Cooper, J.D.; Downes, K.; Yang, J.H.; Howson, J.M.; Stevens, H.; McManus, R.; Wijmenga, C.; et al. Shared and distinct genetic variants in type 1 diabetes and celiac disease. *N. Engl. J. Med.* **2008**, *359*, 2767–2777. [CrossRef] [PubMed]

21. Bao, F.; Yu, L.; Babu, S.; Wang, T.; Hoffenberg, E.J.; Rewers, M.; Eisenbarth, G.S. One third of HLA DQ2 homozygous patients with type 1 diabetes express celiac disease associated transglutaminase autoantibodies. *J. Autoimmun.* **1999**, *13*, 143–148. [CrossRef] [PubMed]

22. Stamnaes, J.; Sollid, L.M. Celiac disease: Autoimmunity in response to food antigen. *Semin. Immunol.* **2015**, *27*, 343–352. [CrossRef] [PubMed]

23. Nilsen, E.M.; Lundin, K.E.; Krajci, P.; Scott, H.; Sollid, L.M.; Brandtzaeg, P. Gluten specific, HLA-DQ restricted T cells from coeliac mucosa produce cytokines with Th1 or Th0 profile dominated by interferon gamma. *Gut* **1995**, *37*, 766–776. [CrossRef] [PubMed]

24. Fina, D.; Sarra, M.; Caruso, R.; Del Vecchio Blanco, G.; Pallone, F.; MacDonald, T.T.; Monteleone, G. Interleukin-21 contributes to the mucosal T helper cell type 1 response in coeliac disease. *Gut* **2008**, *57*, 887–892. [CrossRef] [PubMed]

25. Troncone, R.; Discepolo, V. Celiac disease and autoimmunity. *J. Pediatr. Gastroenterol. Nutr.* **2014**, *59*, S9–S11. [CrossRef] [PubMed]

26. Marietta, E.V.; Gomez, A.M.; Yeoman, C.; Tilahun, A.Y.; Clark, C.R.; Luckey, D.H.; Murray, J.A.; White, B.A.; Kudva, Y.C.; Rajagopalan, G. Low incidence of spontaneous type 1 diabetes in non-obese diabetic mice raised on gluten-free diets is associated with changes in the intestinal microbiome. *PLoS ONE* **2013**, *8*, e78687. [CrossRef] [PubMed]

27. Okazaki, K.; Uchida, K.; Ohana, M.; Nakase, H.; Uose, S.; Inai, M.; Matsushima, Y.; Katamura, K.; Ohmori, K.; Chiba, T. Autoimmune-related pancreatitis is associated with autoantibodies and a Th1/Th2-type cellular immune response. *Gastroenterology* **2000**, *118*, 573–581. [CrossRef]

28. Lohr, J.M.; Faissner, R.; Koczan, D.; Bewerunge, P.; Bassi, C.; Brors, B.; Eils, R.; Frulloni, L.; Funk, A.; Halangk, W.; et al. Autoantibodies against the exocrine pancreas in autoimmune pancreatitis: Gene and protein expression profiling and immunoassays identify pancreatic enzymes as a major target of the inflammatory process. *Am. J. Gastroenterol.* **2010**, *105*, 2060–2071. [CrossRef] [PubMed]

29. Brusco, G.; Muzi, P.; Ciccocioppo, R.; Biagi, F.; Cifone, M.G.; Corazza, G.R. Transglutaminase and coeliac disease: Endomysial reactivity and small bowel expression. *Clin. Exp. Immunol.* **1999**, *118*, 371–375. [CrossRef] [PubMed]

30. Martucci, S.; Corazza, G.R. Spreading and focusing of gluten epitopes in celiac disease. *Gastroenterology* **2002**, *122*, 2072–2075. [CrossRef] [PubMed]

31. Moon, S.H.; Kim, J.; Kim, M.Y.; Park, D.H.; Song, T.J.; Kim, S.A.; Lee, S.S.; Seo, D.W.; Lee, S.K.; Kim, M.H. Sensitization to and challenge with gliadin induce pancreatitis and extrapancreatic inflammation in HLA-DQ8 Mice: An animal model of type 1 autoimmune pancreatitis. *Gut Liver.* **2016**, *10*, 842–850. [CrossRef] [PubMed]

32. Leeds, J.S.; Sanders, D.S. Risk of pancreatitis in patients with celiac disease: Is autoimmune pancreatitis a biologically plausible mechanism? *Clin. Gastroenterol. Hepatol.* **2008**, *6*, 951. [CrossRef] [PubMed]

33. Cebe, K.M.; Swanson, P.E.; Upton, M.P.; Westerhoff, M. Increased IgG4+ cells in duodenal biopsies are not specific for autoimmune pancreatitis. *Am. J. Clin. Pathol.* **2013**, *139*, 323–329. [CrossRef] [PubMed]

34. D'Argenio, V.; Casaburi, G.; Precone, V.; Pagliuca, C.; Colicchio, R.; Sarnataro, D.; Discepolo, V.; Kim, S.M.; Russo, I.; Del Vecchio Blanco, G.; et al. Metagenomics reveals dysbiosis and a potentially pathogenic N. flavescens strain in duodenum of adult celiac patients. *Am. J. Gastroenterol.* **2016**, *11*, 879–890. [CrossRef] [PubMed]

35. Masoodi, I.; Wani, H.; Alsayari, K.; Sulaiman, T.; Hassan, N.S.; Nazmi Alqutub, A.; Al Omair, A.; H Al-Lehibi, A. Celiac disease and autoimmune pancreatitis: An uncommon association. A case report. *Eur. J. Gastroenterol. Hepatol.* **2011**, *23*, 1270–1272. [CrossRef] [PubMed]

36. Kawa, S.; Ota, M.; Yoshizawa, K.; Horiuchi, A.; Hamano, H.; Ochi, Y.; Nakayama, K.; Tokutake, Y.; Katsuyama, Y.; Saito, S.; et al. HLA DRB10405-DQB10401 haplotype is associated with autoimmune pancreatitis in the Japanese population. *Gastroenterology* **2002**, *122*, 1264–1269. [CrossRef] [PubMed]

37. Zen, Y.; Fujii, T.; Harada, K.; Kawano, M.; Yamada, K.; Takahira, M.; Nakanuma, Y. Th2 and regulatory immune reactions are increased in immunoglobin G4-related sclerosing pancreatitis and cholangitis. *Hepatology* **2007**, *45*, 1538–1546. [CrossRef] [PubMed]

38. Miyoshi, H.; Uchida, K.; Taniguchi, T.; Yazumi, S.; Matsushita, M.; Takaoka, M.; Okazaki, K. Circulating naive and CD4+CD25high regulatory T cells in patients with autoimmune pancreatitis. *Pancreas* **2008**, *36*, 133–140. [CrossRef] [PubMed]

39. Jeannin, P.; Lecoanet, S.; Delneste, Y.; Gauchat, J.F.; Bonnefoy, J.Y. IgE versus IgG4 production can be differentially regulated by IL-10. *J. Immunol.* **1998**, *160*, 3555–3561. [PubMed]

40. Yamamoto, M.; Shimizu, Y.; Takahashi, H.; Yajima, H.; Yokoyama, Y.; Ishigami, K.; Tabeya, T.; Suzuki, C.; Matsui, M.; Naishiro, Y.; et al. CCAAT/enhancer binding protein alpha (C/EBPalpha)(+) M2 macrophages contribute to fibrosis in IgG4-related disease? *Mod. Rheumatol.* **2015**, *25*, 484–486. [CrossRef] [PubMed]

41. Ravi, K.; Chari, S.T.; Vege, S.S.; Sandborn, W.J.; Smyrk, T.C.; Loftus, E.V., Jr. Inflammatory bowel disease in the setting of autoimmune pancreatitis. *Inflamm. Bowel Dis.* **2009**, *15*, 1326–1330. [CrossRef] [PubMed]

42. Park, S.H.; Kim, D.; Ye, B.D.; Yang, S.-K.; Kim, J.-H.; Yang, D.-H.; Jung, K.W.; Kim, K.-J.; Byeon, J.-S.; Myung, S.-J.; et al. The characteristics of ulcerative colitis associated with autoimmune pancreatitis. *J. Clin. Gastroenterol.* **2013**, *47*, 520–525. [CrossRef] [PubMed]

43. Chari, S.T. Diagnosis of autoimmune pancreatitis using its five cardinal features: Introducing the Mayo Clinic's HISORt criteria. *J. Gastroenterol.* **2007**, *42*, 39–41. [CrossRef] [PubMed]

44. Otsuki, M.; Chung, J.B.; Okazaki, K.; Kim, M.H.; Kamisawa, T.; Kawa, S.; Park, S.W.; Shimosegawa, T.; Lee, K.; Ito, T.; et al. Asian diagnostic criteria for autoimmune pancreatitis: Consensus of the Japan-Korea Symposium on Autoimmune Pancreatitis. *J. Gastroenterol.* **2008**, *43*, 403–408. [CrossRef] [PubMed]

45. Berkson, J. Limitations of the application of fourfold tables to hospital data. *Biometr. Bull.* **1946**, *2*, 47–53. [CrossRef] [PubMed]

46. Nousia-Arvanitakis, S.; Fotoulaki, M.; Tendzidou, K.; Vassilaki, C.; Agguridaki, C.; Karamouzis, M. Subclinical exocrine pancreatic dysfunction resulting from decreased cholecystokinin secretion in the presence of intestinal villous atrophy. *J. Pediatr. Gastroenterol. Nutr.* **2006**, *43*, 307–312. [CrossRef] [PubMed]

47. Hart, P.A.; Kamisawa, T.; Brugge, W.R.; Chung, J.B.; Culver, E.L.; Czakó, L.; Frulloni, L.; Go, V.L.; Gress, T.M.; Kim, M.H.; et al. Long-term outcomes of autoimmune pancreatitis: A multicentre, international analysis. *Gut* **2013**, *62*, 1771–1776. [CrossRef] [PubMed]

17

Non-Celiac Gluten Sensitivity

Anna Roszkowska [1],*, Marta Pawlicka [1], Anna Mroczek [1], Kamil Bałabuszek [1] and Barbara Nieradko-Iwanicka [2]

[1]   Medical University of Lublin, Radziwillowska 11 Street, 20-080 Lublin, Poland; martamisztal991@gmail.com (M.P.); anna.mroczek94@wp.pl (A.M.); balkam@o2.pl (K.B.)

[2]   Chair and Department of Hygiene, Medical University of Lublin, Radziwillowska 11 Street, 20-080 Lublin, Poland; barbaranieradkoiwanicka@umlub.pl

*   Correspondence: annros7@gmail.com

Abstract: *Background and objectives:* Grain food consumption is a trigger of gluten related disorders: celiac disease, non-celiac gluten sensitivity (NCGS) and wheat allergy. They demonstrate with non-specific symptoms: bloating, abdominal discomfort, diarrhea and flatulence. Aim: The aim of the review is to summarize data about pathogenesis, symptoms and criteria of NCGS, which can be helpful for physicians. *Materials and Methods:* The PubMed and Google Scholar databases were searched in January 2019 with phrases: 'non-celiac gluten sensitivity', non-celiac gluten sensitivity', non-celiac wheat gluten sensitivity', non-celiac wheat gluten sensitivity', and gluten sensitivity'. More than 1000 results were found. A total of 67 clinical trials published between 1989 and 2019 was scanned. After skimming abstracts, 66 articles were chosen for this review; including 26 clinical trials. *Results:* In 2015, Salerno Experts' Criteria of NCGS were published. The Salerno first step is assessing the clinical response to gluten free diet (GFD) and second is measuring the effect of reintroducing gluten after a period of treatment with GFD. Several clinical trials were based on the criteria. *Conclusions:* Symptoms of NCGS are similar to other gluten-related diseases, irritable bowel syndrome and Crohn's disease. With Salerno Experts' Criteria of NCGS, it is possible to diagnose patients properly and give them advice about nutritional treatment.

Keywords: non-celiac gluten sensitivity; irritable bowel disease; gluten; FODMAP; wheat allergy

1. Introduction

Wheat, rice and maize are the most commonly consumed grains worldwide. These products are rich sources of starch—the basic dietary component for the growing human population [1]. Wheat contains gluten. In 1953 Dickie, van de Kamer and Weyers published a study confirming malabsorption after wheat consumption in patients with celiac disease (CD) [2]. Nowadays, gluten intake is considered to be the trigger of gluten related disorders (GRDs). In GRD, the gluten-free diet (GFD) is principal, effective and yet the only treatment method. The gluten-free market is still rising, not only because of growing interest and public awareness of GRDs, but also due to celebrities touting this diet by for weight loss and athletes for improved performance [3], which is debatable as grains should be the main source of energy in the human diet.

2. Materials and Methods

Standard up-to-date criteria were followed for review of the literature data. A search for English-language articles in the PubMed database was performed. The PubMed and Google Scholar databases were searched in January 2019 with phrases: 'non-celiac gluten sensitivity', non-celiac gluten sensitivity', non-celiac wheat gluten sensitivity', non-celiac wheat gluten sensitivity', and gluten sensitivity'. More than 1000 results were found. A total of 67 clinical trials published between 1989 and 2019 was scanned. After skimming abstracts, 66 articles were chosen for this review including 26 clinical trials.

2.1. Gluten Related Disorders (GRDs)

The term "gluten intolerance" includes three different conditions: CD, allergy to wheat (WA) and non-celiac gluten sensitivity (NCGS) [4]. To date, CD and WA comprise for the best known and studied entities, which are mediated by immune system [1]. WA—classified as a classic food allergy is induced by wheat (not only gluten) intake that leads to type I and type IV hypersensitivity. The crucial role in WA disorder play IgE immunoglobulins [1,5]. CD is an autoimmune disease occurring in genetically susceptible individuals with HLA-DQ2 and/or HLA-DQ8 genotypes. CD is characterized by the presence of specific serological antibodies such as: anti-tissue transglutaminase (tTG) IgA, anti-endomysium IgA (EMA) and anti-deamidated gliadin peptides IgG (DPG) [1]. There were reported cases of patients with gluten sensitivity in which allergic and autoimmune mechanisms could not be identified. They were collectively described as NCGS [1]. The NCGS or "non-celiac wheat sensitivity" (NCWS) has been a topic of interest in recent years. This trend is associated with a large number of studies concerning the syndrome [6,7]. The term NCWS is more adequate because of components other than gluten, that may contribute to intestinal and extra-intestinal symptoms [6]. In 1980, Cooper et al. described intestinal gluten-sensitive symptoms in 8 patients in whom CD was ruled out [8]. Further studies led to the definition of NCGS. NCGS is a condition characterized by clinical and pathological manifestations, related to gluten ingestion in individuals in whom CD and WA have been excluded [1,6,9,10]. Leccioli et al. described NCGS as a multi-factor-onset disorder, perhaps temporary and preventable, associated with an unbalanced diet [11].

Interestingly, II MHC haplotype HLA-DQ2 and HLA-DQ8 typical for CD is present only in about 50% of NCGS patients [1]. The main features of GRDs are summarized in Table 1.

Table 1. Comparison of prevalence, pathogenic, and diagnostic features of gluten related disorders (GRDs); non-celiac gluten sensitivity (NCGS), IgA anti-EMA (IgA antibodies against endomysium), IgA anti-tTG (IgA antibodies against transglutaminase), IgG anti-DGP (IgG antibodies against deamidated gliadin peptides).

	Celiac Disease	NCGS	Wheat Allergy
Prevalence	0.5–1.7%	no population studies	0.5–9% in children
Pathogenesis	autoimmune	non-specific immune response	IgE mediated response
DQ2-DQ8 HLA haplotypes	positive in 95% cases	positive in 50% cases	negative
Serological markers	IgA anti-EMA, IgA anti-tTG, IgG anti-DGP, IgA anti-gliadin	IgA/IgG anti-gliadin in 50% cases	specific IgE antibodies against wheat and gliadin
Duodenal biopsy *	Marsh I to IV with domination of Marsh III and IV	Marsh 0-II, but according to some experts Marsh III might also be in NCGS	Marsh 0-II
Duodenal villi atrophy	present	absent	might be present or absent

* Marsh classification.

2.2. Epidemiology of Gluten Related Disorders (GRDs)

CD morbidity, based on serological results, is estimated to be 1.1% to 1.7% worldwide [12,13]. WA among children occurs with a frequency of 0.4–9% [5,14]. Due to an absence of diagnostic markers and population studies, the prevalence of NCGS is not well established [5,6]. Although studies have been conducted by several authors, this problem is still insufficiently explored. Previous data were based primarily on questionnaires for self-reported gluten sensitivity SR-GS/self-reported NCGS. According to several authors, the NCGS prevalence is from 0.6% up to 13% of the general population [15–19]. NCGS was reported more often among women [16–18], adults in the fourth decade of life [19,20] and individuals coming from urban area [18]. Among intestinal symptoms the most frequent in NCGS are: bloating, abdominal discomfort and pain, diarrhea and flatulence.

The most common extra-intestinal symptoms were: tiredness, headache and anxiety [15,16,18,20]. Differentiation between NCGS and functional gastrointestinal (GI) disease—mainly irritable bowel syndrome (IBS)—may be difficult as some of the above-mentioned symptoms overlap with IBS manifestations. Van Gils et al. pointed that 37% of self-reported gluten sensitivity individuals (SR-GS) fulfilled the Rome III criteria for IBS, in contrast to 9% prevalence in the control group [18]. Similar findings were reported by Carroccio et al. IBS symptoms were reported in 44% self-reported NCWS [15]. According to research conducted by Cabrera et al., IBS, eating disorders and lactose intolerance were present more often in SR-GS individuals than in non-SR-GS group (14.3% vs. 4.7%) [16]. Herein, discussed studies indicate that SR-GS/SR-NCGS may correlate with more frequent occurrence of IBS, comparing to the general population. However, the German Society of Allergology and Clinical Immunology emphasized that the publications about NCGS suffer from certain weaknesses: absence of validated diagnostic criteria, suitable biomarkers, frequent self-diagnosis and unconfirmed etiology of reported symptoms. Thus, the prevalence of NCGS cannot be clearly established [21].

2.3. Gluten

Gluten is defined as a family of proteins found in grains (wheat, rye, barley, oats). It includes two main proteins: gliadin and glutenin. Also, similar proteins such as secalin in rye, harden in barley and avenues in oats contribute to the definition of 'gluten' [22]. Gluten proteins are characterized by high proline and glutamine content, moreover, they are resistant to proteolytic enzymes in the gastrointestinal tract. In some individuals these peptides can cross the epithelial barrier and activate immune system: trigger an allergic (WA) or autoimmune response (CD) [5]. Incomplete digestion leads to significant changes in human gut and causes intestinal or extra-intestinal symptoms. Gliadin and other gluten proteins stimulate T-cells. Some authors suggested that amylase-tripsin inhibitors (ATIs) and fermentable oligo-, di-, and mono-saccharides and polyols (FODMAPs) may be associated with NCGS [11]. Another wheat constituent, known as agglutinin-carbohydrate binding protein and exorphins seem to influence immune system and induce damage of intestinal epithelium [11,22].

2.4. Amylase-Tripsin Inhibitors (ATIs)

ATIs are albumin proteins found in wheat representing up to 4% of total proteins in grains [1]. They are highly resistant to intestinal proteases [1] and may induce release of pro-inflammatory cytokines from monocytes, macrophages and dendritic cells through activation of a toll-like receptor-4 in CD and NCGS patients [1,22]. ATIs may provoke activation of innate immune cells and intestinal inflammation [21]. ATIs activate immunological system through effect on toll-like receptor-4 in CD, that was confirmed in the research conducted by Junker et al. on mice deficient in TLR4 or TLR signaling [23]. Authors observed, that their mice models were protected from intestinal and systemic immune responses during oral ATIs intake [23]. Scientists also confirmed, that ATIs stimulate monocytes, macrophages and dendritic cells *in vitro* to produce IL-8, IL-12, TNF, MCP-1 and Regulated on Activation, Normal T-cell Expressed and Secreted (RANTES) [23].

2.5. Fermentable Oligo-, Di- and Mono-Saccharides and Polyols (FODMAPs)

FODMAPs are short-chain sugars with less than 10 carbon atoms in the molecule [24]. The attention of scientists in recent years was drawn to the potential contribution of FODMAPS to pathogenesis of gastrointestinal disorders [25]. The scientists from Monash University in Australia conducted thorough analysis of a group of carbohydrates, which, despite their different structures, produced similar postprandial effects. The most prevalent forms of FODMAP include: fructooligosaccharides (FOS), galactooligosaccharides (GOS), lactose, fructose, polyols, sorbitol and mannitol. Barrett et al. created a list of food products that are good sources of FODMAP (Figure 1) and poor in short chain sugars (Figure 2) [24].

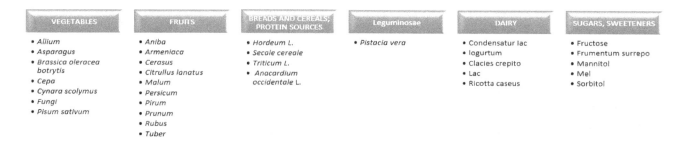

Figure 1. List of products being the source of fermentable oligo-, di-, and mono-saccharides and polyols (FODMAPs).

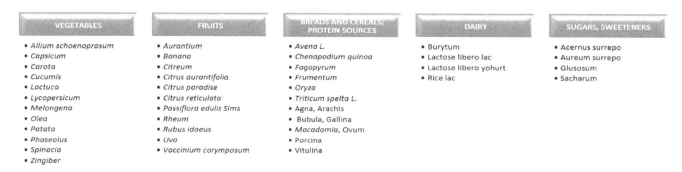

Figure 2. List of products low in FODMAPs.

Compounds belonging to the FODMAP group are not digested nor absorbed in the gastrointestinal tract. They have a strong osmotic effect and undergo rapid fermentation in the intestines, resulting in intestinal liquefaction, excessive gas production, bloating and pain. They may cause or exacerbate symptoms in susceptible patients with inflammatory bowel disease and irritable bowel syndrome (IBS) [24,25]. Numerous studies have confirmed the improvement in patients suffering from ulcerative colitis, Crohn's Disease and IBS following the elimination of short-chain sugars from the diet [26].

Wheat is a rich source of gluten and also contains large amounts of FODMAPs, which play a key role in NCGS development [27]. Some researchers suggest that diet low in FODMAP is beneficial for NCGS patients [25].

Considering the above research results, scientists are leaning towards renaming NCGS to a more recent NCWS [27]. It should be emphasized that a diet poor in FODMAPs should not be used without medical indications, as healthy people do not benefit from such diet [24]. Moreover, it was proven that FOS and GOS, compounds belonging to FODMAPS, alike prebiotic, favor proper colonization of intestines with *Bifidobacteria* and *Lactobacilli* bacteria and limit the proliferation of *Bacteroides* spp., *Clostridium* spp. and *Escherichia coli*. There is evidence that short-chain fatty acids (SCFA)—the product of FODMAP fermentation—have protective properties against colorectal cancer [24,27]. FODMAPs are believed to have a positive effect on lipid metabolism by lowering serum cholesterol, triglycerides and phospholipids [27]. In addition, this diet leads to calcium absorption disorders, lowering its serum levels. People resigning from products that are the source of FODMAP are at risk of vitamin and antioxidants deficiency [27,28]. Therefore, it is suggested to supplement vitamins, pro- and prebiotics when switching to the low FODMAPs diet [24,27].

2.6. The Salerno Experts' Criteria of NCGS

As long as the NCGS biomarker is not available, certain limitations are included in two-step diagnostic protocol introduced in 2015. However, up to date The Salerno Experts' Criteria constitute the only accessible recommendations for diagnosis of NCGS. It should be emphasized that according to currently used criteria, NCGS should not be based only on exclusion diagnosis, which is new in comparison to the former practice [29]. Thus, the guidelines indicate the need of a standardized procedure: 6-week course of gluten-free diet—with the simultaneous, continuous assessment of symptoms and their intensity, followed by measuring the effect of reintroducing gluten after a period of treatment with GFD. A modified version of the Gastrointestinal Symptom Rating Scale (GSRS) was found to be applicable in terms of symptoms evaluation. Although limited, double-blind-placebo-controlled (DBPC) procedure remains to be the golden standard in NCGS investigation, yet, single-blinded procedure is allowed for the purposes of clinical practice [29–31]. The guidelines stress the importance of patient compliance, especially when it comes to shift to GFD, which should be discussed with a dietitian before implementation [29].

Back to the limitations—it is recommended to use gluten in the form of commonly consumed food products, during gluten challenge, rather than in the form of gluten capsules. Nevertheless, there is presumption that ATIs and FODMAPS—as the constituents of grains—interfere with the DPBC results [6,30,32]. Moreover, since the study on patients complaining about IBS-like symptoms, it was revealed that almost two-thirds of questioned patients presented nocebo effect after elimination diet, which seems to have same significant influence on performing DBPC during gluten challenge [29,33].

The fact that numerous symptoms manifested by active NCGS can be either vague or simply mimic other medical conditions, makes the diagnostic process long lasting and complex. For instance, bloating, abdominal pain, and irregular bowel movements are typical symptoms seen in IBS [20]. The overlapping symptoms of IBS, Crohn's disease and GRD are shown in Figure 3.

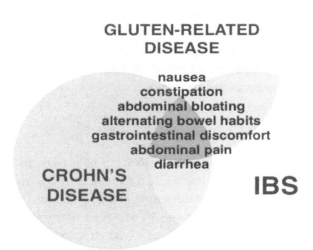

Figure 3. Overlapping symptoms in Crohn's disease, IBS and gluten-related disease.

The similarity between symptomatology of IBS and NCGS may lead to a wrong diagnosis and ineffective treatment [6]. The clinical case described by Vojdani and Perlmutter, presented a 49-year-old woman formerly diagnosed with IBS. The patient complained about abdominal pain, constipation, acid reflux and headache. Following conditions were contemplated and finally excluded: autoimmunological disorders, abnormal level of thyroid hormones, *H. pylori* infection [34]. Consequently, in the course of inappropriate therapy, the patient developed symptoms imitating systemic lupus erythematosus. Furthermore, the patient showed some improvement after corticosteroids administration, which appeared to be confusing for making right diagnosis as well [34]. Ultimately, after years of inappropriate treatment, the NCGS turned out to be the reason for patient's affliction. In addition, a few studies indicate that NCGS can be primary trigger for developing IBS. Virtually, as NCGS and IBS-like symptoms tend to overlap, the diagnostic process is particularly challenging [20,35,36].

Even though the diagnosis within the wide spectrum of bowel diseases was made, in the case of continuous therapy failure, it is crucial to reconsider NCGS as the possible cause. A clinical case of a patient with NCGS overlapping Crohn's disease has been reported. The onset of Crohn's disease is characterized mainly by unspecific symptoms, including diarrhea, weight loss, right lower quadrant abdominal pain, which proceed in a gradual way, with very harmful effects [37]. In the above-mentioned case report, the patient suffered from refractory Crohn's disease for 14 years and elevated IgG class antibodies directed against native gliadin (AGA) were detected, which shed a light on gluten related disorder. Introduction of GFD ceased diarrhea and enabled the patient to gain weight [34]. It is worth highlighting that NCGS patients are twice as likely to have AGA positivity [38].

At present, the linkage between gluten sensitivity, such as CD, and neurological disorders seems to be obvious. So far, numerous studies have unveiled extra intestinal symptoms affecting the peripheral and central nervous system due to celiac sprue. Although not fully understood yet, a wide range of NCGS neurological complications has been reported too. The state-of-the-art knowledge on NCGS revealed its association with transient and subtle cognitive impairment, being called "brain fog" [39]. Some scientists suggest NCGS to worsen symptoms in the context of depression but further examination must be performed to comprehend and determine NCGS relation with depressive disorders [32]. Busby et al. in their meta-analysis pointed out that standardization of methods measuring dietary adherence and mood symptoms is vital in terms of future research. Nevertheless, they admit that the gluten elimination diet may be an applicable treatment for mood disorders in patients suffering from gluten-related diseases [40].

It has not been until recently, when researchers explored that NCGS may be associated with gluten ataxia (GA), as the patients with typical GA symptoms did not meet criteria for CD diagnosis [41]. NCGS symptoms are believed to originate from an innate immune response. Interestingly, autoimmune diseases are reported to be more frequent in this group of patients, comparing to sheer IBS patients [42].

3. Results

Comparison of selected clinical trials concerning NCGS is shown in Table 2. In the study by Capannolo et al. patients with CD and WA were excluded while in the study by Elli et al. patients without CD, WA, IBS were enrolled. The prevalence of NCGS, CD and WA among patients with functional GI symptoms in the study of Capannolo et al. was estimated to be 6.88%, 6.63% and 0.51%. Capannolo et al. indicate that high frequency of visits due to gluten-related symptoms is not associated with high prevalence of GRDs. Ellie et al. established that 14% of patients, suspected to have NCGS because of responding to gluten withdrawal showed a symptomatic relapse during the gluten challenge. It was highlighted that GFD can have a beneficial effect even in the absence of CD or WA. However, there are certain limitations seen in both of compared above research papers. The research of Capannolo et al. was lacking blindness in GFD challenge and missing evaluation of possible influence of other food components. Besides it was conducted before Salerno Criteria were introduced (2015). A choice of timing and gluten dosage shown in the research of Elli et al. was not in line with the timing suggested by Salerno criteria. In addition, the protocol did not make use of a scheduled diet besides GFD. Moreover, a nocebo effect may be presumed, in consistence with symptomatic deterioration observed in the placebo group. Other diet variables in both studies cannot be excluded (ATIs) [43,44].

Table 2. Comparison of selected researches on NCGS.

References	Study Group	Exclusion Criteria	Methods	Findings	Comments
Biesiekierski et al. 2013	IBS patients fulfilling Rome III criteria in NCGS criteria, on GFD for 6 weeks	CD, IBD, age < 16, serious GI disease (cirrhosis), psychiatric disorders, alcohol abuse, NSAIDs and immunosuppressive treatment	GFD for 6 weeks, next 2-weeks diet low in FODMAPs, then 3 days one of the groups—high gluten 16 g, low gluten 2 g gluten or 14 g whey protein, control for 2 weeks washout period and crossover to another group for 3 days. **The primary outcome:** GI symptoms measured by using 100-mm VAS scoring. **The secondary outcome:** Fatigue measured by Daily-Fatigue Impact Scale (D-FIS), gliadin-specific T-cell response, biomarkers.	**The primary outcome:** Gluten-specific responses only in 8% of patients, 16% had worsening of overall GI symptoms in high gluten diet. **The secondary outcome:** Fatigue measured by D-FIS was lower in the low FOTMAPs diet, no significant difference in biomarkers, physical activity or sleep was observed, only one patient had gliadin-specific T-cell response.	**Limitations:** The nocebo effect was present independent of substances which was delivered
Capannolo et al. 2014	Individuals with gluten related symptoms	CD and WA	**NCGS finding:** on the basis of the disappearance of the symptoms within GFD 6 month, followed by 1month GD.	CD patients: 26 (6.63%); WA patients: 27 (6.88%). Patients with **no change of symptoms after GFD 337 (85.9%).** **Symptoms in 74% NCGS patients:** **Intestinal:** abdominal pain, diarrhea, constipation, alternating bowel function, epigastric pain. **Extra intestinal:** malaise, chronic fatigue, headache, anxiety, confused mind, depression, joint/muscle pain, resembling fibromyalgia, weight loss, anemia, dermatitis, rash. **Related disorders in NCGS patients:** lactose intolerance, autoimmune thyroiditis, type 1 diabetes, psoriasis, sarcoidosis	**Limitations:** Lack of blindness in GFD challenge. Missing evaluation of possible influence by other food components
Zanini et al. 2015	Individuals on gluten-free diet (GFD) on their own initiative	CD, non-strict adherence to a GFD, symptomatic on GFD	The primary outcome: the ability of the participants to correctly identify flour containing gluten. GSRS questionnaire was performed	Only 34% (12 participants) correctly identified gluten-containing flour fulfilling the clinical diagnostic criteria for NCGS.	The gluten-free flour used in this test contained FODMAP
Hollon et al. 2015	Individuals with Active CD, CD in Remission, Gluten Sensitivity (GS)	Positive CD serology, abnormal duodenal histopathology, unresponsive to gluten open challenge	**GS finding:** on the basis of the disappearance of the symptoms within GFD; non-blinded gluten challenge (10 g) for a minimum of 2 months before endoscopy	Increase of gut permeability after PT-gliadin ex-vivo administration in all three study groups, and in control group	**Limitations:** Lack of blindness in GFD challenge—possible placebo-response; Lack of GFD challenge in the control group—possible individuals with undiagnosed GS/CD
Shahbazkhani et al. 2015	Individuals with newly diagnosed IBS based on the Rome III criteria	Patients with CD, GFD introduced ever in medical history, self-exclusion of wheat from the diet, IBD, diabetes, concurrent drugs for depression/anxiety, NSAI drugs intake, abnormal levels of: glucose, urea, creatinine, sodium, potassium, hemoglobin, erythrocyte sedimentation rate, thyroid function tests	**GS finding:** IBS diagnosed patients responding to gluten challenge by means of statistically significant worsening of symptoms after gluten meal challenge. Patients previously following strict GFD, continued gluten challenge for 6 weeks	Significant increase for following symptoms after gluten-containing meal challenge: bloating, abdominal pain, stool consistence, tiredness, nausea	**Limitations:** Packets containing gluten meal in the form of powder—not recommended according to Salerno criteria. **Pros:** double-blind randomized placebo-controlled trial

Table 2. *Cont.*

References	Study Group	Exclusion Criteria	Methods	Findings	Comments
Di Sabatino et al. 2015	Suspected NCGS individuals	CD, WA	Individuals were randomly assigned to groups given gluten or placebo for 1 week, each via gastro-soluble capsules. After a 1 week of gluten-free diet, participants crossed over to the other group.	Gluten group: significantly increased overall symptoms (intestinal symptoms: abdominal bloating and pain, extra-intestinal symptoms: foggy mind, depression, aphthous stomatitis) vs. placebo group.	**Limitation:** small study group
Elli et al. 2016	Individuals with functional gastroenterological symptoms with enrolled on 3-week-long GFD	CD, WA, IBS psychiatric disorders, major abdominal surgery, diabetes mellitus, systemic autoimmune diseases, previous anaphylactic episodes, any systemic disorders, pregnant, breast feeding women, GFD in previous 6 months, patients on pharmacological therapy	**Phase 1.** GFD response individuals: questionnaire and next 3-week GFD. Patients with significantly improvement carried on to next phase. **Phase 2. 98 subjects.** GFD response patients—maintain strict GFD and underwent placebo-controlled double-blind gluten challenge with crossover. Patients were randomized to take gluten in capsules or placebo (rice starch) for 7 days. Total duration: 21 days: 7 days on gluten or placebo, 7 days wash-out, 7 days on gluten or placebo.	28 individuals from phase 2 reported a symptomatic relapse and deterioration of quality of life. 14 patients responded to the placebo ingestion. About 14 patients responding to gluten withdrawal showed a symptomatic relapse during the gluten challenge—they are suspected to have NCCS.	**Strengths:** The blinding of patients and doctors, and the crossover design. **Weaknesses:** arbitrary choice of timing and gluten dosage, the protocol did not make use of a scheduled diet besides GFD, other diet variables cannot be excluded (ATIs). Symptomatic deterioration was also observed in placebo group.
Rosinach et al. 2016	Individuals with clinical GI symptoms and clinical and histological remission after GFD	Age < 18, CD, NSAIDs and Olmesartan immunosuppressive treatment in last month, immunosuppressive therapy, parasitic or H. pylori infection, AD, pregnant or breastfeeding women, participation in other randomized controlled trials in the last 4 weeks, serious GI diseases and GI surgery, severe comorbidities, failure to comply with the protocol requirements	Patients were randomly assigned to gluten group (20 g/day, n = 11) and placebo (n = 7). Clinical symptoms were measured by VAS, quality of life using GIQLI. Scientists examined the presence of gamma/delta+ cells and transglutaminase deposits. primary end-point: disease relapse after 6 months	91% of patients with clinical relapse during gluten challenge compared to 28.5% after placebo. Worsening results in clinical scores and GIQLI was observed in patients on gluten diet, but not in the placebo	**Limitations:** a small study group
Carroccio et al. 2017	Individuals with NCWS		Data collecting from a previous study of NCWS.	88% subjects improved after a diagnosis of NCWS; 145 of 148 patients on strict GFD (98%) had reduced symptoms, compared to 30 of 52 patients who was not on GFD. 20 (from 22) subjects who repeated DBPC challenge reacted to wheat. NCWS is a persistent condition.	**Limitations:** not thoroughly discussed exclusion criteria
Skodje et al. 2018	Individuals self-reported NCGS on gluten-free diet (GFD) on their own initiative for at least 6 months	**Exclusion criteria: CD, WA, IBD,** gastrointestinal comorbidity, allergy to nuts and sesame, alcohol abuse, pregnancy, breast feeding, women in fertile age without using contraception, long travel distance, considerable infection, patients on immunosuppressive agents' therapy	GFD for 6 months, next 7 days on one of three diets challenge (gluten 5,7g, fructans 2,1g and placebo), 7 days washout, then crossover to next diet. **The primary outcome:** gastrointestinal symptoms measured by GSRS-IBS. **The secondary outcome:** daily GI symptoms measured by VAS, life quality depends on symptoms by SF-36, depression and anxiety symptoms measured by Hospital Anxiety and Depression Scale, Fatigue measured by Giessen Subjective Complaint List and VAS	**The primary outcome:** overall GSRS-IBS higher in the fructans group (38.6) than in the gluten group (33,1) and placebo (34.3). **The secondary outcome:** overall GI symptoms measured by VAS higher in FODMAPs diet, decreased vitality and greater weakness in the group of patients receiving fructans	**Limitations:** high nocebo response

Table 2. *Cont.*

References	Study Group	Exclusion Criteria	Methods	Findings	Comments
Roncoroni et al. 2019	Individuals with NCGS criteria, complaining about functional GI symptoms	CD, WA, IBD, adult age (<18 years old), positive anti-tissue transglutaminase IgA, psychiatric disorders, major abdominal surgery, diabetes, GFD for previous six months, autoimmune diseases and systemic disorders, pregnancy, breast feeding, experience of anaphylaxis and patients during pharmacotherapy	GFD for 3 weeks, then exposure to diets with gradually increasing the amount of gluten: low-gluten diet (3.5–4 g gluten/day, week 1, n = 22 + 2 dropped out patients), mid-gluten diet (6.7–8 g gluten/day, week 2, n = 14), and a high-gluten diet (10–13 g gluten/day, week 3, n = 8). Patients without GI symptoms on a previous diet were classified into more gluten- containing diet. Patients with GI symptoms were shifted back to a well-tolerated diet. Daily GI symptoms measured by VAS, life quality depends on symptoms by SF-36	Different reactions of patients after the introduction of gluten.	Limitation: a small study group

In 2015, Zanini et al. published a prospective, randomized, double-blind, placebo-controlled study on patients without CD or wheat allergy as seen in Table 2. Scientists observed 35 patients (31 females and 4 males) being on a GFD due to their own initiative because of gastrointestinal symptoms they had had on a diet containing gluten. They were switched to a diet containing gluten. Participants' ability to distinguish between flours containing gluten and gluten-free was assessed, as well as their score in the Gastrointestinal Symptoms Rating Scale (GSRS). In order to participate in the study, patients had to be over 6 months a self-prescribed GFD and have a Gastrointestinal Symptoms Rating Scale (GSRS) below 4. The CD had had to be excluded before the start of the GFD. Before the beginning of the study t-TG antibody levels were measured and patients were instructed how to keep a diet diary. After 3 months, t-TG antibody level was checked again and GSRS questionnaire was performed. The participants received 10-g sachets containing gluten-free or gluten- containing flour labeled A or B. Patients were ordered to add contents to the pasta or soup for 10 days. Then for 2 weeks there was a washout period. Then, the patients received a second sachet with the other label, which they were to consume for 10 days. The primary outcome was the ability of the participants to correctly identify flour containing gluten. The study showed that only 34% (12 participants) correctly identified gluten- containing flour. Two thirds of the participants were not able to properly identify flour containing gluten. Almost half of the participants 17 (49%) misidentified gluten-free flour as gluten-containing flour, but those patients recorded symptoms and their GSRS scores increased on the flour not containing gluten. The gluten-free flour used in this test contained FODMAP [45].

Hollon et al. in their study (Table 2) disclosure ex-vivo gliadin effect on gut permeability in patients with active celiac disease (ACD), remission celiac disease (RCD) and gluten sensitivity (GS). The results of the research indicated that in all four groups, including control group (NG), there is certain response to gluten administration [46]. Researchers reported increased permeability particularly comparing ACD and GS groups to RCD, which is due to gluten induced alteration of intestinal barrier. Furthermore, researchers by means of quantification method investigated changes in following cytokines IL-6, IL-8, IFN-γ, TNF-α, which showed no significant difference, however, in this case a short period of incubation could implicate results. It should be emphasized that lack of blindness in GFD challenge while recruiting GS group along with lack of GFD challenge in the control group are important limitation in discussed study and could impact final results [46].

Shahbazkhani et al. investigated the relationship between dietary habits in IBS patients and consequent symptom fluctuations (Table 2). In particular researchers were interested in gluten impact on wellbeing of IBS patients and weather it may induce IBS-like symptoms. After rigid inclusion and exclusion criteria, strict six-week GFD 72 patients were recruited and divided into two groups: gluten containing group (study group), gluten free group (placebo group). Symptoms were analyzed by means of visual analogue scale (VAS). The results of the research revealed significant worsening of symptoms in a study group after gluten powder challenge. Scientists reported increase of overall symptoms such as satisfaction with stool consistency, tiredness, nausea, bloating in study group comparing to the control one. The results occurred to be statistically significant [47]. Nevertheless, there was limitation such as gluten form—a packet of 100 g powder, which is not recommended anymore by Salerno criteria [29].

According to the study published in Gastroenterology, scientists discovered that FODMAPs are another wheat antigen along with gluten triggering symptoms in patients with NCGS. Biesiekierski et al. conducted a double-blind crossover trial in which participated 37 patients suffering from NCGS and IBD. The following exclusion criteria were applied: age less than 16 years, CD confirmed by genetic tests and duodenal biopsy, alcohol abuse, chronic non-steroidal anti-inflammatory drugs (NSAIDs) and immunosuppressant treatment, uncontrolled psychiatric illness. Patients who had confirmed symptoms of IBS by accomplished the Rome III criteria and symptoms well controlled on a GFD were qualified for the study. Another requirement was to follow the GFD 6 weeks before this clinical trial. The first stage of the study was identical for all participants and the task was consuming for a one week a gluten-free and low FODMAPs diet. After a 2-week washout period, patients were randomly assigned to the three groups: high-gluten, low-gluten and placebo, without introducing FODMAP into the diet. The symptoms of the patients were measured by using 100-mm VAS scoring and Daily-Fatigue Impact Scale (D-FIS). All participants were asked to return to the second stage of this study—trial in which all patients received each diets for 3-days [48]. Gluten-specific responses were found only in 8% of patients. Scientists found a high nocebo effect and reproducibility of induction of symptoms in each arm was low [48].

Biesiekierski et al. noticed that patients with NCGS do not present a statistically significant occurrence of symptoms after introducing gluten into the diet, if at the same time they limit products rich in FODMAP (Table 2). These results may suggest that the symptoms in patients suffering from NCGS may in many cases be associated with intolerance to the contained sugars, but not hypersensitivity to gluten. Surprisingly, the patients involved into study evinced eminently high VAS ratings for their symptoms, despite being on GFD. Furthermore, an anticipatory nocebo response could influence the final results of this DBPC research. It is interesting that all participants eventually returned to GFD at the end of the trail as they 'subjectively describe feeling better' [48].

Scientists from Oslo, Skodje et al., conducted a study in which took part 59 patients on a GFD, in whom CD was excluded (Table 2). Participants were divided into three groups: receiving diet including gluten (5.7 g), fructans (2.1 g) and placebo. The clinical trial lasted 7 days and was preceded by a 1-week washout period. The following symptoms were recorded: pain, bloating, diarrhea, constipation, nausea, dizziness, weakness, sleepiness and tiredness. Participants filled a questionnaire containing 13 questions about their gastrointestinal symptoms and filled VAS. The results were measured by GSRS, Irritable Bowel Syndrome scale (GSRS-IBS), VAS, Short Form-36 (SF-36) and Giessen Subjective Complaint List [49]. Scientists observed that daily symptoms calculated using VAS score were significantly higher in fructans diet. Furthermore, they noticed that overall GSRS-IBS was higher in the FODMAPs group (38.6 g) than in the gluten group (33.1 g) and placebo (34.3 g). More ailments were recorded in the group receiving fructans, compered to two another groups. In addition, it was demonstrated that a diet rich in FODMAPSs caused greater weakness and decreased vitality compared to the placebo and gluten groups. The results of the study indicate that FODMAPs are a trigger factor of gastrointestinal complaints in patients suffering from NCGS [49]. Thus, scientists are leaning towards renaming NCGS to a more recent NCWS [27].

Di Sabatino et al. observed increased severity of intestinal symptoms (abdominal bloating, abdominal pain) and extra intestinal symptoms (foggy mind, depression, and aphthous stomatitis) among subjects with suspected NCGS (excluded CD and WA). Although, this study did not make a significant contribution in development of knowledge about NCGS and had some weaknesses such as lack of a control group, it indicates possible symptoms experienced by NCGS patients (Table 2) [50].

In order to prove that gluten is a trigger factor in patients with NCGS, Rosinach et al. conducted a study in which 18 participants were assigned to gluten or placebo groups. In 10 out of 11 patients, symptoms worsened in response to a gluten-containing diet, 7 of which were withdrawn from the study due to the severity of the symptoms [51]. There was no early termination in the placebo group although in 2 participants symptoms were observed (Table 2) [51].

Carroccio et al. collected and analyzed data from 200 patients examined in previous study with diagnosed NCWS. Their findings are interesting because about 90% of patients who maintained wheat-free diet (WFD) were characterized by significant improvement of IBS symptoms [52]. The authors came to the conclusion that NCWS is a persistent condition and patients with NCWS should therefore be correctly identified and treated with WFD (Table 2) [52].

Roncoroni et al. conducted a study on dietary exposure to different amounts of gluten in patients meeting the criteria of the NCGS [53]. Researchers observed different reactions of patients after the introduction of gluten. Some of them had a worsening of well-being and increased symptoms after a small dose of gluten, others observed this effect after the medium dose and others only after a high dose of gluten (Table 2) [53].

Carrocio et al. in their study in 2011 emphasize the link between particular food ingestion and deteriorating symptoms in a subgroup of IBS patients [54]. It clearly shows alleviation of the symptoms in 22% of IBS patients—whose previous treatment was ineffective—after eliminating gluten from the diet. Moreover, researchers excluded association of DQ2 and DQ8 haplotypes with frequent gluten sensitivity, however, patients presenting food hypersensitivity (FH) to both wheat- and cow's milk-protein were reported to be often DQ2/DQ8 positive. Fecal eosinophil cationic protein (ECP) may be useful while identifying FH in IBS-patients (Table 3) [54].

Carroccio et al. in their study published in 2012 examined individuals with non-celiac WS, diagnosed by DBPC challenge with IBS-like symptoms, compared to CD patients and IBS patients [55]. Authors described presence of two types of WS subjects: WS similar to CD and WS associated with multiple food hypersensitivity. Besides, symptoms such as anemia, weight loss, self-reported wheat intolerance, coexistent atopy, and food allergy in infancy were noticed more often in WS compared to IBS controls. Furthermore, WS individuals were characterized by higher frequency of presence IgG/IgA anti-gliadin in serum, basophil activation (assessed by flow cytometric method) and histology specific eosinophil infiltration of the duodenal and colon mucosa. This study shows the differences between non-celiac WS and other gluten-related disorders (Table 3) [55].

Volta et al. in their study, assessed the level of immunoglobulin distinctive for CD in patients with GS comparing to CD [56]. They revealed that 50% of GS patients presented IgG AGA, whereas IgA AGA was seen only in a few patients in study group. Besides, researchers observed absence of IgA EmA, IgA tTGA, IgG DGP-AGA, which are typical for CD, within GS group (Table 3) [56].

Basing on a study group conducted by Volta et al., Caio et al. continued research on AGA IgG [38]. Scientists aimed to explore GFD impact on AGA IgG titer in AGA IgG positive patients (44 individuals) with NCGS. After six months of GFD AGA IgG disappeared in all the patients (Table 3).

Carrocio et al., in another research conducted in 2015, evaluated and described frequent ANA positivity within NCWS patients group [57]. The study demonstrated ANA positivity occurring along with DQ2/DQ8 haplotypes. As it was previously discussed, DQ2/DQ8 positivity is a distinctive feature of CD rather than NCWS. Thus, researchers highlight the need of intraepithelial intestinal flow cytometric pattern, which is an accurate method identifying seronegative CD patients, in the initial diagnostic biopsy. However, scientists found autoimmune diseases (AD) particularly frequent in study group. Autoimmune thyroiditis was reported to be the most frequent AD and amounted for 22% and 24% in retrospective and prospective groups respectively Table 3) [57].

Infantino et al. similarly to Volta observed frequent IgG AGA occurrence in NCGS patients, however, the author highlights that it is still lacking diagnostic accuracy. Nevertheless, in some cases, it can be helpful in the diagnostic process of NCGS patients [58].

Papers included in Table 3. Indicate IgG AGA and ECP to be helpful diagnostic tool while diagnosing NCGS. Still they have limited application in a large group of NCGS patients and cannot be widely used in NCGS diagnostic protocol [54,58].

Table 3. Researches on potential NCGS biomarkers.

References	Study Group	Exclusion Criteria	Methods	Findings	Comments
Carroccio et al. 2011	Individuals who fulfilled Rome II criteria for IBS	Individuals with organic diseases	Symptom severity questionnaire was analyzed, fecal samples were assayed, and levels of specific immunoglobulin E were measured. Patients were observed for 4 weeks, placed on an elimination diet (without cow's milk and derivatives, wheat, egg, tomato, and chocolate) for 4 weeks, and kept a diet diary. Those who reported improvements after the elimination diet period were then diagnosed with food hypersensitivity (FH), based on the results of a double-blind, placebo-controlled, oral food challenge (with cow's milk proteins and then with wheat proteins).	40 of patients with IBS (25%) were found to have FH. Levels of fecal ECP and tryptase were significantly higher among patients with IBS and FH than those without FH. The ECP assay was the most accurate assay for diagnosis of FH, showing 65% sensitivity and 91% specificity.	Limitations: recruitment of patients not in line with Salerno criteria.
Carroccio et al. 2012	Individuals with non-celiac wheat sensitivity (NCWS),	IgA deficiency, self-exclusion of wheat from the diet, lack of DBPC-challenge method in the diagnosis	A review of the clinical charts of patients with IBS-like presentation, diagnosed with WS challenge in the years 2001-2011.	1/3 IBS patients who underwent DBPC wheat challenge were really suffering from WS. WS group: higher frequency of anemia, weight loss, self-reported wheat intolerance, coexistent atopy, and food allergy in infancy than the IBS controls, higher frequency of positive serum assays for IgG/IgA anti-gliadin and cytometric basophil activation in "in vitro" assay, eosinophil infiltration of the duodenal and colon mucosa. Two groups with distinct clinical characteristics were identified: WS alone (with similar to CD clinical features) and WS with multiple food hypersensitivity (clinical features similar to those found in allergic patients)	Limitations: recruitment of patients not in line with Salerno criteria.
Volta et al. 2012	Individuals with GS (NCGS)	CD, WA	Retrospective evaluation of collected samples from GS (study group) and CD (control group) individuals. Assessment of IgG/IgA AGA, IgA EmA, IgA tTGA, IgG DGP-AGA. HLA DQ2/DQ8 presence was assessed	GS is characterized by IgG AGA positivity (50%), although is less common comparing to CD. IgA AGA are rare. GS patients were lacking EmA, tTGA, and DGP-AGA.	Limitations: not thoroughly described exclusion criteria for study group

Table 3. *Cont.*

References	Study Group	Exclusion Criteria	Methods	Findings	Comments
Caio et al. 2014	Individuals with NCGS with simultaneous AGA IgG positivity	CD, WA	AGA of both IgG and IgA classes were assayed by ELISA in 44 NCGS and 40 CD patients after 6 months of gluten-free diet.	AGA IgG in NCGS patients disappear after introduction of GFD.	
Carroccio et al. 2015	NCWS patients of the retrospective cohort study / NCWS patients of the prospective study	Incomplete clinical charts were excluded from retrospective study; for both studies: EmA in the culture medium of the duodenal biopsies, self-exclusion of wheat from the diet and refusal to reintroduce it before entering the study; other organic gastrointestinal diseases.	NCWS patients—tTG IgG, EmA IgA and IgG negative, absence of intestinal villous atrophy and WA. Patient medical records were reviewed to identify those with autoimmune disease (AD). CD or IBS served as controls. Serum samples were collected from all subjects and ANA levels were measured by immunofluorescence analysis. Participants completed a questionnaire and their medical records were reviewed to identify those with ADs. Individuals were randomly assigned to groups given gluten or placebo for 1 week, each via gastro-soluble capsules. After a 1 week of gluten-free diet, participants crossed over to the other group.	Patients with NCWS were more likely to be ANA positive than both patients with CD and IBS, in both the retrospective and prospective studies. Patients with NCWS showed a frequency of AD similar to CD, but significantly higher than IBS controls, in both the retrospective and prospective studies. NCWS or CD are more likely to be ANA-positive, have DQ2/DQ8 haplotypes and AD compared with patients with IBS.	Limitations: selection bias of the tertiary centers conducting research; evaluation of the duodenal histology; not in line with Salerno criteria
Infantino et al. 2015	Individuals with suspected NCGS	CD, WA	Evaluation of collected samples from GS (study group), CD and healthy (control group) individuals. Assessment of IgG/IgA AGA, IgA EmA, IgA tTGA, IgG/IgA DGP-AGA. HLA DQ2/DQ8 presence was assessed	Statistically significant correlation between AGA IgG and NCGS were found. However, AGA IgG still remains to be weak NCGS marker.	Limitations: recruitment of patients not in line with Salerno criteria; small study group

4. Discussion

Nowadays, a gluten-free diet is fashionable and is promoted by many celebrities. Many people undergo this fashion and despite lack of symptoms, try to reject gluten because they believe it may harm their health. In 2016, as much as USD 15.5 billion was spent on gluten-free food sales. This value is more than twice as high as in 2011. Lack of gluten in food consumed by people who tolerate it well may not bring favorable results.

In a study conducted by Norsa et al., children with CD were tested for at least one year on a GFD diet. As many as 34.8% of children on GFD diet had high concentrations of triglycerides on fasting, 24.1% high concentration of LDL cholesterol and 29.4% increased blood pressure. In 52 out of 114 participants there were available cards with information on blood lipids concentration before GFD introduction. 24% of children on GFD had had LDL cholesterol borderline values. That was much more than before the introduction of the diet (10%). However, these data did not meet the value of statistical significance ($p = 0.09$) [59].

Studies show that gluten may have a positive effect on triglyceride levels. In a clinical trial in which 20 adults with hyperlipidemia took part, a group with a balanced diet and a group with a high gluten content (78 g per day with an average human intake of 10–15 g) were studied. The high gluten diet group had a decreased triglyceride concentration of 19.2% ($p = 0.0003$) compared to the control group after one month of the study [60]. In another study, a group of patients consuming 60 g of gluten per day had a 13% ($p = 0.05$) lower triglyceride concentration compared to the control group [61]. In a study published in 2017, the estimated gluten consumption lead to the protective effect against cardiovascular disease (HR 0.85, 95% CI 0.77-0.93, $p = 0.002$) [62].

Gluten-free products can also be more than twice as expensive as regular products [63]. There are other disadvantages of GFD. The GFD turned out to be poor in trace elements and vitamins, such as zinc, iron, magnesium, calcium, vitamin D, vitamin B_{12}, folate, and fiber [64,65]. Furthermore, Tovoli et. al. compared scores obtained by NCWS and CD individuals using quality of life questionnaire (CDQ) before GFD introduction and after at least one year. NCWS patients still reported intestinal and parenteral symptoms, although symptoms were significantly reduced in comparison to period before GFD. Therefore, other factors influencing NCWS should be investigated [66].

Finally, based on revised research results, it is clear that NCGS still remains to be the subject of uncertainty, especially in terms of other wheat components contribution to its symptoms. There are only a few published forms of research in the last six years. It should be stressed that it is hard to compare the results of each study as obtained methods and criteria significantly vary. Moreover, the timing of onset of each research was of a great importance as some of them were conducted before Salerno criteria were introduced, which led to many interpretations and qualification protocols of patients with NCGS-like symptoms. Further investigations and seeking for biomarkers would play key role in improving of the diagnostic process and patients' follow up.

5. Conclusions

1. Symptoms of non-celiac gluten sensitivity are similar to gluten-related disease, irritable bowel syndrome and Crohn's disease.
2. With Salerno Experts' Criteria of non-celiac gluten sensitivity it is possible to diagnose patients properly and give them advice about nutritional treatment.

Author Contributions: Conceptualization, A.R., M.P., B.N.-I.; Methodology and resources A.M., K.B., B.N.-I.; Visualization A.M., M.P., A.R., K.B.; Writing—Review & Editing A.R., M.P., A.M., K.B., B.N.-I.; Software K.B.; Supervision—B.N.-I.

References

1. Sapone, A.; Bai, J.C.; Ciacci, C.; Dolinsek, J.; Green, P.H.R.; Hadjivassiliou, M.; Kaukinen, K.; Rostami, K.; Sanders, D.S.; Schumann, M.; et al. Spectrum of gluten-related disorders: Consensus on new nomenclature and classification. *BMC Med.* **2012**, *10*, 13. [CrossRef] [PubMed]

2.   Alvey, C.; Anderson, C.M.; Freeman, M. Wheat Gluten and Coeliac Disease. *Arch. Dis Child.* **1957**, *32*, 434–437. [CrossRef] [PubMed]

3.   Jones, A.L. The Gluten-Free Diet: Fad or Necessity? *Diabetes Spectr. Publ. Am. Diabetes Assoc.* **2017**, *30*, 118–123. [CrossRef] [PubMed]

4.   Balakireva, A.V.; Zamyatnin, A.A. Properties of Gluten Intolerance: Gluten Structure, Evolution, Pathogenicity and Detoxification Capabilities. *Nutrients* **2016**, *8*. Available online: https://www.ncbi.nlm.nih.gov/pmc/articles/PMC5084031/ (accessed on 28 January 2019). [CrossRef] [PubMed]

5.   Ortiz, C.; Valenzuela, R.; Lucero, A.Y. Celiac disease, non celiac gluten sensitivity and wheat allergy: Comparison of 3 different diseases triggered by the same food. *Rev. Chil. Pediatría* **2017**, *88*, 417–423. [CrossRef] [PubMed]

6.   Barbaro, M.R.; Cremon, C.; Stanghellini, V.; Barbara, G. Recent advances in understanding non-celiac gluten sensitivity. *F1000Research* **2018**, *7*. [CrossRef] [PubMed]

7.   Catassi, C.; Bai, J.C.; Bonaz, B.; Bouma, G.; Calabrò, A.; Carroccio, A.; Castillejo, G.; Ciacci, C.; Cristofori, F.; Dolinsek, J.; et al. Non-Celiac Gluten Sensitivity: The New Frontier of Gluten Related Disorders. *Nutrients* **2013**, *5*, 3839–3853. [CrossRef] [PubMed]

8.   Cooper, B.T.; Holmes, G.K.; Ferguson, R.; Thompson, R.A.; Allan, R.N.; Cooke, W.T. Gluten-sensitive diarrhea without evidence of celiac disease. *Gastroenterology* **1980**, *79*, 801–806. [CrossRef]

9.   Ludvigsson, J.F.; Leffler, D.A.; Bai, J.; Biagi, F.; Fasano, A.; Green, P.H.; Hadjivassiliou, M.; Kaukinen, K.; Kelly, C.P.; Leonard, J.N.; et al. The Oslo definitions for coeliac disease and related terms. *Gut* **2013**, *62*, 43–52. [CrossRef]

10.   Ierardi, E.; Losurdo, G.; Piscitelli, D.; Giorgio, F.; Amoruso, A.; Iannone, A.; Principi, M.; Di Leo, A. Biological markers for non-celiac gluten sensitivity: A question awaiting for a convincing answer. *Gastroenterol. Hepatol. Bed Bench.* **2018**, *11*, 203–208.

11.   Leccioli, V.; Oliveri, M.; Romeo, M.; Berretta, M.; Rossi, P. A New Proposal for the Pathogenic Mechanism of Non-Coeliac/Non-Allergic Gluten/Wheat Sensitivity: Piecing Together the Puzzle of Recent Scientific Evidence. *Nutrients* **2019**, *9*. Available online: https://www.ncbi.nlm.nih.gov/pmc/articles/PMC5707675/ (accessed on 28 January 2019). [CrossRef] [PubMed]

12.   Tanveer, M.; Ahmed, A. Non-Celiac Gluten Sensitivity: A Systematic Review. *J. Coll Physicians Surg.–Pak. Jcpsp* **2019**, *29*, 51–57. [CrossRef] [PubMed]

13.   Singh, P.; Arora, A.; Strand, T.A.; Leffler, D.A.; Catassi, C.; Green, P.H.; Kelly, C.P.; Ahuja, V.; Makharia, G.K. Global Prevalence of Celiac Disease: Systematic Review and Meta-analysis. *Clin. Gastroenterol. Hepatol. Off. Clin. Pr. J. Am. Gastroenterol. Assoc.* **2018**, *16*, 823–836.e2. [CrossRef] [PubMed]

14.   Elli, L.; Branchi, F.; Tomba, C.; Villalta, D.; Norsa, L.; Ferretti, F.; Roncoroni, L.; Bardella, M.T. Diagnosis of gluten related disorders: Celiac disease, wheat allergy and non-celiac gluten sensitivity. *World J. Gastroenterol.* **2015**, *21*, 7110–7119. [CrossRef] [PubMed]

15.   Carroccio, A.; Giambalvo, O.; La Blasca, F.; Iacobucci, R.; D'Alcamo, A.; Mansueto, P. Self-Reported Non-Celiac Wheat Sensitivity in High School Students: Demographic and Clinical Characteristics. *Nutrients* **2017**, *9*. Available online: https://www.ncbi.nlm.nih.gov/pmc/articles/PMC5537885/ (accessed on 28 January 2019). [CrossRef] [PubMed]

16.   Cabrera-Chávez, F.; Dezar, G.V.A.; Islas-Zamorano, A.P.; Espinoza-Alderete, J.G.; Vergara-Jiménez, M.J.; Magaña-Ordorica, D.; Ontiveros, N. Prevalence of Self-Reported Gluten Sensitivity and Adherence to a Gluten-Free Diet in Argentinian Adult Population. *Nutrients* **2017**, *9*, 81. [CrossRef] [PubMed]

17.   DiGiacomo, D.V.; Tennyson, C.A.; Green, P.H.; Demmer, R.T. Prevalence of gluten-free diet adherence among individuals without celiac disease in the USA: Results from the Continuous National Health and Nutrition Examination Survey 2009–2010. *Scand. J. Gastroenterol.* **2013**, *48*, 921–925. [CrossRef] [PubMed]

18.   Van Gils, T.; Nijeboer, P.; IJssennagger, C.E.; Sanders, D.S.; Mulder, C.J.J.; Bouma, G. Prevalence and Characterization of Self-Reported Gluten Sensitivity in The Netherlands. *Nutrients* **2016**, *8*. Available online: https://www.ncbi.nlm.nih.gov/pmc/articles/PMC5133100/ (accessed on 28 January 2019). [CrossRef]

19.   Aziz, I.; Lewis, N.R.; Hadjivassiliou, M.; Winfield, S.N.; Rugg, N.; Kelsall, A.; Newrick, L.; Sanders, D.S. A UK study assessing the population prevalence of self-reported gluten sensitivity and referral characteristics to secondary care. *Eur J. Gastroenterol. Hepatol.* **2014**, *26*, 33–39. [CrossRef]

20. Volta, U.; Bardella, M.T.; Calabrò, A.; Troncone, R.; Corazza, G.R.; Study Group for Non-Celiac Gluten Sensitivity. An Italian prospective multicenter survey on patients suspected of having non-celiac gluten sensitivity. *BMC Med.* **2014**, *12*, 85. [CrossRef]

21. Reese, I.; Schäfer, C.; Kleine-Tebbe, J.; Ahrens, B.; Bachmann, O.; Ballmer-Weber, B.; Beyer, K.; Bischoff, S.C.; Blümchen, K.; Dölle, S.; et al. Non-celiac gluten/wheat sensitivity (NCGS)-a currently undefined disorder without validated diagnostic criteria and of unknown prevalence: Position statement of the task force on food allergy of the German Society of Allergology and Clinical Immunology (DGAKI). *Allergo J. Int.* **2018**, *27*, 147–151. [PubMed]

22. Biesiekierski, J.R. What is gluten? *J. Gastroenterol. Hepatol.* **2017**, *32* (Suppl 1), 78–81. [CrossRef] [PubMed]

23. Junker, Y.; Zeissig, S.; Kim, S.-J.; Barisani, D.; Wieser, H.; Leffler, D.A.; Zevallos, V.; Libermann, T.A.; Dillon, S.; Freitag, T.L.; et al. Wheat amylase trypsin inhibitors drive intestinal inflammation via activation of toll-like receptor 4. *J. Exp. Med.* **2012**, *209*, 2395–2408. [CrossRef] [PubMed]

24. Barrett, J.S. Extending our knowledge of fermentable, short-chain carbohydrates for managing gastrointestinal symptoms. *Nutr. Clin. Pr. Off. Publ. Am. Soc. Parenter. Enter. Nutr.* **2013**, *28*, 300–306. [CrossRef] [PubMed]

25. Dieterich, W.; Schuppan, D.; Schink, M.; Schwappacher, R.; Wirtz, S.; Agaimy, A.; Neurath, M.F.; Zopf, Y. Influence of low FODMAP and gluten-free diets on disease activity and intestinal microbiota in patients with non-celiac gluten sensitivity. *Clin. Nutr. Edinb Scotl.* **2019**, *38*, 697–707. [CrossRef] [PubMed]

26. Gearry, R.B.; Irving, P.M.; Barrett, J.S.; Nathan, D.M.; Shepherd, S.J.; Gibson, P.R. Reduction of dietary poorly absorbed short-chain carbohydrates (FODMAPs) improves abdominal symptoms in patients with inflammatory bowel disease-a pilot study. *J. Crohns Colitis* **2009**, *3*, 8–14. [CrossRef] [PubMed]

27. Priyanka, P.; Gayam, S.; Kupec, J.T. The Role of a Low Fermentable Oligosaccharides, Disaccharides, Monosaccharides, and Polyol Diet in Nonceliac Gluten Sensitivity. *Gastroenterol. Res. Pract.* **2018**, *2018*, 1561476. [CrossRef] [PubMed]

28. Catassi, G.; Lionetti, E.; Gatti, S.; Catassi, C. The Low FODMAP Diet: Many Question Marks for a Catchy Acronym. *Nutrients* **2017**, *9*, 292. [CrossRef] [PubMed]

29. Catassi, C.; Elli, L.; Bonaz, B.; Bouma, G.; Carroccio, A.; Castillejo, G.; Cellier, C.; Cristofori, F.; de Magistris, L.; Dolinsek, J.; et al. Diagnosis of Non-Celiac Gluten Sensitivity (NCGS): The Salerno Experts' Criteria. *Nutrients* **2015**, *7*, 4966–4977. [CrossRef]

30. Guandalini, S.; Polanco, I. Nonceliac gluten sensitivity or wheat intolerance syndrome? *J. Pediatr.* **2015**, *166*, 805–811. [CrossRef]

31. Volta, U.; Caio, G.; De Giorgio, R.; Henriksen, C.; Skodje, G.; Lundin, K.E. Non-celiac gluten sensitivity: A work-in-progress entity in the spectrum of wheat-related disorders. *Best Pr. Res. Clin. Gastroenterol.* **2015**, *29*, 477–491. [CrossRef] [PubMed]

32. Slim, M.; Rico-Villademoros, F.; Calandre, E.P. Psychiatric Comorbidity in Children and Adults with Gluten-Related Disorders: A Narrative Review. *Nutrients* **2018**, *10*, 875. [CrossRef] [PubMed]

33. Carroccio, A.; Brusca, I.; Mansueto, P.; Pirrone, G.; Barrale, M.; Di Prima, L.; Ambrosiano, G.; Iacono, G.; Lospalluti, M.L.; La Chiusa, S.M.; et al. A cytologic assay for diagnosis of food hypersensitivity in patients with irritable bowel syndrome. *Clin. Gastroenterol. Hepatol. Off. Clin. Pr. J. Am. Gastroenterol. Assoc.* **2010**, *8*, 254–260. [CrossRef]

34. Vojdani, A.; Perlmutter, D. Differentiation between Celiac Disease, Nonceliac Gluten Sensitivity, and Their Overlapping with Crohn's Disease: A Case Series. *Case Rep. Immunol.* **2013**, *2013*, 248482. [CrossRef] [PubMed]

35. Makharia, A.; Catassi, C.; Makharia, G.K. The Overlap between Irritable Bowel Syndrome and Non-Celiac Gluten Sensitivity: A Clinical Dilemma. *Nutrients* **2015**, *7*, 10417–10426. [CrossRef] [PubMed]

36. Catassi, C.; Alaedini, A.; Bojarski, C.; Bonaz, B.; Bouma, G.; Carroccio, A.; Castillejo, G.; De Magistris, L.; Dieterich, W.; Di Liberto, D.; et al. The Overlapping Area of Non-Celiac Gluten Sensitivity (NCGS) and Wheat-Sensitive Irritable Bowel Syndrome (IBS): An Update. *Nutrients* **2017**, *9*. Available online: https://www.ncbi.nlm.nih.gov/pmc/articles/PMC5707740/ (accessed on 27 January 2019). [CrossRef] [PubMed]

37. Torres, J.; Mehandru, S.; Colombel, J.-F.; Peyrin-Biroulet, L. Crohn's disease. *Lancet* **2017**, *389*, 1741–1755. [CrossRef]

38. Caio, G.; Volta, U.; Tovoli, F.; De Giorgio, R. Effect of gluten free diet on immune response to gliadin in patients with non-celiac gluten sensitivity. *BMC Gastroenterol.* **2014**, *14*, 26. [CrossRef]

39. Makhlouf, S.; Messelmani, M.; Zaouali, J.; Mrissa, R. Cognitive impairment in celiac disease and non-celiac gluten sensitivity: Review of literature on the main cognitive impairments, the imaging and the effect of gluten free diet. *Acta Neurol. Belg.* **2018**, *118*, 21–27. [CrossRef]

40. Busby, E.; Bold, J.; Fellows, L.; Rostami, K. Mood Disorders and Gluten: It's Not All in Your Mind! A Systematic Review with Meta-Analysis. *Nutrients* **2018**, *10*, 1708. [CrossRef]

41. Rodrigo, L.; Hernández-Lahoz, C.; Lauret, E.; Rodriguez-Peláez, M.; Soucek, M.; Ciccocioppo, R.; Kruzliak, P. Gluten ataxia is better classified as non-celiac gluten sensitivity than as celiac disease: A comparative clinical study. *Immunol. Res.* **2016**, *64*, 558–564. [CrossRef] [PubMed]

42. Hadjivassiliou, M.; Rao, D.G.; Grìnewald, R.A.; Aeschlimann, D.P.; Sarrigiannis, P.G.; Hoggard, N.; Aeschlimann, P.; Mooney, P.D.; Sanders, D.S. Neurological Dysfunction in Coeliac Disease and Non-Coeliac Gluten Sensitivity. *Am. J. Gastroenterol.* **2016**, *111*, 561–567. [CrossRef] [PubMed]

43. Capannolo, A.; Viscido, A.; Barkad, M.A.; Valerii, G.; Ciccone, F.; Melideo, D.; Frieri, G.; Latella, G. Non-Celiac Gluten Sensitivity among Patients Perceiving Gluten-Related Symptoms. *Digestion* **2015**, *92*, 8–13. [CrossRef] [PubMed]

44. Elli, L.; Tomba, C.; Branchi, F.; Roncoroni, L.; Lombardo, V.; Bardella, M.T.; Ferretti, F.; Conte, D.; Valiante, F.; Fini, L.; et al. Evidence for the Presence of Non-Celiac Gluten Sensitivity in Patients with Functional Gastrointestinal Symptoms: Results from a Multicenter Randomized Double-Blind Placebo-Controlled Gluten Challenge. *Nutrients* **2016**, *8*, 84. [CrossRef] [PubMed]

45. Zanini, B.; Baschè, R.; Ferraresi, A.; Ricci, C.; Lanzarotto, F.; Marullo, M.; Villanacci, V.; Hidalgo, A.; Lanzini, A. Randomised clinical study: Gluten challenge induces symptom recurrence in only a minority of patients who meet clinical criteria for non-coeliac gluten sensitivity. *Aliment. Pharm. Ther.* **2015**, *42*, 968–976. [CrossRef]

46. Hollon, J.; Puppa, E.L.; Greenwald, B.; Goldberg, E.; Guerrerio, A.; Fasano, A. Effect of gliadin on permeability of intestinal biopsy explants from celiac disease patients and patients with non-celiac gluten sensitivity. *Nutrients* **2015**, *7*, 1565–1576. [CrossRef] [PubMed]

47. Shahbazkhani, B.; Sadeghi, A.; Malekzadeh, R.; Khatavi, F.; Etemadi, M.; Kalantri, E.; Rostami-Nejad, M.; Rostami, K. Non-Celiac Gluten Sensitivity Has Narrowed the Spectrum of Irritable Bowel Syndrome: A Double-Blind Randomized Placebo-Controlled Trial. *Nutrients* **2015**, *7*, 4542–4554. [CrossRef]

48. Biesiekierski, J.R.; Peters, S.L.; Newnham, E.D.; Rosella, O.; Muir, J.G.; Gibson, P.R. No effects of gluten in patients with self-reported non-celiac gluten sensitivity after dietary reduction of fermentable, poorly absorbed, short-chain carbohydrates. *Gastroenterology* **2013**, *145*, 320–328.e1-3. [CrossRef]

49. Skodje, G.I.; Sarna, V.K.; Minelle, I.H.; Rolfsen, K.L.; Muir, J.G.; Gibson, P.R.; Veierød, M.B.; Henriksen, C.; Lundin, K.E.A. Fructan, Rather Than Gluten, Induces Symptoms in Patients with Self-Reported Non-Celiac Gluten Sensitivity. *Gastroenterology* **2018**, *154*, 529–539.e2. [CrossRef]

50. Di Sabatino, A.; Volta, U.; Salvatore, C.; Biancheri, P.; Caio, G.; De Giorgio, R.; Di Stefano, M.; Corazza, G.R. Small Amounts of Gluten in Subjects with Suspected Nonceliac Gluten Sensitivity: A Randomized, Double-Blind, Placebo-Controlled, Cross-Over Trial. *Clin. Gastroenterol. Hepatol. Off. Clin. Pr. J. Am. Gastroenterol. Assoc.* **2015**, *13*, 1604–1612.e3. [CrossRef]

51. Rosinach, M.; Fernández-Bañares, F.; Carrasco, A.; Ibarra, M.; Temiño, R.; Salas, A.; Esteve, M. Double-Blind Randomized Clinical Trial: Gluten versus Placebo Rechallenge in Patients with Lymphocytic Enteritis and Suspected Celiac Disease. *PLoS ONE* **2016**, *11*, e0157879. [CrossRef] [PubMed]

52. Carroccio, A.; D'Alcamo, A.; Iacono, G.; Soresi, M.; Iacobucci, R.; Arini, A.; Geraci, G.; Fayer, F.; Cavataio, F.; La Blasca, F.; et al. Persistence of Nonceliac Wheat Sensitivity, Based on Long-term Follow-up. *Gastroenterology* **2017**, *153*, 56–58.e3. [CrossRef] [PubMed]

53. Roncoroni, L.; Bascuñán, K.A.; Vecchi, M.; Doneda, L.; Bardella, M.T.; Lombardo, V.; Scricciolo, A.; Branchi, F.; Elli, L. Exposure to Different Amounts of Dietary Gluten in Patients with Non-Celiac Gluten Sensitivity (NCGS): An Exploratory Study. *Nutrients* **2019**, *11*, 136. [CrossRef] [PubMed]

54. Carroccio, A.; Brusca, I.; Mansueto, P.; Soresi, M.; D'Alcamo, A.; Ambrosiano, G.; Pepe, I.; Iacono, G.; Lospalluti, M.L.; La Chiusa, S.M.; et al. Fecal assays detect hypersensitivity to cow's milk protein and gluten in adults with irritable bowel syndrome. *Clin. Gastroenterol. Hepatol. Off. Clin. Pr. J. Am. Gastroenterol. Assoc.* **2011**, *9*, 956–971.e3. [CrossRef] [PubMed]

55. Carroccio, A.; Mansueto, P.; Iacono, G.; Soresi, M.; D'Alcamo, A.; Cavataio, F.; Brusca, I.; Florena, A.M.; Ambrosiano, G.; Seidita, A.; et al. Non-celiac wheat sensitivity diagnosed by double-blind placebo-controlled challenge: Exploring a new clinical entity. *Am. J. Gastroenterol.* **2012**, *107*, 1898–1907. [CrossRef]

56. Volta, U.; Tovoli, F.; Cicola, R.; Parisi, C.; Fabbri, A.; Piscaglia, M.; Fiorini, E.; Caio, G. Serological Tests in Gluten Sensitivity (Nonceliac Gluten Intolerance). *J. Clin. Gastroenterol.* **2012**, *46*, 680–685. [CrossRef]

57. Carroccio, A.; D'Alcamo, A.; Cavataio, F.; Soresi, M.; Seidita, A.; Sciumè, C.; Geraci, G.; Iacono, G.; Mansueto, P. High Proportions of People with Nonceliac Wheat Sensitivity Have Autoimmune Disease or Antinuclear Antibodies. *Gastroenterology* **2015**, *149*, 596–603.e1. [CrossRef]

58. Infantino, M.; Manfredi, M.; Meacci, F.; Grossi, V.; Severino, M.; Benucci, M.; Bellio, E.; Bellio, V.; Nucci, A.; Zolfanelli, F.; et al. Diagnostic accuracy of anti-gliadin antibodies in Non-Celiac Gluten Sensitivity (NCGS) patients. *Clin. Chim. Acta* **2015**, *451*, 135–141. [CrossRef]

59. Norsa, L.; Shamir, R.; Zevit, N.; Verduci, E.; Hartman, C.; Ghisleni, D.; Riva, E.; Giovannini, M. Cardiovascular disease risk factor profiles in children with celiac disease on gluten-free diets. *World J. Gastroenterol.* **2013**, *19*, 5658–5664. [CrossRef]

60. Jenkins, D.J.; Kendall, C.W.; Vidgen, E.; Augustin, L.S.; van Erk, M.; Geelen, A.; Parker, T.; Faulkner, D.; Vuksan, V.; Josse, R.G.; et al. High-protein diets in hyperlipidemia: Effect of wheat gluten on serum lipids, uric acid, and renal function. *Am. J. Clin. Nutr.* **2001**, *74*, 57–63. [CrossRef]

61. Jenkins, D.J.; Kendall, C.W.; Vuksan, V.; Augustin, L.S.; Mehling, C.; Parker, T.; Vidgen, E.; Lee, B.; Faulkner, D.; Seyler, H.; et al. Effect of wheat bran on serum lipids: Influence of particle size and wheat protein. *J. Am. Coll Nutr.* **1999**, *18*, 159–165. [CrossRef] [PubMed]

62. Lebwohl, B.; Cao, Y.; Zong, G.; Hu, F.B.; Green, P.H.R.; Neugut, A.I.; Rimm, E.B.; Sampson, L.; Dougherty, L.W.; Giovannucci, E.; et al. Long term gluten consumption in adults without celiac disease and risk of coronary heart disease: Prospective cohort study. *BMJ* **2017**, *357*, j1892. [CrossRef] [PubMed]

63. Niland, B.; Cash, B.D. Health Benefits and Adverse Effects of a Gluten-Free Diet in Non–Celiac Disease Patients. *Gastroenterol Hepatol.* **2018**, *14*, 82–91.

64. Vici, G.; Belli, L.; Biondi, M.; Polzonetti, V. Gluten free diet and nutrient deficiencies: A review. *Clin. Nutr. Edinb. Scotl.* **2016**, *35*, 1236–1241. [CrossRef] [PubMed]

65. Hallert, C.; Grant, C.; Grehn, S.; Grännö, C.; Hultén, S.; Midhagen, G.; Ström, M.; Svensson, H.; Valdimarsson, T. Evidence of poor vitamin status in coeliac patients on a gluten-free diet for 10 years. *Aliment. Pharm. Ther.* **2002**, *16*, 1333–1339. [CrossRef]

66. Tovoli, F.; Granito, A.; Negrini, G.; Guidetti, E.; Faggiano, C.; Bolondi, L. Long term effects of gluten-free diet in non-celiac wheat sensitivity. *Clin. Nutr. Edinb. Scotl.* **2019**, *38*, 357–363. [CrossRef] [PubMed]

Permissions

All chapters in this book were first published by MDPI; hereby published with permission under the Creative Commons Attribution License or equivalent. Every chapter published in this book has been scrutinized by our experts. Their significance has been extensively debated. The topics covered herein carry significant findings which will fuel the growth of the discipline. They may even be implemented as practical applications or may be referred to as a beginning point for another development.

The contributors of this book come from diverse backgrounds, making this book a truly international effort. This book will bring forth new frontiers with its revolutionizing research information and detailed analysis of the nascent developments around the world.

We would like to thank all the contributing authors for lending their expertise to make the book truly unique. They have played a crucial role in the development of this book. Without their invaluable contributions this book wouldn't have been possible. They have made vital efforts to compile up to date information on the varied aspects of this subject to make this book a valuable addition to the collection of many professionals and students.

This book was conceptualized with the vision of imparting up-to-date information and advanced data in this field. To ensure the same, a matchless editorial board was set up. Every individual on the board went through rigorous rounds of assessment to prove their worth. After which they invested a large part of their time researching and compiling the most relevant data for our readers.

The editorial board has been involved in producing this book since its inception. They have spent rigorous hours researching and exploring the diverse topics which have resulted in the successful publishing of this book. They have passed on their knowledge of decades through this book. To expedite this challenging task, the publisher supported the team at every step. A small team of assistant editors was also appointed to further simplify the editing procedure and attain best results for the readers.

Apart from the editorial board, the designing team has also invested a significant amount of their time in understanding the subject and creating the most relevant covers. They scrutinized every image to scout for the most suitable representation of the subject and create an appropriate cover for the book.

The publishing team has been an ardent support to the editorial, designing and production team. Their endless efforts to recruit the best for this project, has resulted in the accomplishment of this book. They are a veteran in the field of academics and their pool of knowledge is as vast as their experience in printing. Their expertise and guidance has proved useful at every step. Their uncompromising quality standards have made this book an exceptional effort. Their encouragement from time to time has been an inspiration for everyone.

The publisher and the editorial board hope that this book will prove to be a valuable piece of knowledge for researchers, students, practitioners and scholars across the globe.

List of Contributors

Laura Airaksinen, Pilvi Laurikka and Katri Lindfors
Celiac Disease Research Center, Faculty of Medicine and Health Technology, Tampere University, 33520 Tampere, Finland

Heini Huhtala
Faculty of Social Sciences, Tampere University, 33520 Tampere, Finland

Kalle Kurppa
Tampere Centre for Child Health Research, Tampere University Hospital and Tampere University, 33521 Tampere, Finland
Department of Pediatrics, Seinäjoki Central Hospital and University Consortium of Seinäjoki, 60220 Seinäjoki, Finland

Teea Salmi
Celiac Disease Research Center, Faculty of Medicine and Health Technology, Tampere University, 33520 Tampere, Finland
Department of Dermatology, Tampere University Hospital, 33521 Tampere, Finland

Päivi Saavalainen
Research Programs Unit, Immunobiology, and Haartman Institute, Department of Medical Genetics, University of Helsinki, 00014 Helsinki, Finland

Katri Kaukinen
Celiac Disease Research Center, Faculty of Medicine and Health Technology, Tampere University, 33520 Tampere, Finland
Department of Internal Medicine, Tampere University Hospital, 33521 Tampere, Finland

Federica Gaiani and Gian Luigi de'Angelis
Gastroenterology and Endoscopy Unit, University Hospital of Parma, University of Parma, via Gramsci 14, 43126 Parma, Italy
Interdepartmental Center Biopharmanet-tec, Parco Area delle Scienze, University of Parma, 43124 Parma, Italy

Sara Graziano
Interdepartmental Center SITEIA.PARMA, Parco Area delle Scienze, University of Parma, 43124 Parma, Italy

Fatma Boukid, Barbara Prandi, Arnaldo Dossena, Mariolina Gullì and Stefano Sforza
Interdepartmental Center SITEIA.PARMA, Parco Area delle Scienze, University of Parma, 43124 Parma, Italy

Department of Food and Drug, Parco Area delle Scienze, University of Parma, 27/A-43124 Parma, Italy

Lorena Bottarelli
Interdepartmental Center Biopharmanet-tec, Parco Area delle Scienze, University of Parma, 43124 Parma, Italy
Department of Medicine and Surgery, Unit of Pathological Anatomy, University Hospital of Parma, via Gramsci 14, 43126 Parma, Italy

Amelia Barilli
Department of Medicine and Surgery, Unit of General Pathology, University of Parma, Via Volturno 39, 43125 Parma, Italy

Nelson Marmiroli
Interdepartmental Center SITEIA.PARMA, Parco Area delle Scienze, University of Parma, 43124 Parma, Italy
Department of Chemistry, Life Sciences, and Environmental Sustainability, University of Parma, Parco Area delle Scienze 11a, 43124 Parma, Italy

Aarón D. Ramírez-Sánchez, Iris Jonkers and Sebo Withoff
Department of Genetics, University of Groningen, University Medical Center Groningen, 9700 RB Groningen, The Netherlands

Ineke L. Tan
Department of Genetics, University of Groningen, University Medical Center Groningen, 9700 RB Groningen, The Netherlands
Department of Gastroenterology and Hepatology, University of Groningen, University Medical Center Groningen, 9700 RB Groningen, The Netherlands

B.C. Gonera-de Jong
Department of Pediatrics, Wilhelmina Hospital Assen, 9401 RK Assen, The Netherlands

Marijn C. Visschedijk
Department of Gastroenterology and Hepatology, University of Groningen, University Medical Center Groningen, 9700 RB Groningen, The Netherlands

Mahmoud Slim
Division of Neurology, The Hospital for Sick Children, The Peter Gilgan Centre for Research and Learning, 686 Bay St., Toronto, ON M5G 0A4, Canada

Fernando Rico-Villademoros and Elena P. Calandre
Instituto de Neurociencias, Universidad de Granada, Avenida del Conocimiento s/n, 18100 Armilla, Granada, Spain

Cristina Capittini, Annalisa De Silvestri and Carmine Tinelli
Scientific Direction, Clinical Epidemiology and Biometric Unit, Fondazione IRCCS Policlinico San Matteo, 27100 Pavia, Italy

Chiara Rebuffi
Grant Office and Scientific Documentation Center, Fondazione IRCCS Policlinico San Matteo, 27100 Pavia, Italy

Dimitri Poddighe
Department of Medicine, Nazarbayev University School of Medicine, Nur-Sultan City 010000, Kazakhstan

Elizabeth S. Mearns, Kelly J. Thomas Craig, Stefanie Puglielli and Allie B. Cichewicz
IBMWatson Health, Cambridge, MA 02142, USA

Aliki Taylor
Takeda Development Centre Europe Ltd., London WC2B 4AE, UK

Daniel A. Leffler
Takeda Pharmaceuticals International Co, Cambridge, MA 02139, USA

David S. Sanders and Marios Hadjivassiliou
Royal Hallamshire Hospital and University of Sheffield, Sheffield S10 2RX, UK

Benjamin Lebwohl
Department of Medicine, Celiac Disease Center, Columbia University Medical Center, New York, NY 10032, USA

Jesús Gilberto Arámburo-Gálvez and Oscar Gerardo Figueroa-Salcido
Unidad Academica de Ciencias de la Nutrición y Gastronomia, Universidad Autónoma de Sinaloa, Culiacán, Sinaloa 80019, Mexico
Posgrado en Ciencias de la Salud, División de Ciencias Biológicas y de la Salud, Universidad de Sonora, Hermosillo, Sonora 83000, Mexico

Itallo Carvalho Gomes and Tatiane Geralda André
Programa de Maestría en Ciencias en Enfermeria, Facultad de Enfermería, Los Mochis, Sinaloa 81220, Mexico

Carlos Eduardo Beltrán-Cárdenas, Feliznando Isidro Cárdenas-Torres and Francisco Cabrera-Chávez
Unidad Academica de Ciencias de la Nutrición y Gastronomia, Universidad Autónoma de Sinaloa, Culiacán, Sinaloa 80019, Mexico

María Auxiliadora Macêdo-Callou and Élida Mara Braga Rocha
Faculdade de Juazeiro do Norte, Juazeiro do Norte, Ceará 63010-215, Brazil

Elaine Aparecida Mye-Takamatu-Watanabe and Vivian Rahmeier-Fietz
Universidade Estadual de Mato Grosso do Sul, Dourados, Mato Grosso do Sul 79804-970, Brazil

Noé Ontiveros
Division of Sciences and Engineering, Department of Chemical, Biological, and Agricultural Sciences (DC-QB), Clinical and Research Laboratory (LACIUS, URS), University of Sonora, Navojoa 85880, Sonora, Mexico

Alina Popp
University of Medicine and Pharmacy "Carol Davila" and National Institute for Mother and Child Health "Alessandrescu-Rusescu", Bucharest 020395, Romania
Faculty of Medicine and Health Technology, Tampere University and Tampere University Hospital, 33520 Tampere, Finland
"Carol Davila" University of Medicine and Pharmacy, 020021 Bucharest, Romania
Pediatrics Department, "Alessandrescu-Rusescu" National Institute for Mother and Child Health, 020395 Bucharest, Romania

Markku Mäki
Faculty of Medicine and Health Technology, Tampere University and Tampere University Hospital, 33520 Tampere, Finland

Tsvetelina Velikova and Iskra Altankova
Clinical Immunology, University Hospital Lozenetz, 1407 Sofia, Bulgaria

Martin Shahid, Kossara Drenovska and Snejina Vassileva
Department of Dermatology, Faculty of Medicine, Medical University—Sofia, 1431 Sofia, Bulgaria

Ekaterina Ivanova-Todorova and Kalina Tumangelova-Yuzeir
Laboratory of Clinical Immunology—University Hospital St. Ivan Rilski, 1431 Sofia, Bulgaria

Lars-Petter Jelsness-Jørgensen
Department of Health Science, Østfold University College, N-1757 Halden, Norway
Department of Gastroenterology, Østfold Hospital Trust Kalnes, N-1714 Grålum, Norway

Tomm Bernklev
Department of Research and Innovation, Vestfold Hospital Trust, N-3103 Tønsberg, Norway
Faculty of Medicine, Institute of Clinical Medicine, University of Oslo, N-0318 Oslo, Norway

Knut E. A. Lundin
K.G. Jebsen Coeliac Disease Research Centre, University of Oslo, N-0318 Oslo, Norway
Department of gastroenterology, Oslo University Hospital Rikshospitalet, N-0372 Oslo, Norway

Ludovico Abenavoli and Francesco Luzza
Digestive Physiopathology Unit, Department of Health Sciences, Magna Graecia University of Catanzaro, 88100 Catanzaro, Italy

Stefano Dastoli, Luigi Bennardo, Maria Passante, Martina Silvestri and Steven Paul Nisticò
Dermatology Unit, Department of Health Sciences, Magna Graecia University of Catanzaro, 88100 Catanzaro, Italy

Luigi Boccuto
JC Self Research Institute, Greenwood Genetic Center, Greenwood, SC 29646, USA
Clemson University School of Health Research, Clemson University, Clemson, SC 29634, USA

Ilaria Proietti and Concetta Potenza
Dermatology Unit "Daniele Innocenzi", Department of Medical-Surgical Sciences and Biotechnologies, Sapienza University of Rome, Polo Pontino, 04110 Terracina, Italy

Thomas Julian
Medical School, University of Sheffield, Sheffield S10 2TN, UK

Daniel Vasile Balaban and Mariana Jinga
"Carol Davila" University of Medicine and Pharmacy, 020021 Bucharest, Romania
Gastroenterology Department, "Dr. Carol Davila" Central Military Emergency University Hospital, 010825 Bucharest, Romania

Antonella Riva
Research and Development Unit, Indena, 20139 Milan, Italy

Florentina Ionita Radu
Gastroenterology Department, "Dr. Carol Davila" Central Military Emergency University Hospital, 010825 Bucharest, Romania
Faculty of Medicine, Titu Maiorescu University, 004051 Bucharest, Romania

Marios Hadjivassiliou, Richard A Grünewald, Panagiotis Zis, Iain Croall, Priya D Shanmugarajah and Ptolemaios G Sarrigiannis
Academic Departments of Neurosciences and Neuroradiology, Sheffield Teaching Hospitals NHS Trust, Sheffield S10 2JF, UK

Nick Trott
Departments of Dietetics, Sheffield Teaching Hospitals NHS Trust, Sheffield S10 2JF, UK

Graeme Wild
Departments of Immunology, Sheffield Teaching Hospitals NHS Trust, Sheffield S10 2JF, UK

Nigel Hoggard and David S Sanders
Departments of Gastroenterology, Sheffield Teaching Hospitals NHS Trust, Sheffield S10 2JF, UK

Mariangela Rondanelli
IRCCS Mondino Foundation, 27100 Pavia, Italy
Department of Public Health, Experimental and Forensic Medicine, University of Pavia, 27100 Pavia, Italy

Milena A. Faliva, Clara Gasparri, Gabriella Peroni, Maurizio Naso, Giulia Picciotto and Mara Nichetti
Endocrinology and Nutrition Unit, Azienda di Servizi alla Persona "Istituto Santa Margherita", University of Pavia, 27100 Pavia, Italy

Catherine Klersy
Clinical Epidemiology & Biometry Unit, IRCCS Fondazione Policlinico San Matteo; Viale Golgi 19, 27100 Pavia, Italy

Giulia De Marchi, Maria Cristina Conti Bellocchi, Valeria Zuliani, Luca Frulloni and Rachele Ciccocioppo
Gastroenterology Unit, Department of Medicine, AOUI Policlinico G.B. Rossi, University of Verona; Piazzale L.A. Scuro, 10, 37134 Verona, Italy

Giovanna Zanoni and Monica Brentegani
Immunology Unit, Department of Pathology and Diagnostics, AOUI Policlinico G.B. Rossi, Piazzale L.A. Scuro, 10, 37134 Verona, Italy

Tariq A. Alalwan and Simone Perna
Department of Biology, College of Science, University of Bahrain, Sakhir Campus, Bahrain

Elena Betti
Clinica Medica I, Department of Internal Medicine, IRCCS Policlinico San Matteo Foundation, Piazzale Golgi, 19, 27100 Pavia, Italy

Paola Capelli
Pathology Unit, Department of Pathology and Diagnostics, AOUI Policlinico G.B. Rossi, Piazzale L.A. Scuro, 10, 37134 Verona, Italy

Vittoria Infantino
University of Bari, Department of Biomedical Science and Human Oncology, 70121 Bari, Italy

Anna Roszkowska, Marta Pawlicka, Anna Mroczek and Kamil Bałabuszek
Medical University of Lublin, Radziwillowska 11 Street, 20-080 Lublin, Poland

Barbara Nieradko-Iwanicka
Chair and Department of Hygiene, Medical University of Lublin, Radziwillowska 11 Street, 20-080 Lublin, Poland

Index

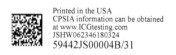

Printed in the USA
CPSIA information can be obtained
at www.ICGtesting.com
JSHW062346180324
59442JS00004B/31